MW00844269

Advances in Tissue Banking

Vol. 2

Advances in Tissue Banking

Vol. 2

Editor-in-Chief

G O Phillips
The North Wales and Oswestry Tissue Bank, UK

Volume II Editor

D M Strong
Puget Sound Blood Center, USA

Regional Editors

R von Versen (Europe)
German Inst. for Cell and Tissue Replacement, Germany

A Nather (Asia Pacific)
Nat'l Univ. Hospital Bone Bank, Singapore

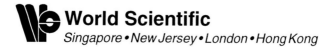

World Scientific
Singapore • New Jersey • London • Hong Kong

Published by

World Scientific Publishing Co. Pte. Ltd.

P O Box 128, Farrer Road, Singapore 912805

USA office: Suite 1B, 1060 Main Street, River Edge, NJ 07661

UK office: 57 Shelton Street, Covent Garden, London WC2H 9HE

British Library Cataloguing-in-Publication Data
A catalogue record for this book is available from the British Library.

ADVANCES IN TISSUE BANKING (Vol. 2)

ISBN 981-02-3534-8

Printed in Singapore.

ADVANCES IN TISSUE BANKING

International Advisory Board

PREFACE

The response to this new series "Advances in Tissue Banking" has been excellent. It has fulfilled all our expectations. Sales have been very satisfactory, high-quality papers have been forthcoming and independent comments have confirmed that we are fulfilling a need. As I write these comments for Volume II, the material for Volume III is almost complete.

This present volume is a very special one, we believe. We are most grateful to our North American Editor, Dr. Michael Strong for editing and undertaking the main responsibility for this volume, dedicated to the memory of Dr. Kenneth Sell. It would be amiss of me if I did not acknowledge here also the special contribution made to the final preparation of this volume by Ms. Mary West, Personal Secretary to Dr. Strong. Her meticulous typing and organisation have made the preparation of this volume quite painless. Thank you Mary and Michael.

The subject matter for this volume illustrates how extensive has been the influence of Dr. Sell on the wider field of tissue banking, covering blood transfusion; bone marrow and stem cell transplantation; immunology and the role of immunology in musculoskeletal transplantation; various aspects of cryopreservation of organs; cartilage and tendons; organ perfusion preservation; the history and long term follow-up of osteochondral allografts, both frozen and fresh; neuro-surgical applications; cardiovascular applications; and the use of skin and newer biological membranes for wound coverage.

All these areas are covered here by specialists who all can trace the influence of Kenneth Sell in the development of their subject. I am confident that all connected with tissue banking will be consulting this book for a view of this field from an American perspective, mainly.

I first met Dr. Kenneth Sell at a meeting organised by my good friend Dr. Nicholas Triantafyllou in Athens, Greece, in the early 1970s. His enthusiasm for his subject and life generally was infectious. That meeting effectively marked the birth of the International Atomic Energy Agency's programme in "Radiation and Tissue Banking". New programmes in tissue banking have been launched in 27 countries, producing, at the last count, more than 110 000 grafts used in clinical practice. This programme will be described in Volume III, which again owes a debt of gratitude to Dr. Sell. As will be demonstrated in Volume III, it is this programme, above any other influence, which led to the development of tissue banking in the Asia and Pacific Region, and lately in Latin America.

Finally, may I again thank WORLD SCIENTIFIC, particularly Ms. Joy Marie, Editor, for that unfailing courtesy and professionalism. To the tissue banking community, let me say, thank you for your support and please keep the articles coming in.

Glyn O. Phillips
Editor-in-Chief

CONTENTS

Chapter 1

THE CONTRIBUTION OF KENNETH W. SELL TO THE PROGRESS OF TISSUE BANKING

It was with great sadness that we learned of the death of Dr. Kenneth Sell this past year. Dr. Sell made many contributions to the field of transplantation and tissue banking in particular. It was through his leadership that many scientists, physicians and practitioners in tissue banking were introduced to the fields of Tissue Banking, Transplantation and Immunology. In 1975, Dr. Sell organised a tissue bank symposium honouring the 25th Anniversary of the US Navy Tissue Bank. For this meeting, he brought together physicians and scientists from around the world to discuss a variety of topics including: the development and progress of tissue banking; clinical results of transplantation of stored tissues and organs; techniques of viable low temperature tissue preservation; techniques of viable tissue and organ preservation; and the logistical and legal problems of tissue banking. Presentations were made by leaders who had established tissue banks during the previous 25 years, but also included practitioners of allotransplantation who relayed the benefit of tissue banking. (*Tissue Banking for Transplantation*, K.W. Sell and G.E. Friedlaender, eds., Grune & Stratton, Inc., New York, 1976.)

In honour of Dr. Sell's contributions to the field of tissue banking, a symposium was organised in 1997 to pay tribute to him, and to recount the many accomplishments that have occurred both during his participation in the field and thereafter. Many of the participants in the 1997 symposium had been contributors in the 1975 symposium. The fields of tissue banking and tissue transplantation have made great strides since that time, many as a result of Dr. Sell's leadership and his mentoring of several of the participants who presented at this meeting and contributed to this volume.

Dr. Sell's interest in tissue banking was initiated during his service at the US Navy Tissue Bank. It is therefore of interest to review briefly the history of that organisation and how it has played a leading role in the establishment of standards and the practice of tissue banking today. The Navy Tissue Bank was established by Dr. G.W. Hyatt who conceived of the idea during his fellowship at the Lahey Clinic. In 1949, he returned to the orthopaedic service of the Naval Hospital in Bethesda, Maryland, and convinced the department chairman to purchase a small freezer for storing surplus bone collected from orthopaedic surgical cases. It soon became evident that a four-foot cubic freezer could not adequately store bone in sufficient quantity for all the cases needing bone grafts. By late 1949, the increased Navy-wide interest in bone banking led the Navy to establish a bone bank as a specialty activity of the Naval Medical School. Provisions were made to establish a centre for the procurement, processing, storage and shipment of tissues to all medical facilities of the Navy.

Dr. Hyatt's experience with freeze-dried plasma during World War II led to the development of a freeze drying process for bone and solved the logistical difficulties of transporting tissue throughout the Naval Medical system. The successful experimental use of freeze-dried bone in animals prompted the tissue bank to undertake a clinical research project in which 14 patients at the Naval Hospital were grafted with freeze-dried allogeneic bone. The results from this project indicated that freeze drying offered many advantages over freezing alone.

As the demand for bone increased it was evident that an alternative source was needed, and following lengthy legal consultations and the advice of surgeons and physicians, procedures were established to aseptically recover bone and tissue from cadavers. This concept became reality in May 1951, when the tissue bank opened a new surgical suite and performed the first post-mortem recovery of tissue under aseptic conditions.

This chapter includes the biography of Dr. Sell, along with a recent update on his legacy as provided by the current Commanding Officer of the United States Naval Medical Research Institute. The 1975 meeting in Washington D.C., organised by Dr. Sell, resulted in the gathering of North American Tissue bankers and became the nucleus around which the American Association of Tissue Banks (AATB) was formed. Since that time, the AATB has been a leader in establishing standards, accreditation processes, and working with the Food and Drug Administration in the most current regulatory efforts of tissue banking in the United States. Dr. Michael Joyce, an orthopaedic surgeon, is the newly elected President of the AATB and provides his insights into that organisation's present and future activities.

D.M.S.

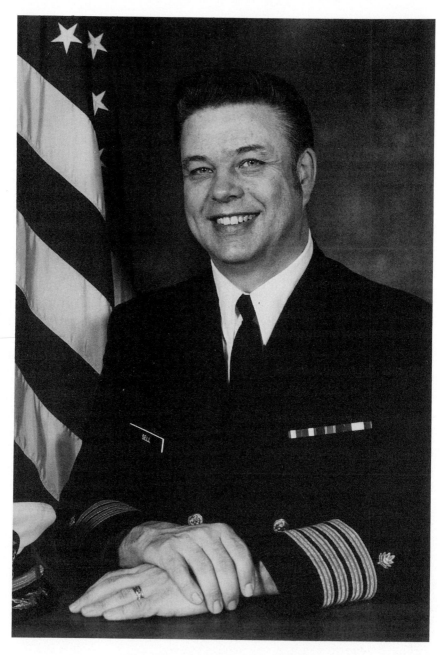

Kenneth W. Sell, M.D., Ph.D.
1931–1996

1.1 KENNETH W. SELL — REFLECTIONS ON A SUCCESSFUL LIFE

L.A. KIESOW

Clinical Research and Technology Center
Legacy Health System
Legacy Holladay Park Medical Center
PO Box 3950
Portland, OR 97208-3950
USA

1. Wednesday, 29 April 1931 —According to the *Bismarck Tribune* of Bismarck, North Dakota

It is always challenging to trace the beginnings of a person's life regardless of how well or how little you knew him. The lack of shared personal experience and our general knowledge about history leads us only to very common conclusions. Yes, Kenneth Sell was born only eighteen months after the stock market crashed in '29 and the world entered a deep economic crisis. What happened in Valley City, North Dakota, at that time, and what concerned the people living there can only be guessed — unless we consult the local newspaper of the day, and that is what I have done.

The *Bismarck Tribune* reported mostly fair weather, promising rising temperatures to a comfortable 22 degrees Fahrenheit for the following day. Proudly calling itself "North Dakota's Oldest Newspaper", the *Bismarck Tribune* was delivered daily by carrier for an annual subscription fee of $7.20 — "to be paid in advance". The front page of the 29 April issue notes that Secretary of Commerce, Robert P. Lamont, urged higher wages and shorter hours to compensate for the decrease in buying power. He also said that "a governmental program contemplating expenditures of as high as a million dollars could not materially affect a situation where only private industry and private initiative would combat the loss of jobs effectively". The paper also reports that President Hoover received the King and Queen of Siam with a friendly handclasp at the White House. It further noted that this was the first time in American History that an absolute monarch crossed the threshold of the White House and stayed there as the personal guest of the President, and also, "the Queen smiled at the people grouped around the north entrance".

The Tribune also reported, as an exiting event, that a Californian built the most powerful radio set to tune in to the stars. Doctor Dunham, an astronomer from the Carnegie Institution assembled at the Mount Wilson Observatory a photo-electric cell as a detector tube with the most powerful amplifying tubes ever built. The device — a radio spectroscope — was designed to tune in to the light-waves from stars millions of miles away and the amplifying tubes were expected to register a delicate galvanometer by which the temperature of the stars would be recorded.

The remainder of the paper is devoted to society news and to lengthy reports on sports, particularly boxing. The comics are not missing and they are followed by "The Tribune's Grain and Livestock Report" which, judging by its length and details, must have been of considerable importance to readers.

Like any good newspaper now or then, the Tribune of 29 April 1931 reported the events of the day which most likely addressed the public interest of the time and place. The Tribune did not take note of the fact that this was also the day Kenneth W. Sell was born in Valley City to parents of Icelandic and German descent. It could not predict that he would grow up and be educated to become a remarkable and accomplished physician and scientist who would make many significant contributions to the field of medicine.

2. Someone asked why I would make biographical remarks about Kenneth W. Sell?

This question puzzled me. Yes, I knew Ken for more than a quarter of a century, but I knew nothing about his childhood, only a few anecdotes about his education and early professional life. But then again, I always felt I knew him well, that we understood each other. We had similar opinions and ideas, and shared similar beliefs in human values and responsibilities.

The real answer to the question, however, may in part stem from the fact that we were true contemporaries and must have had similar experiences growing up. I am only three months older than Ken and both of us were the only child. Our parents, while living in different countries and on different continents many thousands of miles apart, guided us through the same epoch of history. Our identical age made us witnesses to similar events, and our points of reference, different as they must have been, must have led us to similar conclusions and left similar imprints on our development.

Our education and training followed identical tracks and we were both achievers. We did not have to work too hard to be good at what we did, or better, what we were required to do. This allowed us to keep some distance from the actual substance of learning and to muse and form opinions about it. At the same time this was the environment that gave us time and opportunity to develop not only a love for medicine but also for the medical sciences — loves and commitments we shared for the rest of our lives.

Ken and I knew each other for nearly 30 years. We were often amused by the things we did in the same way — then and in the past. As one example, we both knew our future spouses during our school years. In later years the intensity of personal contact varied greatly, ranging from daily to very sporadic. But during all that time we always held a high regard for each other as physicians and scientists, and as people. We helped each other and learned from each other. We criticised each other honestly and patted each other's shoulder when appropriate. We laughed together, sometimes about the clever things we did, sometimes about how foolishly we had acted.

We had a common mentor, John R. Seal, whom we respected and who coached us and helped us along our career paths for many years; sometimes with a visible, and sometimes an invisible hand. We both believed firmly in the value of and the need for research physicians who are trained to advance the frontiers of medicine and we believed in the importance of scientific apprenticeship in the training of medical research scientists. All in all, both of us were a peculiar blend of dreamer and realist, often referred to today as visionaries. I believe we lived mainly in the future, and looked at the present as the beginning of the past. And this is why I feel comfortable talking and writing about Ken's life today.

3. Individuals perform research — You'll just have to find them

Ken Sell was perhaps the most successful architect of research infrastructure I ever met. But then, he also knew that it is the individual scientist who is the backbone of scientific achievement and discovery. This led Ken to a neverending search for scientific talent, particularly among young physicians, and this search was met with extraordinary success. Not only this, almost everyone who joined Ken's team embarked on remarkable careers in medicine or medical sciences, or both, and many of these success stories were participants in the 1997 symposium organised in his honour.

In his quest for scientific talent Ken was greatly helped by being the deeply moral and ethical man he was. He was genuinely interested in his fellow men and he was someone who was committed to helping other individuals in the most unselfish way. It was never difficult for him to recognise talent and to mentor it. He could launch careers, and was committed to providing the protective umbrella so essential for individual careers to unfold, mature and flourish. Ken would develop the best in people by being an example and role model. He would stimulate intellectual competition by entering into it himself. He would never tire in challenging his co-workers and colleagues to competitive teamwork and there were many examples where the initially weakest member of the team eventually became the strongest and most successful contributor, often enough with Ken's invisible assistance.

Some developments were not of Ken Sell's personal design but came nevertheless to his aid. One such example was the Berry Plan during Ken's years in the Navy. Intended to offer deferrals from the draft to young physicians in training, it became to Ken an instrument to find talented individuals to join his research teams while serving in the Navy and he learned quickly to play this instrument with the skill and perfection of a virtuoso. A long list of names joined his research teams in this way, and after their successful initiation spent several productive years in medical research under Ken's personal tutelage or under the guidance of his senior staff. Many successful careers in medicine and the medical sciences began this way and came to fruition in later years.

Ken Sell led by example and his boundless energy. In this he was supported by an all too likable and dynamic personality. He was a wise and honest man who understood his fellow men all too well, both in failure and success. He would easily side with the underdog and the underprivileged, elevating them to high stature and accomplishment. But he would not hesitate to admonish the arrogant and the "know-it-all", often with his buoyant and towering personality that could also be stern, or with a well-placed joke, and never ever without the twinkle in his eye. He was an honest and truthful man who would not hesitate to admit to his own weaknesses. I remember him interrupting himself in the midst of one of his wonderful lectures in front of a large audience and at a point where others may want to appear sovereign and brilliant by saying, "I just don't know why I am so terribly nervous today?"

Well Ken, you had no reason to be nervous, not then or ever. You inspired and led by being who you were: towering, yet modest; stern, but likable; friendly, but serious; personable, but distant; and most of all, honest and always ready to offer a helping hand. You rightfully and proudly presided over the two families to whom you were truly a father. One was your personal family and the other — much larger one — consisting of your students, co-workers and professional colleagues.

4. An architect of research environments

What are the essential elements for the creation of an environment that fosters innovative and productive research? As was said before, it requires the most qualified and dedicated people who have to be molded into successful research teams. But there are many more quintessential features that a leader of research has to offer before he can be an effective guide through new and uncharted territories of scientific discovery. Here again, Kenneth W. Sell knew what was needed and provided it in his superb and congenial way as just another hallmark of his career.

Very early in his career as a Navy physician, he encountered the unifying and guiding star of his whole research career. Resulting from his assignments and the subsequent deepening interest in tissue banking and tissue transplantation he became aware of the significance of the immune response for successful transplantation outcomes. Following his belief that research apprenticeship is the most direct way to the acquisition of scientific skills and knowledge, he was successful in obtaining Navy-sponsored out-service training in one of the finest immunological research laboratories in the world at that time. He trained with Dr. Coombs in Cambridge, England, one of the most outstanding scientists in the newly emerging field of immunology. There he received his Ph.D. in immunopathology, and upon his return to the Naval Hospital in Bethesda, began his fulminating career as a medical research scientist. Now he has acquired the sound foundation for all his future scientific endeavours. He possessed the tools of the most rapidly unfolding field in medicine and he could combine them with his brilliant mind and wonderful imagination. He set out to conquer a small world … and he did.

Very soon Ken's application of immunological principles and methodologies were no longer limited to areas of his original interests, i.e. tissue banking and tissue transplantation. They rapidly expanded into other fields of medical research and clinical investigation, thereby beginning a process that would be typical for him for the rest of his life. The application of immunology as a guiding principle of research was greatly assisted by Ken's rapidly increasing role as a leader at the Naval Medical Research Institute. In very short order immunology became the driving force of intense research activities in parasitic diseases, wound infections, intracellular parasitic infections, burn injuries and infections, Gram-negative sepsis and septic shock, organ preservation and transplantation, and in bone marrow transplantation and its clinical complications. Yes, even decompression sickness and the bends were investigated as potential immunological disorders and antibodies against substances of abuse were looked at for their potential as curative or preventive measures in cases of substance abuse and dependency.

Ken seeded ideas for immune-biology based research everywhere at any time. He brought interdisciplinary teams together for workshops constantly asking them to present new ideas, their work in progress and research results, and to critique it all. Everyone who participated — and few were given a choice — became aware of and knowledgeable in other fields of biomedical sciences and the resulting cross-fertilisation was highly productive. Ken, however, was no longer the virtuoso of a single instrument in this scientific orchestra, he was truly its conductor. Human dynamo that he was, he kept everything and everyone in perpetual motion. While guiding and mentoring his associates and co-workers, he was constantly canvassing the scene for research opportunities. Not just opportunities for the pursuit of new research ideas, but also for new funding support, for new research facilities, and for new research collaborations. All these became the building blocks that were part of a complex and masterfully-designed research network. In it, everything new and innovative could be subjected to scientific investigation in a legally feasible and financially well-supported manner. What could not be done 'in-house' was simply subcontracted, or as we now call it 'out-sourced'. A whole division came to reside at Georgetown University, and the American Institute for Biological Sciences was established. The news that Secretary of Defense Harold Brown intended to close the Uniformed University of the Health Sciences in Bethesda had not even reached the press when Ken already held the blueprints of the University in his hands, and we were examining how the Naval Medical Research Institute would best fit into the buildings soon to become vacant.

In Ken's pursuit of scientific research and discovery, it did not matter where something happened or who did it as long as it really happened. It could happen at Harvard or Georgetown University, at the National Institutes of Health in Bethesda, at Massachusetts General in Boston, or at the University of London. As long as it was good research, Ken Sell would lend his support. It also did not matter if the individuals who were engaged in this research were wearing the Navy uniform, were civil servants or academicians. As long as they did the best possible research, in his opinion they were the right people for the job. In fact a next door neighbour of mine had been working for many years at Georgetown University in close proximity of two of our Navy physician investigators. It came as quite a surprise when I told him that both of these gentlemen were actually uniformed Naval officers.

This research clockwork was kept in motion by a good-humoured man who apparently could draw from endless reserves of energy. I remember asking his wife Marlys once: when does he ever sleep? She answered: in the evening, on the floor, in front of the fireplace.

Granted, to be a true architect of a successful research and the creator of ideal research environments is something that Ken learned, mastered and began to practice during his years at the Naval Medical Research Institute. However, he continued applying these skills wherever he went thereafter. First the National Institutes of Health and later Emory University in Atlanta became subsequent beneficiaries of his earlier experience. But organisations and societies benefitted from this experience as well, since he either created or helped create them for the sole purpose of serving as a forum for or protectorate of medical research and development.

Yet, the greatest beneficiaries of all were those of us who had the privilege to work with Ken. Yes, he dwarfed us all, but at the same time he lifted us to heights of success and accomplishment that only few of us would have reached without his example and tutorship.

5. 2 January 1991 — A visit with Ken Sell at Emory University in Atlanta

Late in 1990, I accepted a position in Portland, Oregon, and needed advice for the transition from the Federal Government to the private business world and to academia. Nothing was more natural than calling Ken and to accept the immediate invitation to "come on down for a day and we'll talk", and that was what I did.

I met Ken in his office at Emory's Department of Pathology. A large office, maybe a little too dark, with a large desk and armchair close to the window and a conference table with comfortable seating to one side of the room. Ken was on the phone, and had someone present in the room for a discussion that had been interrupted by the call. The phone call was clearly about a clinical matter in the department, and the other person in the room appeared to be a petitioner of sorts; as a matter of fact, a slightly nervous or depressed petitioner. Ken waved me to take my coat off and make myself comfortable at the conference table while he finished his phone conversation. He then devoted his full attention to the person sitting right next to his desk, and continued a conversation that apparently dealt with space or space allocation. Only later in my new job in Portland did I learn about the full significance of departmental space allocations, making it often more of an emotional rather than a logical issue. The petitioner may have needed more space, he no doubt wanted more space, and I watched the master at his best convincing the man that he really had enough space. In fact, if he had perhaps one or two more people working in the space he currently used, it would certainly make him more efficient and possibly even a little more productive, because recently Ken had been wondering a bit about the progress of the man's work, etc, etc. The man left the office, not perfectly happy perhaps, but appearing grateful, with Ken beaming at him, a twinkle in his eyes and one eyebrow fluttering while his fatherly hand patted the man's shoulder. Job well done, Ken.

Then he turned his full attention to me, took my hands, shook them vigorously and sat down next to me to describe the plan for the rest of the day. First, discussions to be continued at his other office at the Cancer Center — I definitely had to see it! This would be followed by lunch at the Faculty Club with a long-standing junior associate and friend of his, whom I also knew for many years. Then more discussions, and before I departed I definitely had to see his restored Atlanta home.

We began talking about Ken's life, and particularly about his initial experiences at Emory with many well-remembered details. He knew exactly how helpful they would be to me, the 'novice elect' in a similar environment. We were interrupted by a phone call from someone who, as Ken quickly explained, was considered for a faculty position in his department. Ken answered a variety of questions with great care, speaking in his usual fast manner with a friendly, reassuring and warm voice. Immediately after hanging up, he called his secretary to make arrangements for the prospective faculty member's forthcoming visit. He gave the name of the Hotel where the visitor should stay, defining the floor and room that should be reserved. He was concerned that the person will be properly received, and specified what should be in the room to welcome the visitor and accommodate him comfortably. He dictated in great detail what he expects to happen during the visit and then came back to the conference table. There he explained to me who the person was, where he came from, what his achievements were and what he, Ken Sell, plans to accomplish by bringing this person on faculty in his department. These explanations were generously interlaced and expanded with experiences and observations intended to make me understand and appreciate the differences between the private, academic world and the Federal Government and how differently they operate.

According to plan we have to change our location and move to the Cancer Center. However, before we did that each of us had to grab some pictures and the components of a stereo system to take to his other office. Ken explained — what I already knew — that he likes to work in a pleasant office environment and loves to listen to music for relaxation.

At the Cancer Center, he proudly showed me his second office and explained with great care the Center and its programmes and functions.

As always, I was impressed by Ken's amazing knowledge of the smallest detail and by his ability to answer every question that came to my mind. Then it was time to move to the Faculty Club for lunch and to meet our common acquaintance. On the way to the Club, Ken expressed his concerns about the academic future for our common friend here at Emory. He was obviously worried, and had no simple solution for this particular problem. But when our friend arrived at the luncheon table, Ken was once again his buoyant self. He invited him immediately to talk about his latest research findings, and beamed like a proud father while interjecting comment and explanation, and pointing out the difficulties of the research and the significance of the progress achieved. How wonderful to see an old friend so unchanged and still so much the person you remember.

We returned to Ken's office for more discussion and advice, and finally moved on to his home to meet Marlys, his wife, and have a bite to eat before he took me to the airport. On the way to his home, however, we engaged in a hunt for a convenient bank drive-in window that had to be close to a gas station, since Ken was "driving on fumes" and had to cash a check before he could purchase gasoline. But during this drive I learned about the story of the Sells' transition to Atlanta, the purchase of their beautiful old home and the restoration of the house. This, of course, was done in the best tradition by Ken himself and, as he sheepishly explained, it took so long and caused so much continued commotion that he was at times afraid he would loose Marlys over the project. He obviously didn't, because she was there for a warm welcome and to assume her role as the most gracious hostess. She served a delightful light supper, and then there was time remaining to exchange the latest updates about our families and also to show me the house. Then time came for the ride to the airport, a friendly embrace, a handshake and a final farewell.

Little did I know at the time that this was the last farewell from a greatly admired and dear friend.

Some facts about the career of Kenneth W. Sell, M.D., Ph.D.

Education

Bismarck High School (Valedictorian, 1949)

B.A., University of North Dakota, Grand Forks, ND (Valedictorian; Magna Cum Laude, 1953)

B.S. (Medical), University of North Dakota (Magna Cum Laude, 1954)

M.D., Harvard University, 1956, Boston, MA

Ph.D. (Immunopathology), 1965, University of Cambridge, England

Positions Held

Director, US Navy Tissue Bank, 1965, Bethesda Naval Hospital, Bethesda, MD

Chairman, Department of Experimental and Clinical Immunology, 1971, Naval Medical Research Institute, Bethesda, MD

Scientific Director, 1977, National Institute of Allergy and Infectious Diseases, National Institutes of Health, Bethesda, MD

Professor, Department of Pathology and Laboratory Medicine, 1985, Emory University School of Medicine, Atlanta, GA

Director, Winship Cancer Center, 1985, Emory University School of Medicine, Atlanta, GA

Professor and Chairman, Department of Pathology and Laboratory Medicine, 1985, Emory University School of Medicine, Atlanta, GA

Professor Emeritus, Department of Pathology and Laboratory Medicine, 1996, Emory University School of Medicine, Atlanta, GA

Board Certifications
Diplomat, National Board of Medical Examiners
Board of Pediatrics
Board of Pathology (Blood Banking)

Teaching Appointments
Emory University School of Medicine
Georgetown University Medical School
Foundation for Advanced Education in the Sciences
Uniformed Services University of the Health Sciences

Hospital Appointments
Medical Staff, Pathology, Emory University Hospital, Atlanta, GA
Medical Staff, Pathology, Grady Memorial Hospital, Atlanta, GA
Medical Staff, Pathology, Crawford Long Hospital, Atlanta, GA
Medical Staff, Pathology, Henrietta Egleston Hospital for Children, Atlanta, GA and Wesley Woods Hospital, Atlanta, GA
Pathology Section, Emory Clinic, Atlanta, GA

Military Service
July 1956–September 1977, US Navy Medical Corps
Intern, Bethesda Naval Hospital, Bethesda, MD
Resident, Pediatrics, Bethesda Naval Hospital
Pediatric Staff, Bethesda Naval Hospital
Assistant Director, US Navy Tissue Bank, Bethesda Naval Hospital
Director, US Navy Tissue Bank, Bethesda Naval Hospital

Chairman, Department of Clinical and Experimental Immunology, Naval Medical Research Institute, Bethesda, MD

Director, Clinical Bone Marrow and Kidney Transplant Service, Naval Medical Center, Bethesda, MD

Commanding Officer, Naval Medical Research Institute

Member of 31 Academic and Professional Societies including:
American Academy of Pediatrics
American Association of Blood Banks
American Association for Cancer Research
American Association of Immunologists
American Association of Pathologists
American Association of Tissue Banks, Founding Member, President
American Council on Transplantation, Founding Member
American Society for Microbiology

Special Honors and Other Scientific Recognition
Bausch and Lomb Award in Science
Campbell Award for Highest Overall Average, University of North Dakota Medical School
Legion of Merit, United States Navy
Certificate of Merit, Surgeon General, United States Navy
Navy Meritorious Service Medal
Public Health Service Special Recognition Award
American Association of Tissue Banks, Distinguished Service Award
Naval Medical Research Institute, Bethesda, MD, Honored as Most Distinguished Alumnus of First Fifty Years

Editorial Boards
Cryobiology
Transplantation Proceedings
In Vitro
Experimental Hematology
Annals of Clinical and Laboratory Science
Emory University Journal of Medicine

Committee Appointments
Served on 52 committees

Bibliography
Encompasses 224 journal publications and five books

1.2 BRIEF HISTORY OF THE UNITED STATES NAVY TISSUE BANK AND TRANSPLANTATION PROGRAMME. CAPTAIN KENNETH SELL'S LIVING LEGACY

T.J. CONTRERAS, JR.

Commanding Officer

P.J. BLAIR

Immune Cell Biology Research Program

D.M. HARLAN

Head, Combat Casualty Care Department
Immune Cell Biology Research Program
Naval Medical Research Institute
8901 Wisconsin Avenue
Bethesda, MD 20889-5607, USA

1. Introduction

The Navy has had a vested interest in clinical transplantation since 1950 when Dr. George Hyatt founded the Navy Tissue Bank in Bethesda, Maryland. The initial purpose of the Tissue Bank was rather modest, to store frozen bone for clinical and research purposes. From this tiny acorn, however three grand oaks have sprung: the Immune Cell Biology (ICBRP), Bone Marrow (BMRP), and Transfusion and Cryopreservation (TCRP) Research Programmes, all world-class research teams each pursuing different aspects of the transplantation field. These programmes have remained in close proximity to the National Naval Medical Center and have never lost sight of the fact that they continue the Navy Tissue Bank's long-standing resolve to relieve the pain and suffering of military personnel and their beneficiaries. Captain Kenneth W. Sell, MC, USN served as both Director of the Navy Tissue Bank from 1965 to 1974 and as Commanding Officer of the Naval Medical Research Institute (NMRI) from 1974 to 1977, and played an instrumental role in the earliest stages of the Navy's transplantation efforts.

In 1960, with Drs. R. Stevenson and V. Perry, Dr. Sell began a new era in tissue bank history by introducing surface antigen typing to the field of tissue banking. These investigators along with Dr. T.I. Malinin, Dr. Harold T. Meryman and other Navy scientists, were instrumental in the establishment of the International Society for Cryobiology in 1963. Dr. Meryman is currently serving as Programme Director of the TCRP at NMRI. Following Captain Sell as Director of the Navy Tissue Bank, between 1974 and 1979, were several individuals. Lieutenant Commander John Curry, MC, USNR, Commander Richard Cahill, MC, USN, and Dr. Richard Wistar all held the directorship for short periods of time. In 1979 Commander D. Michael Strong, MSC, USN began his tour as Tissue Bank Director. He was relieved by Captain James N. Woody, MC, USN, in 1982. Captain Woody served until 1986. By 1985, the scope of research undertaken by the Navy Tissue Bank had grown too diverse to continue as a single programme. Consequently, the diverse programmes representing the Navy Tissue Bank begin transition into the research programmes we know today under the direction of Commander Thomas J. Contreras, Jr., Research Area Manager for Combat Casualty Care, Naval Medical Research and Development Command (NMRDC). In 1985 the Navy Bone Marrow Registry Programme, now the BMRP, was established. In 1986 this program split and the ICBRP was established to pursue bone marrow growth factor research. In 1994, Dr. Meryman rejoined NMRI and the TCRP was established.

Much has been written about the early history and major accomplishments of Dr. Sell and the Navy Tissue Bank (Sell and Friedlaender, 1976). With this lauded history in mind and their eyes set clearly on the needs of the sailors and marines in the field, investigators within these research programmes continue to strive to new research heights. Indeed, the evolutionary research being conducted at NMRI today stem directly from Dr. Sell's earlier studies addressing the problems of bone marrow failure and unwanted immune responses.

2. Bone Marrow Research to Serve the Combat Casualty

Hematopoietic growth factors can speed the recovery of the "stunned" bone marrow of any military combatant exposed to ionising irradiation or chemical warfare agents. During the 1991 Gulf War, when military intelligence suspected that chemical weapons might be used against allied forces, Navy investigators within the ICBRP tested, then received Food and Drug Administration (FDA) approval for a novel growth factor therapy to treat the large number of anticipated casualties. This opportune effort was cited in the Congressional Record for its potential life saving impact. Unfortunately, in many casualty scenarios, the bone marrow is completely destroyed when exposed to ionising irradiation or chemical agents. Here, the only viable option is bone marrow transplantation. However, despite the remarkable efforts of the BMRP, matched donors can at most be found for 70% of certain populations. In a military mass casualty scenario, the logistics of finding suitable matched donors would be immense. Recognising these severe limitations, a team of NMRI scientists lead by Drs. Thomas Davis and Kelvin Lee of the Stem Cell Biology Branch of the ICBRP, developed a system whereby an individual's stems cells could be harvested from peripheral blood, stored, and then expanded outside the body. In collaboration with investigators from the Army and the private industry, this team developed a self-contained bioreactor that can expand 650-fold the total number of bone marrow cells and increase

100-fold the number of stem cells within a two week period. Applying this technology, military physicians could treat combat casualties with otherwise fatal acute bone marrow failure without the need for a matched donor. This patent protected technology was field-tested aboard the Space Shuttle Discovery (STS-63) in February 1995 and again on the Space Shuttle Endeavor (STS-69) in September 1995 and received the 1996 Federal Laboratory Consortium Award for Excellence in Technology Transfer.

For decades scientists and clinicians attempting to treat illnesses or victims of trauma or burns by transplanting skin, tissues, organs or cells have been frustrated by significant problems that continue to limit the field. First and foremost, there has always been a severe problem with an insufficient number of donor tissues and organs. It was the recognition of this fact that led the Navy to establish the world's first tissue bank to store some of the tissues that could be frozen and later thawed and yet remain functional. From the onset, however, it was also evident that only a limited number of tissues could be cryopreserved. To address this problem Dr. Meryman and his colleagues have pursued the advancement of tissue cryopreservation. Just as important is the fact that most tissues once transplanted live but a short time in the new host because the host's immune system recognises the transplant as foreign (non-self) and destroys it. Thus, massive efforts have been undertaken by Navy scientists, both at NMRI and the Naval Blood Research Laboratory, Boston, MA, under the scientific direction of Captain (retired) C. Robert Valeri, MC, USN, and many other investigators — including several Nobel laureates — to better understand those factors responsible for the immune-mediated rejection of transplanted tissues.

Great advances have been made by many in the immunology field making it clear that individuals have very specific tissue types. Furthermore, it has been clearly shown that the closer the organ donor matches the intended recipient, the likelihood for organ rejection is diminished. In the broadest possible sense, the recognition that tissue typing is of utmost importance in limiting rejection episodes is the fundamental premise underlying the establishment of the Navy Bone

Marrow Registry by NMRDC in 1985 under the directorship of Commander Strong and Captain James Woody at NMRI. The current director of the now Bone Marrow Research Programme is Captain Robert Hartzman, MC, USN. Patients with illnesses amenable to treatment with a bone marrow transplant are "lucky" in one sense because as opposed to other transplanted tissues, a bone marrow donor can be a good Samaritan without suffering undue pain or significant medical consequence. This is unquestionably NOT true for heart, liver, lung, or pancreas transplant donors. Bone marrow transplantation is complicated by the fact that not only can the host's immune system reject the transplanted bone marrow, but donor immune cells within the transplanted bone marrow can attack the new host in what is called graft versus host disease. In recognition of these special characteristics surrounding bone marrow transplantation, the Bone Marrow Registry was established to precisely type willing potential donors and to store that information in a large national registry. The basic goal, now dramatically realised in the many lives saved because of the registry, was to quickly and unerringly identify a matched donor for a particular bone marrow type required for the transplant. This registry currently contains over three million typed potential donors and can find a suitable donor for up to 70% of patients in need, although an increased emphasis is now being placed on minority donor recruitment to improve the likelihood of matching patients of African or Asian ancestry.

3. Controlling the Immune Response to Aid Battlefield Casualties

Unfortunately, for individuals in need of a solid organ graft, an identically-matched donor organ is only very rarely available. Most of us are not fortunate enough to have an identical twin, and even if we did our twin could not serve as a heart, lung, liver, or pancreas donor (for obvious reasons). Individuals in need of one of these organs can only hope to receive a graft from an unrelated cadaveric source. Unfortunately many others die while awaiting a transplant. Then, even if the transplanted tissue is closely matched, the patient must take powerful immune-suppressing, anti-rejection medications for the rest of their lives. If the anti-rejection medications are stopped for any reason, the transplanted organ is almost invariably attacked by the immune system and destroyed. To complicate matters further, anti-rejection medications in use currently are expensive and are associated with significant side effects. Moreover, these immune-suppressing drugs weaken the immune response not only to the transplanted organ but also to infectious agents and tumours. These factors have consequently created a tremendous interest in investigating the immune system and how it is regulated.

Out of this interest, programmatic changes were initiated in 1986 that led to the establishment of the ICBRP at NMRI in 1990 under the direction of then Commander Carl H. June, MC, USN. He served as the Programme Director from 1990 to 1995. The current Programme Director of ICBRP is Captain David M. Harlan, MC, USN.

In 1987, LCDR June and his colleagues made the pioneering observation that optimal stimulation of T cells required not only the recognition of a foreign antigen, but also required the simultaneous signalling via another T cell receptor called CD28, also known as the "T cell costimulatory receptor." He proposed the costimulatory receptor served as an "on-off" switch for any immune response. A 1991 *New York Times* article entitled "Biologists Discover New Immune Switch" described this fundamental discovery as "the holy grail of immunology". The significance of this "on-off" switch is the potential provided to clinicians to both augment desired immune responses, such as those needed to ward off bacterial and viral infections or to fight cancerous tumours, and to prevent undesired immune responses, such as those involved in transplant rejection and in autoimmune diseases. The military relevance of this research is clear as it supports combat casualty care by providing effective therapies for injuries sustained on the battlefield such as weapon-induced bone marrow failure, severe burns or organ failure, especially in mass casualty scenarios.

Recently, Captain David Harlan and his colleagues, Lieutenant Commander Allan Kirk, MC, USNR and Dr. Thomas Davis of the ICBRP, Dr. Stuart Knechtle at the University of Wisconsin, and a team of Navy's commercial partners, via a Cooperative Research and Development Agreement (CRADA), tested a novel medical therapy that appears to prevent the rejection of transplanted organs — even if they are badly mismatched. The new therapy appears to "re-educate" the immune system to recognise the foreign tissue as self, thereby not to reject the transplanted organ. If proven successful in humans, this therapy would prevent the expense and serious side effects associated with current anti-rejection drugs. For the study, recently published in *The Proceedings of the National Academy of Sciences* (Kirk *et al*, 1997), the scientists transplanted mismatched kidneys into primates and treated them with the new therapy for 28 days following the transplant. No other drugs were administered, including anti-rejection drugs. The primates remained robust with virtually no side effects for up to eight months following the transplant. These significant findings portend the ability to successfully transplant even mismatched organs and possibly organs from specially-raised animals (xenografts). This work may not only overcome the organ donor shortage but save thousands of lives each year. Another clear potential use of this therapy would be the first effective treatment of combat injuries involving limb loss and extensive burns. In 1997, Drs. June and Harlan were awarded a Federal Laboratory Consortium Award for Excellence in Technology Transfer for the extensive partnering between ICBRP investigators, industry and academia in performing this work. The ICBRP thus received the prestigious award for two consecutive years.

4. Navy Leading the Way in Transplantation Research

Standing on the shoulders of the memorable founders of and long-time contributors to the Navy Tissue Bank, today's investigators at the Naval Medical Research Institute follow in their great tradition. From the humble beginnings of the Navy Tissue Bank in 1950 to the world-class research being conducted today, the focus has always been and will continue to be on the needs of sailors, marines, soldiers and airmen in the field of battle. Researchers at NMRI hope to develop new medical therapies to revolutionise combat casualty care. Therapies being developed today promise to do just that and more. When it comes to transplantation research, the eyes of the world's leading clinicians are looking toward NMRI in expectation of the next pivotal discovery in transplantation research. Although the fundamental medical breakthroughs described in this manuscript are clearly militarily applicable, they may very well change the practice of medicine itself for the benefit of all mankind. Captain Sell would smile with great pride to see how his noteworthy efforts have led to such grand outcomes.

5. References

KIRK, A.D., HARLAN, D.M., ARMSTRONG, N.N., DAVIS, T.A., DONG, Y., GRAY, G.S., HONG, X., THOMAS, D., FECHNER, J.H. JR. and KNECHTLE, S.J. (1997). CTLA4-Ig and anti-CD40 ligand prevent renal allograft rejection in primates, *Proc. Natl. Acad. Sci. USA* **94(16)**, 8789–8794.

SELL, K.W. and FRIEDLAENDER, G.E. (1976). *Tissue Banking for Transplantation*, Greene and Stratton, New York.

1.3 AMERICAN ASSOCIATION OF TISSUE BANKS — THE PRESENT AND FUTURE

M.J. JOYCE

Cleveland Clinic Foundation
Department of Orthopaedics
9500 Euclid Avenue, A41
Cleveland, OH 44195
USA

1. The Present

What does the future hold for the American Association of Tissue Banks (AATB) in the field of tissue banking? We are indebted to Dr. Ken Sell and express our gratitude for the vision that he had as one of its founding fathers. Not only was Dr. Sell a three-time President of the AATB, he continued his role in his later years on the Board of Governors as a representative of accredited tissue banks. We are indebted to him and he presents to all of us an example of an individual member interested in tissue banking.

As the incoming President of the AATB, I would like to present the immediate and future issues that confront the AATB. I do this from a relatively well-rounded perspective. I am an orthopaedic surgeon involved in limb salvage and essentially my vocation includes being a major user of allograft musculoskeletal tissue. I am indeed the closest to the recipient patient and interact with their concerns about potential transfer of disease and efficacy of the tissue being used. My involvement in being a tissue banker started during my orthopaedic training both as a resident and fellow with Dr. Henry Mankin, and was further stimulated by the need for readily available musculoskeletal tissue in the early 1980s. I have been a Medical Director and Administrator for the Musculoskeletal Tissue Bank both at Case Western Reserve University in the past and currently at the Cleveland Clinic Foundation. I personally have been on more than 100 procurements functioning not only as the Medical Director, but also in years past as the Tissue Bank Coordinator with hands-on experience. In recent years I have become a recipient of freeze dried bone powder for periodontal problems. Although the dentist appreciated that I was a tissue banker, my informed consent was done with the instruments in my mouth and the dentist, with bloody gloves, showing me the label on the demineralised bone powder. There will come a day when the circle will be complete: that of being a donor. If I may take a line from the "Lion King", I would call this the circle of tissue banking. I hope that most of us would feel comfortable in completing the circle.

In 1993, Dr. Charles Cuono presented his paradigm programme. His goal was to have us accept the change from the status quo and not be so rigid in our set perceptions with regards to tissue banking. His goal was to build momentum for changes and to create an attitude of acceptance for eventual changes in the field of tissue banking. He emphasised the need for science in tissue banking. In 1997, Dr. Randolph May organised a strategic planning committee. The mission statement of the AATB remains true to its endeavours such that the AATB promotes the safety, quality and availability of tissues and cells for transplantation. The Food and Drug Administration (FDA) interim rule has now become the FDA final rule and further emphasises the importance of the AATB maintaining a role in accreditation. There are a number of external pressures that directly or indirectly effect the AATB. The FDA clearly has a mutual and distinct interaction with the AATB. The increased use and advertisement of bone substitutes such as hydroxyapatite, tricalcium phosphates and the modified corals have created a polarisation in the choices that the user and the recipient have in contrast to allograft musculoskeletal tissues. New technologies are evolving, but the manufacturers often prefer to use xenografts as their base carrier for bone growth factors. With tissue engineering there is the eventual probability of growing a femur from an osteoprogenitor cell culture on a matrix.

In the United States, there is also the change in reimbursement patterns for medical needs and a further emphasis to for allograft tissue to be cost effective. Competition for the medical dollar in the milieu of managed care and capitation is another concern. There are internal pressures within the organisation of the AATB in which accredited regional banks collide head on regarding issues of market share and access to donors. Appropriate questions revolve around the degree of support that members and accredited banks receive from the AATB and also the converse question regarding the degree of support that the AATB receives from the accredited banks. One may have visions for the AATB, but unfortunately it takes money to implement these new programmes.

2. The Future

As we enter into the 21st century, a crucial question confronts the AATB. Is this a trade organisation or is the AATB an organisation representing bankers, users and indirectly recipients — being the vocal spokesperson for the common points that all of us agree with regards to the mission statement? Any changes in the nature of the AATB will be viewed by the FDA with a cautious eye. In recent years we have gained a mutual respectful relationship with the FDA. Will this change if the AATB is viewed as a trade organisation only?

For the current time the AATB remains the leader in accreditation of US tissue banks. There is clearly an increasing burden of accreditation to the association itself. We recognise and appreciate the many hours of hard work of both the Accreditation Committee and Standards and Procedures Committees. We give thanks to the irrespective Chairpersons Dr. James Forsell and Dr. Richard Kagan. In the recent years this has required a well-trained full-time inspector, Dr. Emanuel

Tayo, as well as national office support staff. This creates a uniform approach to accreditation. There has been increased association liability risk especially with regards to legal decisions and the financial burden to the association for those opinions. Although the AATB accreditation consumes a significant amount of the activities of the AATB, accreditation is not the major net revenue producer. However, all our members should support the concept that AATB will be the accrediting organisation for tissue banks in the United States at least for the current time and especially with the current approach that the FDA has taken.

In recent years the AATB has become significantly involved with governmental interaction including a number of tissue-related congressional endeavours. There has been active involvement on the part of a number of members in addition to the presence of AATB and Jeanne Mowe, our Executive Director. We are greatly indebted to Jeanne Mowe for the continuity of the AATB and for the respect shown to the AATB by these governmental agencies. We have been involved in a mutual education process and communication with regards to this governmental interaction.

The AATB is confronted with a key issue: is the AATB an organisation of accredited tissue banks or is it an organisation of individual professional members involved in tissue banking? Certainly there is need for an organisation which carries the concern of donors, recipients and safety of tissue. However, who represents the public as regards to donors and recipients as a whole? Can there be a unique blend with regards to this polarisation? Truly the AATB must maintain its mission statement with respect to safety in the way of setting standards and accrediting tissue banks, maintaining quality of cells and tissues that are banked and released, and also focusing on the availability of tissues and cells.

As AATB grows, it has taken up the issue of both cells and tissues. A small number of accredited reproductive tissue banks have voiced an interest in maintaining their council affiliation with the AATB. The AATB recognises that it is not the leader concerning the areas of marrow transplantation and use of fetal tissues. Historically, at one time the

AATB represented ocular tissues, but the uniqueness of ocular tissues and the conflicts of standards being established for musculoskeletal tissue donors, have led the ocular council to break away from the AATB. Will this also be the situation with reproductive tissue and cells?

Currently the AATB is wrestling with some modification in governance. The role of President has essentially become a full-time job. It is difficult for those Presidents with full-time jobs to maintain the necessary day-to-day activities of the AATB. We have been privileged to have Jeanne Mowe as our Executive Director over many years, an individual who has maintained the forward progress of the AATB and to whom all Presidents and members of the Board of Governors are deeply indebted. In the recent years there has been an increased awareness of the importance of having a Chief Executive Officer to work with the Executive Director. The CEO would be involved with the daily interactions especially in the area of governmental affairs, accreditation and as a readily available individual who could address timely accredited bank issues. There has been a major interest in preserving those councils that represent unique tissues in the way of reproductive cells, skin and musculoskeletal tissue. Accredited banks have requested to have increased representation on the Board of Governors. Special groups such as certified tissue bank specialists and physicians and Medical Directors should also be represented.

This proposed change of governance, has caused controversy. Do the individual members elect the Board of Governors? Do accredited tissue banks elect the Board of Governors? What part does the financial issue play in the role of representation and voting? We recognise that small banks are paying a larger sum for accreditation in the way of percentage of business, but we do recognise that large banks are paying substantial sums of money to the AATB. There is a current proposal to have a voting Board of Governors of 13 individuals with accredited bank representatives making up six of these slots with these individuals being nominated and voted on only by accredited tissue banks. There will be a physician representative nominated and voted for only by physicians, one certified tissue bank specialist nominated and voted on by the CTBS group, two members at large nominated and voted on by the individual membership, one Musculoskeletal Council representative nominated and voted on by the Musculoskeletal Council, one Reproductive Council representative nominated and voted on by the respective council and one Skin Council representative nominated and voted by the respective council. There will be no past President on the Board of Governors. The CEO would be a non-voting member. The majority of the Board will still be elected by individual members in contrast to the accredited tissue banks. This scheme will be such that each accredited tissue bank will have one vote for each of the six accredited tissue bank positions. The question arises concerning who elects the Executive Committee on the Board of Governors. These positions would be the President, the Vice President, Secretary and Treasurer. These representatives will come from within the group of 13 on the Board of Governors. Should the Board of Governors elect their own Executive Committee including that of the President or should this be something accomplished by the individual members of the AATB? The goal of the AATB is to overcome any inertia and become a working board with the impetus on the shoulders of the President while the CEO maintains the drive to complete tasks according to a set time line. The CEO will maintain continuity such that there will be no need for a past President. Obviously certain changes in the by-laws will need to be implemented. It has been felt by a number of members who have been actively involved in AATB matters that the Board members themselves know who has been available in a timely fashion, who has the ingenuity to put forth working proposals, who has performed tasks diligently and who has leadership qualities. Decisions must be made concerning issues of the makeup of the Board of Governors, the CEO and revenues from accreditation to the AATB.

There is indeed a universal appreciation that the structure of the AATB must adapt to the present situation. The current role of the AATB is much different from what it was one or even two decades ago. However, its mission statement remains the same. As the future evolves and we head towards the next millennium, the AATB's priorities will remain the same in the way of (1) setting standards, (2) providing inspection and accreditation, (3) involvement in tissue banking governmental affairs, (4) education and training, and (5) promoting the AATB and specifically promoting the safety and use of allograft tissue.

Chapter 2

PROGRESS IN BLOOD TRANSFUSION AND MARROW TRANSPLANTATION

2.1 The Red Blood Cell Transfusion Trigger
C.R. Valeri (*Naval Blood Research Laboratory, Boston, USA*)

2.2 Marrow Transplantation from Donors Unrelated to Patients: The Role of the Department of Defense
R. Hartzman (*Naval Research Institute, Kensington, USA*)

2.3 Marrow and Peripheral Blood Stem Cell Transplantation
P. McSweeney and R. Storb (*Fred Hutchinson Cancer Research Center, Seattle, USA*)

In 1960, Dr. Sell joined the Navy Tissue Bank and became involved in studies looking at new applications in tissue banking that same year. Navy investigators initiated studies on bone marrow retrieval from cadaver donors and on bone marrow storage, including cryopreservation and storage in nutrient media for as long as two weeks. The successful use of frozen, thawed autologous bone marrow was first reported by Navy scientists in 1963. Further advances in the recovery of bone marrow from cadaver donors were published by Navy scientists in the early 1980s utilising vertebral bodies from cadaver donors as a source of bone marrow. Bone marrow from such donors has now become a prominent interest in both organ transplantation and bone marrow transplantation. In organ transplantation, this has been a source of cells for the studies now being carried out on the induction of tolerance and the mixed chimeric state.

During the 1970s, many Navy physicians were sent to Seattle by Dr. Sell to learn about bone marrow transplantation at the Fred Hutchinson Cancer Research Center, where many of the modern approaches to bone marrow transplantation were developed. The clinical research conducted at this centre led to a Nobel prize for Dr. E. Donnell Thomas and his team. Dr. Reiner Storb, a member of that team and a presenter at the 1975 conference organised by Dr. Sell as well as at the 1997 Symposium in his honour, provides an update on the field of bone marrow and peripheral blood stem cell transplantation.

The Navy has also contributed to the establishment of the National Marrow Donor Program (NMDP) in the United States. In 1979, I was contacted by Dr. Robert Graves then looking for an unrelated bone marrow donor for his daughter, who was suffering from leukemia. He had discovered that the United States did not have a registry to identify such donors and was interested in determining how one could be established. Over the course of the next several years, Dr. Graves and I worked in collaboration with Senator Paul Laxalt in the United States Senate in the establishment of the NMDP. Funding was obtained in 1984 and the first unrelated bone marrow transplant from the registry occurred in 1987 in Seattle. Both Dr. Contreras, who contributed to the first chapter, and Dr. Hartzman who contributes to this chapter, have been instrumental in managing the Navy's contribution to the NMDP. As Dr. Hartzman reports in this chapter, the US Navy continues to participate in this ongoing programme which now has over 2.5 million donors registered.

It was also during the 1970s that much research was conducted on the effects of septic and haemorrhagic shock. The Navy had conducted experiments in Vietnam to understand the consequences of these clinical problems and as a result research was conducted to improve the delivery of healthcare to casualties in the field. Dr. Robert Valeri, who established the Navy's blood research programme in Boston, was also a collaborator with investigators in Bethesda to understand the consequences of haemorrhagic shock. His contribution to this chapter is a reminder of the consequences of anemia and the importance of maintaining an adequate blood volume.

D.M.S.

2.1 THE RED BLOOD CELL TRANSFUSION TRIGGER

C.R. VALERI

Naval Blood Research Laboratory
Boston University School of Medicine
615 Albany Street
Boston, MA 02118
USA

1. Foreword

Ken Sell was a visionary who left his footprints in the sand. The Greek philosophers asked "Who are you and what are you going to do about it?" Ken knew who he was, and this symposium is, in part, a testimony to what he has done.

2. Introduction

The number of blood transfusions administered in the United States has decreased significantly since 1983 when association with the human immunodeficiency virus (HIV) became known (Surgenor *et al*, 1988, 1990; Wallace *et al*, 1995; Consensus Conference, 1988; Dodd, 1992; Schreiber *et al*, 1996; Holland, 1996). A restrictive transfusion practice was instituted and this policy has been kept in place even though most of the published data supporting it have been gathered from retrospective studies and are inconclusive (Kitchens, 1993; Viele and

Weiskopf, 1994; Lunn and Elwood, 1970; Goldman *et al*, 1977; Czer and Shoemaker, 1978; Rawstron, 1980; Friedman *et al*, 1980; Carson *et al*, 1988; Salem-Schatz *et al*, 1990; Mangano *et al*, 1990; Carson and Willett, 1993; Nelson *et al*, 1993; Hebert *et al*, 1995; Carson *et al*, 1996).

The benefits of a red blood cell transfusion include: an increase in oxygen carriage and delivery to tissues; increase in carbon dioxide carriage and delivery to the lungs; regulation of acid-base balance; increase in red blood cell volume, plasma volume and total blood volume; and restoration of haemostasis (Valeri, 1993a, 1993b). Clearly, there are potential risks: haemolytic transfusion reactions, transfusion-related graft-versus-host disease, non-haemolytic febrile transfusion reactions, transmission of disease, immune suppression, and post-transfusion infection (Dodd, 1992; Schreiber *et al*, 1996; Holland, 1996; Valeri, 1993a, 1993b; Triulzi *et al*, 1992; Vamvakas *et al*, 1996; Jeter and Spivey, 1995; Klein, 1996). Other factors to be considered must include: patient pathophysiology; the clinical situation — whether for elective, urgent or emergency reasons; the disease for which the patient is being transfused; and whether transfusion is required before, during or after surgery. The patient's cerebrovascular and cardiovascular, as well as haemodynamic, pulmonary and haematologic status, are also important determinants.

Before the association between donor blood and HIV infection was made, a haematocrit value of 30% and a haemoglobin concentration of 10 g/dl served as the clinical threshold for a red blood cell transfusion, i.e. the "transfusion trigger" (Finch and Lenfant, 1972). Anaemic patients with cardiopulmonary and cerebrovascular insufficiency were generally transfused to greater extents than anaemic patients without these comorbid conditions (Valeri, 1986; Woodson, 1974).

Oxygen carriage by the blood is determined from the haemoglobin concentration/haematocrit value and the percent saturation of the arterial blood. In an anaemic patient who does not have cardiopulmonary and cerebrovascular insufficiency, blood flow will increase to compensate for any decrease in oxygen carriage. However, when blood flow is impaired because of cardiac dysfunction, coronary artery disease, or cerebrovascular disease and failure of pulmonary function to properly oxygenate the blood, the haemoglobin concentration and haematocrit value affect the morbidity and mortality (Carson *et al*, 1996).

The decision to transfuse or not is usually based on measurements of the haematocrit value and haemoglobin concentration in the patient's peripheral venous blood. However, these measurements do not give a true indication of the red blood cell deficit because they yield inaccurate estimates of the red blood cell volume, plasma volume and total blood volume (Valeri, 1993a, 1993b). The only way to get accurate measurements of the red blood cell volume is to employ tests using radioactive labelling of autologous red blood cells with chromium-51 (51-Cr) or technetium-99m (99mTc) (Valeri *et al*, 1973; Jones and Mollison, 1978).

Most anaemic patients are hypovolemic (Valeri *et al*, 1973). Whereas in a normovolemic patient, a red blood cell transfusion should increase the red blood cell volume, decrease the plasma volume, increase the peripheral venous haematocrit value and the haemoglobin concentration, it may not produce the same response in a hypovolemic anaemic patient. In the hypovolemic anaemic patient, there may be increases in both plasma volume and red blood cell volume but not in the peripheral venous haematocrit or haemoglobin concentration (Valeri, 1993a, 1993b; Valeri and Altschule, 1981; Biron *et al*, 1972; Valeri *et al*, 1986). For this reason, measurements of the peripheral venous haematocrit value and haemoglobin concentration alone are not enough to accurately estimate the therapeutic effectiveness of a red blood cell transfusion.

The role of red blood cells in the carriage and delivery of oxygen to tissues, the carriage and delivery of carbon dioxide to the lungs, and the regulation of acid-base balance is well established. However, the role of red blood cells in the regulation of plasma volume has been recognised only recently (Valeri and Altschule, 1981; Biron *et al*, 1972; Valeri *et al*, 1986). In most patients without renal insufficiency, a reduction in the red blood cell volume is usually associated with a reduction in the plasma volume and the total blood volume (Valeri, 1993a, 1993b; Valeri and Altschule, 1981; Biron *et al*, 1972).

2.1. Central blood volume, peripheral blood volume and total blood volume

The term "normovolemic haemodilution state", commonly used by anaesthesiologists and critical care physicians, is a misnomer because it reflects the central blood volume and not the total blood volume (Stehling and Zauder, 1991). Clinicians usually assess the restoration of blood volume from measurements of mean arterial pressure, heart rate, pulmonary artery wedge pressure, cardiac output, arterial pO_2, pCO_2, pH, and urine output (Valeri and Altschule, 1981; Fisher et al, 1991; Cordts et al, 1992) — measurements that assess only the central blood volume. The peripheral blood volume is the volume of blood in the muscles, bones, skin and, importantly, the gastrointestinal tract.

In anaemic patients, mortality is usually associated with a failure to restore perfusion and oxygen delivery to vital organs, and morbidity with a failure to restore perfusion and oxygen delivery to both vital organs and non-vital organs such as the gastrointestinal tract and the extremities. In hypovolemic anaemic patients, a reduction in perfusion to the gastrointestinal tract may produce intestinal ischaemia with entry of bacteria from the gut into the circulation producing endotoxin-mediated multiple organ dysfunction (Deitch and Berg, 1987; Marik, 1993; Ivatury et al, 1996).

Extensive studies in patients with traumatic injuries exhibiting hypovolemic anaemia with significant reductions in red blood cell, plasma and total blood volumes have shown that although transfusions of red blood cells increased both red blood cell and plasma volumes, they produced only minimal increases in the haematocrit value and haemoglobin concentration (Valeri and Altschule, 1981; Biron et al, 1972). The increased plasma volume seen in these hypovolemic anaemic patients following a red blood cell transfusion was a consequence of recruitment of extravascular proteins via the lymphatic circulation into the systemic circulation (Valeri, 1993a, 1993b; Valeri and Altschule, 1981; Biron et al, 1972; Valeri et al, 1986). Traumatised, hypovolemic anaemic patients had normal central red blood cell volumes and significantly reduced peripheral red blood cell and total red blood cell volumes

(Valeri and Altschule, 1981). When red blood cells were transfused to these patients, a significant increase in the peripheral red blood cell volume was observed, but no increase in the central red blood cell volume was observed during the 24-hour post-transfusion period (Valeri and Altschule, 1981).

2.2. Transfusion trigger

With the current practice of relying solely on measurements of peripheral haematocrit level and haemoglobin concentration to identify the red blood cell transfusion trigger, many patients may be deprived of transfusion therapy to reduce morbidity and mortality.

When trying to interpret published data on the transfusion trigger, it is important to understand that most patients requiring transfusions are hypovolemic and anaemic and thus exhibit false increases in haematocrit levels and haemoglobin concentrations. Therefore, these measurements should not be the only consideration in defining the transfusion trigger.

In recent years, the clinical use of erythropoietin to treat normovolemic anaemic patients with renal disease has been shown to produce considerable improvement in the well-being of these patients (McMahon and Dawborn, 1992). Erythropoietin is usually administered to normovolemic anaemic patients with renal disease to achieve a haematocrit value of 30–35% and a haemoglobin concentration of 10–12 g/dl. Human recombinant erythropoietin has also been recommended to reduce the requirement for allogeneic blood transfusions in surgical patients. Human recombinant erythropoietin is recommended for anaemic patients with hemoglobin concentrations greater than 10 g/dl and less than 13 g/dl undergoing elective surgery and patients at high risk for significant perioperative blood loss (Cazzola *et al*, 1997).

The limitations of the haematologic and haemodynamic measurements underscore the importance of clinical judgment in deciding who needs a red blood cell transfusion. Tachycardia, shortness of breath, pallor, decreased tissue turgor, postural hypotension, light-headedness-dizziness, decreased appetite, weakness, and fatigue are important signs and symptoms to be taken into account. A patient should be properly apprised of the potential risks and benefits of a transfusion, and in some instances even be allowed to play a role in this important decision.

For thousands of years it has been a common belief among physicians that blood letting was a useful way of treating a wide variety of illnesses, a belief that persisted despite the common sense observations of a few observant physicians that this form of treatment made the patient worse, not better (King, 1961). Indeed, the first recorded instance of a successful blood transfusion was in a 15-year old boy who was moribund from 20 successive blood lettings over a two-week period but who was immediately revived following transfusion (Greenwalt, 1997). The present policy of allowing sick patients, particularly elderly patients, in the peri-operative period to develop greater degrees of anaemia without correction by blood transfusion may some day receive the same harsh verdict in history that blood letting as therapy finally received 100 years ago (Greenwalt, 1997). Has the sin of commission now become the sin of omission? We believe so.

3. Summary

The benefits of a haematocrit range of 30–35% include improved oxygen delivery and enhanced haemostasis, which will help minimise complications in patients at high risk for ischaemia and peri-operative non-surgical bleeding. In these settings, the conservative transfusion practice using a lower haematocrit range should be replaced with a more aggressive approach. The known risks of blood transfusion would appear to be sufficiently low and the benefits sufficiently high to justify maintaining a haematocrit value of at least 30%. An even higher haematocrit value of 35% may be desirable in patients who have overt cardiopulmonary disease or are at high risk for myocardial ischaemia. Many retrospective studies have been conducted to persuade us that a conservative transfusion trigger is a safe and prudent practice, but retrospective studies are not what we need. What is needed is a series of well-designed, prospective, randomised trials to evaluate the impact of a more aggressive transfusion policy on peri-operative mortality, morbidity and non-surgical bleeding in patients with known cardiopulmonary disease or who are at high risk for myocardial and cerebrovascular ischaemia.

4. Acknowledgements

The authors acknowledge the editorial assistance of Ms. Cynthia A. Valeri and Ms. Gina Ragno and the secretarial assistance of Ms. Marilyn Leavy.

5. References

BIRON, P.E., HOWARD, J., AETSCHULE, M.D. and VALERI, C.R. (1972). Chronic deficits in red-cell mass in patients with orthopaedic injuries (stress anemia), *J. Bone Joint Surg. (Am)* **54**, 1001–1014.

CARSON, J.L., POSES, R.M., SPENCE, R.K. and BONAVITA, G. (1988). Severity of anaemia and operative mortality and morbidity, *Lancet* **1**, 727–729.

CARSON, J.L., DUFF, A., POSES, R.M., BERLIN, J.A., SPENCE, R.K., TROUT, R., NOVECK, H. and STROM, B.L. (1996). Effect of anaemia and cardiovascular disease on surgical mortality and morbidity, *Lancet* **348**, 1055–1060.

CARSON, J.L. and WILLETT, L.R. (1993). Is a hemoglobin of 10 g/dL required for surgery? *Med.Clin.North Am.* **77**, 335–347.

CAZZOLA, M., MERCURIALI, F. and BRUGNARA, C. (1997). Use of recombinant human erythropoietin outside the setting of uremia, *Blood* **89**, 4248–4267.

CONSENSUS CONFERENCE (1988). Perioperative red blood cell transfusion, *JAMA* **260**, 2700–2703.

CORDTS, P.R., LAMORTE, W.W., FISHER, J.B., DELGUERCIO, C., NIEHOFF, J., PIVACEK, L.E., DENNIS, R.C., SIEBENS, H., GEORGIO, A., VALERI, C.R. and MENZOIAN, J.O. (1992). Poor predictive value of hematocrit and hemodynamic parameters for erythrocyte deficits after extensive elective vascular operations, *Surg. Gynecol. Obstet.* **175**, 243–248.

CZER, L.S. and SHOEMAKER, W.C. (1978). Optimal hematocrit value in critically ill postoperative patients, *Surg. Gynecol. Obstet.* **147**, 363–368.

DEITCH, E.A. and BERG, R.D. (1987). Bacterial translocation from the gut: A mechanism of infection, *J. Burn Care Rehab.* **8**, 475–482.

DODD, R.Y. (1992). The risk of transfusion-transmitted infection, *N. Engl. J. Med.* **327**, 419–421.

FINCH, C.A. and LENFANT, C. (1972). Oxygen transport in man, *N. Engl. J. Med.* **286**, 407–415.

FISHER, J.B., DENNIS, R.C., VALERI, C.R., WOODSON, J., DOYLE, J.E., WALSH, L.M., PIVACEK, L., GIORGIO, A., LAMORTE, W.W. and MENZOIAN, J.O. (1991). Effect of graft material on loss of erythrocytes after aortic operations, *Surg. Gynecol. Obstet.* **173**, 131–136.

FRIEDMAN, B.A., BURNS, T.L. and SCHORK, M.A. (1980). An analysis of blood transfusion of surgical patients by sex: A question for the transfusion trigger, *Transfusion* **20**, 179–188.

GOLDMAN, L., CALDERA, D.L., NUSSBAUM, S.R., SOUTHWICK, F.S., KROGSTAD, D., MURRAY, B., BURKE, D.S., O'MALLEY, T.A., GOROLL, A.H., CAPLAN, C.H., NOLAN, J., CARABELLO, B. and SLATER, E.E. (1977). Multifactorial index of cardiac risk in noncardiac surgical procedures, *N. Engl. J. Med.* **297**, 845–850.

GREENWALT, T.J. (1997). A short history of transfusion medicine, *Transfusion* **37**, 550–563.

HEBERT, P.C., WELLS, G., MARSHALL, J., MARTIN, C., TWEEDDALE, M., PAGLIARELLO, G. and BLAJCHMAN, M. (1995). Transfusion requirements in critical care. A pilot study, *JAMA* **273**, 1439–1444.

HOLLAND, P.V. (1996). Viral infections and the blood supply, *N. Engl. J. Med.* **334**, 1734–1735.

IVATURY, R.R., SIMON, R.J., ISLAM, S., FUEG, A., ROHMAN, M. and STAHL, W.M. (1996). A prospective randomized study of end points of resuscitation after major trauma: Global oxygen transport indices versus organ-specific gastric mucosal pH, *J. Am. Coll. Surg.* **183**, 145–154.

JETER, E.K. and SPIVEY, M.A. (1995). Noninfectious complications of blood transfusion, *Hematol. Oncol. Clin. North Am.* **9**, 187–204.

JONES, J. and MOLLISON, P.L. (1978). A simple and efficient method of labelling red cells with 99mTc for determination of red cell volume, *Br. J. Haematol.* **38**, 141–148.

KING, L.S. (1961). The blood-letting controversy: A study in the scientific method, *Bull. Hist. Med.* **35**, 1–13.

KITCHENS, C.S. (1993). Are transfusions overrated? Surgical outcome of Jehovah's Witnesses, *Am. J. Med.* **94**, 117–119.

KLEIN, H.G. (1996). New insights into the management of anemia in the surgical patient, *Am. J. Med.* **101**, 12S–15S.

LUNN, J.N. and ELWOOD, P.C. (1970). Anaemia and surgery, *Br. Med. J.* **3**, 71–73.

MANGANO, D.T., BROWNER, W.S., HOLLENBERG, M., LONDON, M.J., TUBAU, J.F. and TATEO, I.M. (1990). Association of perioperative myocardial ischemia with cardiac morbidity and mortality in men undergoing noncardiac surgery, *N. Engl. J. Med.* **323**, 1781–1788.

MARIK, P.E. (1993). Gastric intramucosal pH. A better predictor of multiorgan dysfunction syndrome and death than oxygen-derived variables in patients with sepsis, *Chest* **104**, 225–229.

McMAHON, L.P. and DAWBORN, J.K. (1992). Subjective quality of life assessment in hemodialysis patients at different levels of hemoglobin following use of recombinant human erythropoietin, *Am. J. Nephrol.* **12**, 162–169.

NELSON, A.H., FLEISHER, L.A. and ROSENBAUM, S.H. (1993). Relationship between postoperative anemia and cardiac morbidity in high-risk vascular patients in the intensive care unit, *Crit. Care Med.* **21**, 860–866.

RAWSTRON, R.E. (1980). Anaemia and surgery: a retrospective clinical study, *Aust. N. Z. J. Surg.* **39**, 425–432.

SALEM-SCHATZ, S.R., AVORN, J. and SOUMERAI, S.B. (1990). Influence of clinical knowledge, organizational context, and practice style on transfusion decision making. Implications for practice change strategies, *JAMA* **264**, 476–483.

SCHREIBER, G.B., BUSCH, M.P., KLEINMAN, S.H. and KORELITZ, J.J. (1996). The risk of transfusion-transmitted viral infections, *N. Engl. J. Med.* **334**, 1685–1690.

STEHLING, L. and ZAUDER, H.L. (1991). Acute normovolemic hemodilution, *Transfusion* **31**, 857–868.

SURGENOR, D.M., WALLACE, E.L., HALE, S.G. and GILPATRICK, M.W. (1988). Changing patterns of blood transfusions in four sets of United States hospitals, 1980–1985, *Transfusion* **28**, 513–518.

SURGENOR, D.M., WALLACE, E.L., HAO, S.H. and CHAPMAN, R.H. (1990). Collection and transfusion of blood in the United States, 1982–1988, *N. Engl. J. Med.* **322**, 1646–1651.

TRIULZI, D.J., VANEK, K., RYAN, D.H. and BLUMBERG, N. (1992). A clinical and immunologic study of blood transfusion and postoperative bacterial infection in spinal surgery, *Transfusion* **32**, 517–524.

VALERI, C.R., COOPER, A.G. and PIVACEK, L.E. (1973). Limitations of measuring blood volume with iodinated I 125 serum albumin, *Arch. Int. Med.* **132**, 534–538.

VALERI, C.R. (1986). Clinical importance of the oxygen transport function of preserved red blood cells. In: *Proc. 12th Katzir-Katchalsky Meeting on Oxygen Transport in Red Blood Cells.* C. Nicolau, ed., Pergamon Press Ltd., Oxford, England, Vol. 54, pp 37–55.

VALERI, C.R., DONAHUE, K., FEINGOLD, H.M., CASSIDY, G.P. and ALTSCHULE, M.D. (1986). Increase in plasma volume after the transfusion of washed erythrocytes, *Surg. Gynecol. Obstet.* **162**, 30–36.

VALERI, C.R. (1993a). Physiology of blood transfusion. In: *Surgical Intensive Care.* P. S. Barie and G. T. Shires, eds., Little, Brown and Co., pp 681–721.

VALERI, C.R. (1993b). Transfusion medicine and surgical practice. In: *Bulletin of the American College of Surgeons.* Vol. 78, pp 20–24.

VALERI, C.R. and ALTSCHULE, M.D. (1981). *Hypovolemic Anemia of Trauma: The Missing Blood Syndrome.* Chemical Rubber Company, Boca Raton, FL.

VAMVAKAS, E.C., CARVEN, J.H. and HIBBERD, P.L. (1996). Blood transfusion and infection after colorectal cancer surgery, *Transfusion* **36**, 1000–1008.

VIELE, M.K. and WEISKOPF, R.B. (1994). What can we learn about the need for transfusion from patients who refuse blood? The experience with Jehovah's Witnesses, *Transfusion* **34**, 396–401.

WALLACE, E.L., CHURCHILL, W.H., SURGENOR, D.M., AN, J., CHO, G., MCGURK, S. and MURPHY, L. (1995). Collection and transfusion of blood and blood components in the United States, 1992, *Transfusion* **35**, 802–812.

WOODSON, R.D. (1974). Red cell adaptation in cardiorespiratory disease. In: *Clinics in Haematology, Anemia and Hypoxia*. L. Garby, ed., pp 627–628.

2.2 MARROW TRANSPLANTATION FROM DONORS UNRELATED TO PATIENTS: THE ROLE OF THE DEPARTMENT OF DEFENSE

R.J. HARTZMAN

Bone Marrow Research Department
C.W. Bill Young Marrow Donor Recruitment
and Research Program
Naval Medical Research Institute
5516 Nicholson Lane
Kensington, MD 20895, USA

1. Summary

The National Marrow Donor Program (NMDP) was created in 1986 through the effort of families, the medical community and Federal support. NMDP provides a life saving resource for thousands of Americans who need a marrow transplant and do not have a closely matched sibling available as the donor of healthy marrow. The programme provides for clinical support, donor recruitment and transplant matching, and focussed practical medical research and development to improve unrelated donor marrow transplantation.

The Department of Defense, with the Navy as the Executive Agent, has played a key national role in the development of unrelated donor marrow transplantation. At the request of Congress, the Navy initiated Federal funding of an organisation which today has become the National Marrow Donor Program (NMDP). Within the Navy, the

Naval Medical Research Institute's Bone Marrow Research Department has primary responsibility for NMDP programmes, with oversight by the Naval Medical Research and Development Command, and Office of Naval Research. In 1989, the overall Federal oversight for the programme was transferred to the Department of Health and Human Services.

This report focusses on the role of the Naval Medical Research Institute in the development of the NMDP and the national effort to make unrelated donor marrow transplantation a reality. This would not have been possible in the Navy without the support of the Naval Medical Research and Development Command, Office of Naval Research, Navy Bureau of Medicine and Surgery, and Navy Surgeons General, and Chiefs of Naval Operations. The Navy programme operates as Executive Agency under a policy of the Assistant Secretary of Defense (Health Affairs), and has been generously supported by hundreds of thousands of volunteers from the Department of Defense and hundreds of Commands and Commanding Officers from all branches of the Armed Services, Reserves and National Guard.

This report does not focus on the millions of individuals and family members, the NMDP and NMDP member organisations staff, committee and Board members, medical organisations, Department of Health and Human Services (HHS), and US Congress, who have made this national effort possible.

The NMDP, coordinated through a centre in Minneapolis, is a consortium of over 200 institutions including many major teaching hospitals and blood banks. The programme is sponsored by all three US national blood bank organisations: the American Association of Blood Banks, the America's Blood Centers, and the American Red Cross.

In 1998, the NMDP consists of:
• Over three million volunteers willing to provide marrow to a stranger and 600 000 from non-US donor centres that are part of the NMDP network.

- National Marrow Donor Program national coordinating centre in Minneapolis.
- 111 transplant centres at major hospitals
  The medical, technical and scientific expertise to perform marrow and stem cell transplants, work with patients and the NMDP to search for matched donors, and develop unrelated donor transplantation.
- 114 marrow collection centres (hospital based)
  The technology to safely collect marrow for transplantation from volunteer donors.
- 100 donor centres (most at blood banks)
  The commitment to (1) support drives for volunteer donors; (2) maintain confidential donor information; (3) work with the NMDP and transplant centres to find the correct volunteer; (4) support the volunteer donor through all aspects of marrow and stem cell donation.
- Clinical and research laboratories
  Laboratories to test blood samples from volunteers and implement high-volume low-cost DNA-based testing; laboratories to provide research level (high resolution testing including DNA sequencing) to evaluate the role of HLA matching on marrow transplant outcome.
- Formal and informal relationships with many national and international organisations.

The NMDP and the national effort to develop unrelated donor marrow transplantation are supported by two Federal agencies:

(1) Department of Health and Human Services (Health Resources and Services Administration) for overall programme oversight and development
   (a) Policy and programme oversight
   (b) Support for NMDP structures, committees and directors
   (c) Donor recruitment
   (d) Improved patient access, physician education

and

(2)   Department of Defense with the Navy as Executive Agent
       (a) Providing the primary scientific and technical structure
           and support for precise and cost-effective HLA testing for
           all donors, and to determine the role of matching in
           transplant outcome;
       (b) Providing for enhancements in communication and data
           handling supporting effective donor and patient matching
           and rapid identification of donors;
       (c) Providing for HLA typing volunteers with an emphasis on
           minorities to improve timely access to all patients; and
       (d) The C.W. Bill Young Marrow Donor Recruitment and
           Research Program, the Department of Defense Marrow
           Donor Program; the Program's C.W. Bill Young/DoD
           Marrow Donor Center (one of the 100 marrow donor
           centres in the NMDP network), and the 150 000 DoD
           volunteers who have been registered through the DoD
           programme and have been extensively HLA typed. 10%
           of all NMDP marrow donations (more than 600 to date,
           two to four each week) are from DoD volunteers.

The Navy was selected to initiate this Federal programme due to
its long-standing expertise in the development of transplantation
technologies because of military contingency needs. In January 1998,
over three million volunteer marrow donors are listed on the files of
the National Marrow Donor Program (600 000 of these from non-US
members of the NMDP donor centres). The NMDP has facilitated over
6000 transplants at the rate of more than three marrow transplants
per day. Key technologies have been developed and demonstrated,
and unrelated donor marrow transplantation has become an accepted
mode of therapy for over 60 otherwise fatal diseases. Numerous
improvements are being made in all aspects of unrelated donor marrow
transplantation from tissue typing, matching of donors and patients
to medical sciences, to continually increase the likelihood of success
of each transplant.

As a major part of the DoD and National programme, the Department of Defense instituted in 1990 the C.W. Bill Young Marrow Donor Recruitment and Research Program, the Department of Defense Marrow Donor Program. The Navy is the Executive Agent for this DoD programme and for DoD support of the National Marrow Donor Program. The C.W. Bill Young/DoD Marrow Donor Program supports the development of the National effort, plays a key role in technology development both within the DoD and the nation, and responds to military contingency requirements for medical response to marrow toxic injury.

As of January 1998, 150 000 DoD volunteers have enrolled in the C.W. Bill Young/DoD Marrow Donor Program and been listed on the NMDP registry. These DoD volunteers are the single greatest source of unrelated donor transplants, 600 to date, at a current donation rate of two to three marrow donations each week. The national development of DNA-based testing for Human Leukocyte Antigen (HLA) typing was led by this Navy program. This is the central technology for effective unrelated donor marrow transplant matching.

In 1989, primary administrative responsibility for the civilian National Marrow Donor Program was transferred from the Navy to the Department of Health and Human Services, initially the National Heart, Lung and Blood Institute of the National Institutes of Health and subsequently to the Health Resources and Services Administration of HHS. The Navy has continued to play a major role in the development of unrelated donor marrow transplantation and the development of improved NMDP capabilities for these transplants.

2. Background

The Navy initiated its role in the evolution of transplantation technology in the mid 1950s with the development of the Navy Tissue Bank at the Naval Medical Research Institute largely through the foresight of Captain George Hyatt. The Tissue Bank was developed to respond to military casualties caused by burns, fractures and other serious wounds in the Korean conflict.

The Navy Tissue Bank developed and demonstrated all critical technologies for transplantation of skin, dura and bone from cadaveric donors. Today, there are tissue banks throughout the world, each with its origin in the US Navy Tissue Bank.

In the 1960s, when transplantation of kidneys and bone marrow were only in their early stages of development, the Navy began its key role in the development of tissue typing technologies. The expansion of the role of the Navy Tissue Bank was the vision of Captain Kenneth Sell.

The development of traditional tissue banking for non-viable tissues was primarily to support casualties with surgical wounds and burns. The expansion pioneered by Dr. Sell focussed primarily on transplantation of viable organs, initially the kidney and bone marrow. Transplantation of viable organs required a more complete understanding of physiology and biochemistry than the previous focus on non-viable organ transplantation. The focus of the Navy's work in viable organ and marrow transplantation was the immune system and its influence on graft acceptance, rejection and graft-versus-host disease. The needs of successful viable organ transplantation removed almost all limits on the need to understand the full range of laboratory and clinical research questions.

Bone marrow transplantation was uniformly fatal without a correctly tissue typed and closely-matched donor and patient. Marrow transplants were attempted in the 1950s and early 1960s without knowing the requirements for matching. These early marrow transplants were not successful until the end of the 1960s at the time when testing for the HLA genes became well enough understood to detect the most common of these genes.

Initially, marrow donors could only be from tissue type (HLA) matched siblings because the technology was too rudimentary and time consuming to discern more subtle genetic differences. Some of the early development in HLA testing was supported in part through the Navy Tissue Bank in both intramural Navy programmes and extramural support including: (1) the development of serologic typing; (2) development of cellular-based typing for HLA (called HLA-D typing); (3) primed lymphocyte typing and T cell cloning; (4) a wide variety of assays for cellular immune response; and (5) technology to type the DNA from an individual's chromosomes.

At first, tissue typing was performed using sera from post-partum women as the test reagents (women make antibodies toward the HLA types of their child's types that come from the father) (serologic typing). Then *in vitro* methods testing human cells from donors and patients were introduced with refinements leading to cloning of human immune cells (cellular typing). With the simplification in testing of nucleic acid sequences, it became possible to directly type the DNA of the genes encoding the HLA types. (HLA antigens are proteins on the surface of cells and these HLA proteins are critical components of the immune response.) The Navy has played a key role in the development of this technology, and is today providing the scientific and technical support to transform all HLA typing to high-precision, low-cost technology throughout the US.

For 10 years beginning from the early 1970s, the Navy conducted a clinical research programme in marrow and kidney transplantation at the National Naval Medical Center in Bethesda, Maryland. The Navy continued its research in all aspects of transplantation, including the fundamental investigations of immune responses and regulation of the immune and haematopoietic systems. Hundreds of important discoveries were published.

In the early 1980s, marrow transplantation became regularly successful as a cure for certain deadly cancers of the blood-forming system.

HLA testing progressed to the point where the correctly-matched sibling could be routinely identified with relative ease. The technology of HLA typing became more widely used. From clinical experience, it became known that cancer patients receiving platelet transfusions became rapidly sensitised to the HLA types found on platelets following platelet transfusions required to prevent bleeding following chemotherapy. This knowledge of sensitisation to HLA through platelets and the discovery that platelet donations matched for the patient's HLA type could be successfully transfused in sensitised patients led the National Institutes of Health (NIH) to support the development of HLA-matched platelet transfusions. NIH supported HLA typing of platelet donor volunteers in a number of US cities, and by 1985, over 60 000 platelet donor volunteers have been HLA typed as part of this programme.

Although marrow transplant success was beginning to become routine, only 30% of patients needing marrow transplants were fortunate enough to have a brother or sister who matched them. 70% of patients who could be potentially cured of a deadly disease by a marrow transplant could not receive a marrow transplant because there was no donor.

3. Beginning of Unrelated Donor Marrow Transplantation in the US

In the 1980s parents began to search for volunteers and a few successful transplants were performed using unrelated donors who had been HLA typed as platelet donor volunteers through a National Institutes of Health volunteer platelet donor programme, from volunteers recruited by families, or from laboratory volunteers. But it was obvious to families desperately searching for matched volunteers that a national programme was essential. Families then asked for help from Congress.

In 1984, the National Institutes of Health held a consensus conference which concluded that it was premature to start a coordinated national effort in unrelated donor marrow transplantation because of the very limited experience. However, the conference did support the development of elements of a national programme to determine the feasibility of further studies. Congress requested that the Navy institute a national programme.

The Navy issued a Request for Proposals in 1985, awarded the first grant to establish the national programme to a consortium of the three largest national blood programmes, the Red Cross, the American

Association of Blood Banks, and the Council of Community Blood Centers (today named America's Blood Centers) with a board of directors, which included families, medical and scientific experts. The programme developed its structure and began recruiting volunteers, initially from lists of volunteers who had already been registered as volunteer platelet donors primarily through the National Institutes of Health funding to support HLA-matched platelet donations for cancer patients with low platelet counts following chemotherapy. In addition, there were approximately 50 donor centres associated with the programme that were given support and these centres could raise funds for marrow donor drives either in conjunction with platelet donor drives or independently.

The first marrow transplant occurred in Minneapolis in December 1987. (Parenthetically, the donor and patient from that first transplant met each other for the first time in October 1997.)

The NMDP provides a sound national structure through its standards and well-documented policies and procedures. There are established and fair policies for evaluating and adding new donor centre and transplant centre members and for monitoring and improving the effectiveness of the entire system of finding donors and performing transplants. There is a system within NMDP to directly support patients seeking transplants (Office of Patient Advocacy) and a committee that oversees this operation and recommends improvements in NMDP operations from the patient's perspective.

Prior to the development of the NMDP in 1986, there were only a few thousand potential donors available and there was no national coordination of marrow donations.

Since 1986, the number of marrow transplants has steadily increased with more being performed each year. Every element of the national system, including the science of matching donor and patient as well as transplantation medicine have greatly improved.

After the programme was initially established, the National Institutes of Health accepted transfer of the primary administrative responsibility from the Navy in 1989. In 1994 the HHS transferred primary responsibility to the Health Resources and Services Administration.

In 1990, the Congress asked the DoD and Navy to take on a larger role in expanding donor recruitment, expanding diversity through emphasis on American minority volunteer recruitment, for technology development in HLA testing, and development of military contingency capability. A DoD formal policy was developed with concurrence from the Secretaries of each Service. The programme was formally named the C.W. Bill Young Marrow Donor Recruitment and Research Program.

Today the NMDP file lists over three million volunteers — potential donors who are informed, HLA-typed and formally registered. The number of potential donors continues to grow, increasing by over 350 000 each year.

The inclusion of American minorities in this process is one of the most important goals of the NMDP. Today 35% of all newly-added potential donors are from American minorities. As of January 1998, 665 000 potential donors are from American minorities: African American, Asian/Pacific Islander, Hispanic of American Indian/Alaska Native.

Because of this programme the likelihood that an American patient will have at least one volunteer matched in the preliminary search of the NMDP file is over 80%. When searches were initiated by the programme in 1987, there was an 8% chance that a patient would have a donor.

Today, because of an emphasis on donor recruitment from American minorities, as stated in the Transplant Amendments Act of 1990, over 66% of American minority patients (59% to 76%) have preliminary matches on the NMDP registry. This lower percentage of matches for minorities is because of: (1) a lower number of minorities than Caucasians are registered (27.2% of the 2.5 million volunteers where the racial group of the donor is registered according to the Office of Management and Budget guidelines); and (2) because of the extraordinary complexity of genetic (HLA) types from these individuals.

In the 12 months to 1 January, 1998, 1282 transplants were performed with marrow from unrelated donors provided through the National Marrow Donor Program. Although this is a significant milestone, approximately 3500 patients seek donors (progress to requesting advanced matching from NMDP-registered volunteer donors) each year through the NMDP. Each year at least 6000 patients have diseases which could be cured by marrow transplantation from unrelated donors, and likely many more than this number of patients could benefit once scientific and medical developments permit an expansion of diseases treatable by this therapy. Many of those patients not receiving marrow from one of these unrelated donors have been assisted by the NMDP and its Office of Patient Advocacy to find an alternative therapy.

The number of unrelated donor transplants increased by nearly 10% over the previous year (1282 vs. 1174). In addition, over 100 Americans received marrow from volunteer donors registered in foreign donor centres cooperating with the NMDP. Continuous increases in the number of transplants have been powered by the steady improvement in the success of these clinical procedures; the number of available HLA-typed volunteers; the increased sophistication of HLA matching; and the increasing effectiveness of the coordinated efforts of nearly 200 American institutions.

Because of the Navy and related NMDP research programmes supported by Congress, a revolution in technology is unfolding. The capability of directly typing the transplant genes is becoming a practical reality. When this programme began its first transplant in 1987, only expensive and inaccurate matching procedures were available. Typing for each donor cost hundreds of dollars. First, the existing technology was streamlined to reduce the basic cost. Then, the technology was transformed to use the new approach to test the DNA of the donors while maintaining a low cost.

Much of the science and technology of clinical marrow transplantation is being driven by the National Marrow Donor Program and the cooperating transplant centres, the Navy and HHS. From the beginning of the programme, it was known that the technology of transplant matching would undergo major changes. So samples of blood were maintained on all donors and patients in a repository in San Francisco. Those samples are now being tested using DNA-based methods that were not available when the transplants were performed. Critical information is becoming available, possible only because of a nationally-coordinated system supported by the Federal government. Only in this way will we be able to uncover which of the complex array of HLA genes are critical to successful transplant outcome, cure, and which of these genes are less critical.

NMDP donors are typed for their transplant matching genetic types (HLA) using increasingly sophisticated technology. New technology takes advantage of scientific advances permitting the programme to directly type the DNA of the genes in the cells of a donor or patient that code (are the blueprint for) their HLA tissue types.

Of the three main HLA antigens, HLA-A, HLA-B and HLA-DR, all testing of DR has been performed by DNA technology for the past several years. This past year (1997), for the first time, the technology has advanced sufficiently to type the HLA-A and HLA-B genes in relatively high capacity and allow the initiation of pilot programmes to prove the reliability of large-scale testing.

DNA-based testing is at least ten times more precise and reliable than the technology it replaces. DNA technology is particularly essential for testing American minorities. HLA types in many minorities is more complex than in Caucasians, and some of these complex HLA types have only recently been resolved because of the introduction of DNA testing by this programme and its Navy support. Today 750 000 NMDP donors have been tested with this advance-level HLA typing to speed the process of completing searches and performing transplants.

Allogeneic (donation from a second person) marrow transplantation requires every skill in medical science and technology. The science and medical technology continue to improve to this day. At first only a small percentage of patients were cured. Cure rates for transplants using unrelated donors were initially lower than the cure rates where brothers or sisters are used. But as expected, these transplant success rates are now providing a similar success rate where similar diseases are treated.

Improvements in medical care of transplant patients and concurrent advances in the ability to manipulate marrow and immune cells are making unrelated donor marrow transplantation more successful and significant in the evolution of medical science.

4. Navy, C.W. Bill Young Marrow Donor Recruitment and Research Program

Accomplishments:
* Starting from 1986, it supported the development of all administrative, technical and scientific structures of the National Marrow Donor Program.
* Supported the continuous improvements for the national computer-based information and communication system for NMDP providing the basis for linking: (a) NMDP national coordinating centre in Minneapolis; (b) 100 donor centres serving over three million potential donors; (c) 111 hospital-based transplant centres; (d) 40 HLA typing laboratories and two test sample repositories; and (e) international cooperating marrow donor registries.
* Starting from 1988, the Navy laboratory acted as a test bed to demonstrate the feasibility of a laboratory performing large-scale DNA-based testing of HLA reliably (Ng *et al*, 1996). This was accomplished using technology previously reported in the scientific literature by using sequence specific oligonucleotide probe (SSOP) testing (Tiercy *et al*, 1993). Increasing the scale of this low-volume scientific system to maintain and improve reliability while increasing capacity — where more than a million volunteers could be tested at low cost — was a key national accomplishment. The staff and committees of the National Marrow Donor Program and laboratories contracted by the NMDP with Navy funding and technical support played critical parts in this national

development. The Navy laboratory provided a technical advisory system for these laboratories and provided a system of hidden quality control samples to provide the basis for continual improvements in the quality of DNA-based HLA typing.

- This same DNA technology demonstration provides a basis for the technology to convert a broad range of medical laboratory tests to utilise highly accurate and cost-effective DNA-based diagnostic technology — applicable to infectious disease testing and genetic testing in addition to Navy-proven use for HLA testing.
- Developed and implemented improved Human Leukocyte Antigen (HLA) typing technology using a new DNA-based methodology. As of 1997, all DoD donors are typed for HLA by the new DNA technology for HLA-A, B and DR.
- Virtually all HLA-DR testing in the US is now performed by standards of DNA-testing developed by the Navy in conjunction with NMDP. The Navy provides a national clinical research technology support system for DNA typing of HLA for unrelated donor marrow transplantation: (a) technical advisory system for civilian laboratories; (b) quality control for the national system including evaluation of hidden control samples; (c) national standards; and (d) software for computer-based data analysis.
- Support of civilian HLA typing using DNA technology; over 600 000 DNA typings by contract laboratories. The Navy laboratory has performed over 150 000 DNA typings.
- Large-scale HLA Class I typing by DNA is being implemented, led at the national level by this programme.
- The Navy programme, the C.W. Bill Young/DoD Marrow Donor Program, is the largest contributor in the world for the identification of new HLA types. This is made possible by integrating donor testing and research DNA sequence evaluation of unusual results.
- Over 100 DoD families have received unrelated donor marrow transplants through the NMDP.
- The Navy's C.W. Bill Young/DoD Marrow Donor Center provides several hundred donor recruitment drives on military bases each

year, most in support of specific DoD families and Base Commanders supporting these families. Over 25 000 DoD volunteers are added to the DoD and NMDP donor files each year.

- This Navy/DoD programme and its volunteers have provided marrow for over 600 transplants from DoD donors, one to six each week, the largest single source of marrow donations from the 100 NMDP Donor Centers.
- 150 000 DoD donors have registered with the programme and been HLA typed as of January 1998.
- The C.W. Bill Young DoD Program has provided support of civilian donor recruitment with emphasis on minorities, as required by legislation. Of the three million volunteers listed on the NMDP file, the Navy programme has contributed to an increase of 1 500 000 NMDP volunteers (including those recruited directly by DoD and the support of NMDP civilian volunteer recruitment) and, of these, an increase of nearly 600 000 American minority volunteers (including those recruited directly by DoD).
- The NMDP has provided donors for over 6200 transplants to January 1998 and over 1200 in 1997. These unrelated donor transplants are the critical national resource for the medical and scientific development of unrelated donor marrow transplantation.

The Naval Medical Research Institute's Bone Marrow Research Department, C.W. Bill Young Marrow Donor Recruitment and Research Program with NMRDC, and the Office of Naval Research continue to provide critical scientific, technical and medical capabilities required for the full development of unrelated donor marrow transplantation. One area of primary focus is improving the sophistication and uniformity of HLA testing for all donors and patients and a system to streamline donor and patient matching. This will be paired with the development of a wide range of transplant technology developments. These developments are necessary to make unrelated donor transplantation rapidly available to treat an increasing number of diseases or marrow failure.

5. References

NG, J., HURLEY, C.K., CARTER, C., BAXTER-LOWE, L.A., BING, D., CHOPEK, M., HEGLAND, J., LEE, T.D., LI, T.C., HSU, S., KuKURUGA, D., MASON, J.M., MONOS, D., NOREEN, H., ROSNER, G., SCHMECKPEPER, B., DUPONT, B., HARTZMAN, R.J. (1996). Large-scale DRB and DQB1 oligonucleotide typing for the NMDP registry: Progress report from year 2, *Tissue Antigens* **47**(1), 21–26.

TIERCY, J.M., ROOSNEK, E., SPEISER, D., CROS, P., ALLIBERT, P., MACH, B. and JEANNET M. (1993). Replacement of HLA Class II serology by the HLA-DR microtitre plate oligotyping assay: A one-year experiment in unrelated bone marrow donor selection, *Br. J. Haematol.* **85**(2), 417–418.

2.3 MARROW AND PERIPHERAL BLOOD STEM CELL TRANSPLANTATION

P.A. McSWEENEY and R. STORB

Fred Hutchinson Cancer Research Center
and
University of Washington School of Medicine
1124 Columbia Street, M318
Seattle, WA 98104
USA

1. Introduction

The last decade has seen rapid increase in the use of haematopoietic stem cell transplantation as a treatment for a variety of malignant and non-malignant diseases. This has been largely due to improvements in supportive clinical care, haematopoietic engraftment rates, and the prevention of graft-versus-host disease (GVHD) which have resulted in lower morbidity and mortality after stem cell transplantation and thereby improved outcomes. An important advance for autologous transplants has been the use of peripheral blood stem cell (PBSC) grafts that allow for rapid haematopoietic reconstitution after high dose therapy has been given. As a result, PBSC grafts are now being explored for allogeneic stem cell transplantation. In addition, basic research has produced new pharmaceutical and recombinant agents which are increasingly important for further advances in stem cell transplantation.

This review will provide a broad summary of the basic principles, results of treatment, newer developments, and possible future directions of marrow and peripheral blood stem cell transplantation.

2. Background

Initially, most transplants were performed on younger patients with leukaemia or aplastic anaemia, and involved the almost exclusive use of HLA-identical siblings as marrow donors (Thomas et al, 1975). Due to its success, the use of allogeneic stem cell transplantation (allografting) broadened to include a variety of additional severe haematological diseases (Table 1), including genetically-based diseases of the haematopoietic and immune systems, and transplants have been increasingly performed in older patients up to the age of 65 years. Improvements in the prevention of GVHD have encouraged the use of partially HLA-matched family donors and, increasingly, HLA-matched unrelated donors. A great increase in the use of autologous stem cell transplantation (autografting) as a treatment for haematologic malignancy and solid tumours has also occurred. Because of the rapid

Table 1. Diseases treated by stem cell transplantation.

Malignant	Non-malignant
Chronic Leukaemias (CML/CLL)	Aplastic Anaemia
Acute Leukaemias (AML/ALL)	Immunodeficiency Syndromes
Multiple Myeloma	Fanconi Anaemia
Myelodysplastic Syndromes	Inborn Errors of Metabolism
Myeloproliferative Disorders	Beta Thalassemia
Breast Cancer*	Sickle Cell Anaemia
Ovarian Cancer*	Autoimmune Diseases*
Neuroblastoma	
Various Sarcomas*	
Germ Cell Tumour*	

*Autologous transplants almost always used.

recovery of haematopoiesis after treatment, the use of PBSC transplants has largely supplanted the use of bone marrow transplants in autografting performed for myeloma, lymphoma and solid tumours. The main conceptual basis underlying stem cell transplantation for malignancy is that it allows treatment with supralethal doses of chemotherapy and/or radiation in an attempt to overcome tumour resistance. However, it has become increasingly clear that allografts have important anti-tumor activity (graft-versus-leukaemia [GVL] effect) separate from the conditioning regimens. In the treatment of nonmalignant diseases such as aplastic anaemia, the replacement of a defective haematopoietic or immune system is the goal and, therefore, less intensive therapy may be adequate to achieve stable engraftment of donor cells. After allografting, long-term haematopoietic function and, to a large extent, immunological function are reconstituted from so-called stem cells transferred with the graft. After infusion into the blood stream, these immature pluripotential cells home to the marrow micro-environment and give rise to long-term multilineage haematopoiesis. The marrow micro-environment is not destroyed by conditioning programmes and remains of host origin (Simmons *et al*, 1987).

2.1. Source of haematopoietic progenitor cells

Historically, most transplants involved using marrow "harvested" under general anaesthesia from the donor's pelvis (Thomas and Storb, 1970). Recently, there has been an increasing use of haematopoietic progenitor cells collected from the blood by leukapheresis. The term "stem cell transplant" is increasingly used, and can be applied to transplants using either source of haematopoietic progenitors. After treatment with chemotherapy and/or recombinant growth factors, such as granulocyte colony-stimulating factors (G-CSF) or granulocyte/macrophage colony-stimulating factors (GM-CSF), much larger numbers of haematopoietic progenitors circulate in the blood than usual, and these cells can be easily collected by leukapheresis procedures. Transplantation of PBSC has been associated with more rapid haematopoietic recovery than seen after transplantation of bone marrow (Langenmayer *et al*, 1995). Pretreatment of donors with G-CSF may also enhance the rate of haematopoietic recovery after marrow transplants, although this approach is less well studied. As a result, over the last five years PBSC have become the predominant stem cell source used for autografting. Studies are now in progress to evaluate the benefits using PBSC for allografting. One concern with this approach is that, because large numbers of T cells are infused with unmodified PBSC products, this may increase the risk of GVHD, particularly chronic GVHD (Storb *et al*, 1983; Storek *et al*, 1997).

Allografting donors are usually HLA-identical siblings. Approximately 25–30% of patients have such a donor, and in a small percentage of cases, phenotypically HLA-matched or other suitable HLA-non-identical family donors can be identified. Occasionally, an identical twin donor is available, and this is ideal from an immuno-logical standpoint in terms of transplant safety. For patients lacking suitable related donors, phenotypically HLA-matched unrelated donors identified through national or international donor registries can be used. The use of unrelated donor transplants is limited by the availability of suitable HLA-matched donors in the registries, the time required to perform a donor search, and an increased risk of complications associated with these transplants. As a result, these transplants have only rarely been offered to patients above 50 years.

Autologous transplants usually require the cryopreservation and storage of one's own stem cells. Since these transplants are almost always performed for malignancy, the graft may be treated *in vitro* in an attempt to remove tumour cells. This may involve attempts to kill or physically remove malignant cells using monoclonal antibodies or chemotherapy reagents, or more recently by enriching for the critical haematopoietic repopulating cells present in the graft. Techniques that rely on the latter approach and the use monoclonal antibodies against a cell surface glycoprotein, CD34 (Civin *et al*, 1984; Krause *et al*, 1996), have been increasingly used to purge tumour cells from autografts (Schiller *et al*, 1995) and removing T cells from allografts to prevent GVHD (Bensinger *et al*, 1996). Because CD34+ cells, which comprise

1–2% of bone marrow cells, contain the critical pluripotent stem cell population but not mature haematopoietic cells, future attempts at graft "engineering" to enhance transplant results will most likely depend on the *ex vivo* isolation of CD34+ cells.

2.2. Conditioning regimens

A frequently used regimen before allografting for malignancy has been a combination of cyclophosphamide (CY) and fractionated total body irradiation (TBI). Fractionation of TBI reduces radiation-induced side effects such as interstitial pneumonia and cataracts without significant loss of anti-leukaemic activity. An anti-tumour dose response relationship was found for TBI as demonstrated by the lower rates of relapse in patients who received high TBI doses (15.75 Gy) as opposed to lower TBI doses (12 Gy), as shown in Fig. 1 (Clift *et al*, 1991). However, because of the greater toxicity associated with a higher dose of TBI and an

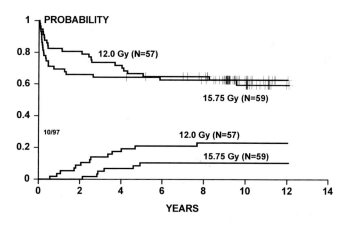

Fig. 1. Outcome after allogeneic marrow transplantation using HLA-matched sibling donors for illustrating effects of radiation dose on overall survival (upper curves) and relapse (lower curves). Patients were treated in Seattle at the Fred Hutchinson Cancer Research Center and randomised to receive cyclophosphamide 120 mg/kg and either TBI 12 Gy (2 Gy × 6) or TBI 15.75 Gy (2.25 Gy × 7) (Clift *et al*, 1991). Although long-term survival is similar, recipients of the higher radiation dose had a higher mortality early after transplant due to treatment toxicities.

Table 2. Agents most frequently used in high-dose chemotherapy regimens*.

Busulfan
Cyclophosphamide
Etoposide
Melphalan
Thiotepa
Bischlorethylnitrosurea (BCNU)
Carboplatin
Cytosine Arabinoside

*Drugs are usually combined into a
two to four drug regimen.

associated increase in transplant-related mortality, there was
no improvement in long-term survival and a higher risk of early
mortality. In other attempts to increase the anti-leukaemic effect of
conditioning regimens, investigators have replaced CY with other
agents to be used in conjunction with TBI, or alternatively have
constructed chemotherapy-based regimens with the omission of TBI
(Table 2). For autologous transplants where host immunosuppression
is not required, numerous multi-drug regimens of varying intensity
have been used, particularly in the treatment of solid tumours and
lymphoma. Studies to date have not demonstrated superior anti-tumour
efficacy of newer regimens as compared to the basic TBI-based
regimens, although in CML patients it was found that a busulfan/CY
regimen was associated with less morbidity than CY/TBI (Clift et al,
1994). A major difficulty in assessing the efficacy of the multitude of
different regimens that have been tested is the paucity of randomised
trials that have been performed specifically to address this issue.

The lack of improved efficacy from intensifying regimens illustrates
a dilemma posed by the use of high-dose therapy. Obtaining increased
anti-tumour effects requires exposing the patient to higher short-term
and long-term regimen-related toxicities, yet it has not resulted in
overall treatment gains. With the maximally-tolerable regimens used

currently, more advanced chemotherapy-refractory malignancies are infrequently eradicated. Improvements in conditioning regimens will depend heavily on specific targeting of tumour cells through the use of monoclonal antibodies or other hematopoietic cell specific reagents (Matthews *et al*, 1995), or through the use of as yet undiscovered but more effective cytotoxic agents with less toxicity.

2.3. Recombinant cytokines

Increasingly, new cytokines are identified that act on haematopoietic and immune cells. A large number of these molecules have already been tested in *in vitro* or *in vivo* studies (Table 3). Potential therapeutic effects from using these agents include stimulating haematopoietic recovery after transplant, "mobilisation" of haematopoietic progenitors into the blood for collection by leukapheresis, and stimulation of immune recovery and anti-tumor activity after transplant. Cytokines currently approved for clinical use include G-CSF, GM-CSF, erythropoietin, *α*-interferon and interleukin-2 (IL-2). GM-CSF (Nemunaitis *et al*, 1990) and probably also G-CSF, may improve outcome of patients with graft failure after transplant. These two factors can enhance the rate of granulocyte recovery after marrow and PBSC grafting and reduce the duration of hospitalisation. However, beneficial effects on survival from the routine post-transplant use of these expensive reagents are less clear, and they may adversely affect survival in some settings (Anasetti *et al*, 1993). Recently identified cytokines of major research interest include thrombopoietin, for it's platelet-stimulating properties, and Flt-3 ligand for stimulating production of dendritic cells *in vivo* and *in vitro*. To date, most of the studies with these cytokines have reported on using these agents as single factors. It is likely that over the next decade there will be many trials to test combinations of these factors in order to obtain enhanced biological activity. For example, a combination of GM-CSF and IL-2 may be synergistic in stimulating immune responses after transplant, and is being tested as post-transplant immunotherapy to try and prevent relapse of malignancy (Herrera *et al*, 1997).

Table 3. Cytokines with a potential clinical application in stem cell transplantation.

Haematopoietic Growth Factors*	Immunomodulatory Factors*
GM-CSF	Alpha interferon
G-CSF	Interleukin-2
Erythropoietin	M-CSF
Interleukin-1	Gamma interferon
Interleukin-3	Interleukin-4
Interleukin-6	Interleukin-7
Interleukin-8	Interleukin-10
Interleukin-11	Interleukin-12
Stem cell factor	
Thrombopoietin	
FLT3/FLK2 ligand	
Leukemia inhibitory factor	
Oncostatin	

GM-CSF = granulocyte-macrophage colony-stimulating factor
G-CSF = granulocyte colony-stimulating factor
M-CSF = macrophage colony-stimulating factor

*Many of these factors are pleiotropic with stimulatory effects on both haematopoietic and immune cells.

3. Results of Clinical Stem Cell Transplantation

The following section summarises results primarily of HLA-matched family donor transplants and autologous transplants. The choice of whether to perform an allograft or an autograft is affected by a number of factors. These include disease type, patient age, the likelihood of obtaining a tumour-free or healthy autologous stem cell graft, physician preference and physician expertise. Allogeneic transplants are offered by some centres to patients up to the age of approximately 65 years, although in practice relatively few allografts are performed over the age of 55 years. The safety and success of performing autografts up to the age of 65 years has been well demonstrated.

Table 4. Results of allogeneic stem cell transplantation and conventional chemotherapy as treatment for haematological malignancies.[a]

	Transplant		Chemotherapy[b]
	Relapse-Free Survival (%)	Probability of Relapse (%)	Relapse-Free Survival (%)
CML			
Chronic phase	60–70	17	Incurable
Accelerated phase	40–50	15–20	Incurable
Blast crisis	15–20	70	Incurable
AML			
CR1[c]	50	22	20–30
1st Relapse/CR2[c]	25–34	45	< 10
Refractory	15	80	Incurable
ALL			
CR1[c]	54	35	40 (adults)
CR2	35	45	< 5
Refractory	15	80	Incurable
Lymphoma (HD, Aggressive NHL)			
CR2[c]	40	20	< 10
Refractory[c]	15	70–80	Incurable
CLL			
Less advanced	60	10–20	Incurable
More advanced	20	unknown	Incurable
Myelodysplasia			
No excess blasts	60	< 10	Incurable
With excess blasts	32	50	Incurable

AML = acute myeloid leukaemia, ALL = acute lymphoblastic leukaemia, CML = chronic myeloid leukaemia, CLL = chronic lymphocytic leukaemia, HD = Hodgkin's disease, NHL = non-Hodgkin's lymphoma, CR = complete remission

[a]Figures are approximate survival estimates compiled from references listed in this manuscript. Note that some variation in outcomes have been reported, both with transplantation and with conventional therapy that may not be reflected in these comparisons.

[b]Patients failing conventional chemotherapy almost always die as a result of malignancy.

[c]Similar overall disease-free survivals have been shown with autologous BMT but relapse rates are higher, and transplant-related mortality lower.

3.1. Transplants for haematologic malignancy

Stem cell transplantation has had its greatest application in the treatment of haematologic malignancies for which the vast majority of transplants have been performed (Bortin et al, 1992). In Table 4, outcomes after allografting for various haematologic malignancies are summarised and compared to outcomes after conventional chemotherapy.

CML and Myelodysplastic Syndromes

Allografting is the only demonstrated curative treatment for almost all patients with chronic myeloid leukaemia (CML) and myelodysplastic syndromes in which the stem cell compartment of the marrow is inherently abnormal. Currently, more allografts are performed for CML than any other disease. Disease phase has been a major determinant of outcome after transplants for CML (Fig. 2). Excellent results have been obtained when patients were transplanted in the chronic phase using conditioning regimens of either TBI/CY or busulfan/CY (Clift et al, 1994). The results were best when transplants were performed in

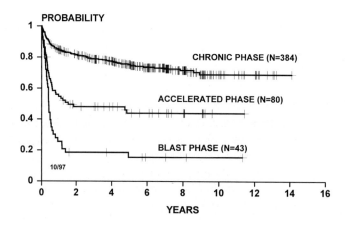

Fig. 2. Survival after allogeneic transplantation from HLA-matched siblings for CML showing survival according to disease phase at transplant. Patients received regimens containing CY/TBI or Bu/CY (Clift et al, 1994). Seattle data as of 1997.

the chronic phase within the first one to two years after diagnosis with five-year relapse-free survivals of 70% and five-year survivals of >80%. For this reason patients with CML who have HLA-matched sibling donors available are usually advised to undergo allografting soon after diagnosis. For patients with myelodysplastic syndromes, approximately 30–40% were cured (Anderson *et al*, 1993). Better results were found in patients with less advanced myelodysplasia, with five-year disease-free survivals of approximately 60%, and disease relapse was rare (Anderson *et al*, 1996). In contrast, patients whose disease had shown evolution into acute leukaemia have had a much poorer disease-free survival of only 15–20%, with a relapse risk of approximately 50% (Anderson *et al*, 1996).

Acute Leukaemia

For patients with acute myeloid leukaemia (AML) in first remission, approximately 50–60% of patients have been cured by allografting and with a risk of relapse of 25% (Champlin R. for the Advisory Committee of the International Bone Marrow Transplant Registry, 1987; Clift *et al*, 1987). Although allografting in younger patients with suitable donors is usually advised for AML in first remission, refinements in determining the prognosis of different AML subtypes (based primarily on bone marrow cytogenetic analysis) may ultimately allow selection of patients for transplant who have a poor prognosis if treated only with standard AML chemotherapy. Advances in patient selection are important because the risk of transplant-related mortality is about 20–25% and the likelihood of success drops with disease progression. However, poor prognosis features also predict for inferior results after transplant (Ferrant *et al*, 1997; Gale *et al*, 1995). For patients with AML beyond first remission, cure cannot be achieved using conventional dose chemotherapy. For patients in first relapse or second remission, allografting has resulted in disease-free survivals of approximately 30% (Clift *et al*, 1987). 10–15% of patients with multiply-relapsed AML, or AML refractory to induction chemotherapy have been cured after allografting (Biggs *et al*, 1992; Thomas *et al*, 1977). Similar results have been reported with the use of allografting for acute lymphoblastic leukaemia (ALL) for the same disease stages (Thomas *et al*, 1977). In contrast to AML most patients with ALL in first remission are not offered transplants because conventional chemotherapy can cure approximately 70% of children and 35–40% of adults with ALL (Durrant *et al*, 1997; Gale and Hoelzer, 1989). Transplants in first remission are indicated when poor prognostic features for relapse are present at diagnosis such as the Philadelphia chromosome (Sebban *et al*, 1994). The overall outcomes for allogeneic and autologous transplantation have been similar for acute leukaemia in first complete remission. However, the transplant-related complications and mortality are greater after allografting and a higher risk of relapse is present after autografting. In general, an allograft is usually preferred over autografting for acute leukaemia when an HLA-identical sibling donor is available, particularly for patients beyond first remission and for those with ALL.

Multiple Myeloma and Lymphoproliferative Disorders

Stem cell transplants have been used to treat many patients with multiple myeloma, lymphoma, and to a lesser extent, chronic lymphocytic leukaemia (CLL). Transplant is usually employed as salvage therapy after failure of initial conventional therapy. As seen with acute leukaemia, relapse of these malignancies is more frequent after autografting, but toxicity is greater after allografting. Multiple myeloma has proven to be particularly difficult to treat because transplants for advanced disease have been associated a high risk of transplant-related mortality and with a high risk of disease progression (Bensinger *et al*, 1997, 1996a, 1996b). Because myeloma is incurable with conventional therapy, newer approaches include the use of autografting and allografting early in the course of the disease at a time when patients should tolerate transplant better and disease resistance to therapy should be less. Autografting early in the course of the disease appears to improve survival (Attal *et al*, 1996), although a curative effect of autografting has not been demonstrated. Outcomes of transplants for Hodgkin's lymphoma and non-Hodgkin's lymphoma have been very similar (Appelbaum *et al*, 1984). High-dose therapy followed by autografting has been superior to conventional chemotherapy as treatment for relapsed non-Hodgkin's lymphoma (Bosly *et al*, 1992; Philip *et al*, 1995). Results of allografting and autografting have been similar (Chopra *et al*, 1992; Jones *et al*, 1991) except for low grade non-Hodgkin's lymphomas, where allografting appears to have curative potential, whereas autografting does not. Transplant prognosis correlates with disease stage and responsiveness to conventional chemotherapy at the time of transplant. Allografting, and possibly autografting in selected cases, can cure patients of CLL (Khouri *et al*, 1994; Michallet *et al*, 1996; Rabinowe *et al*, 1993). In several series, high complete remission rates have been reported and relapse occurred in approximately 10–20% of patients. Overall, allografting for these lymphoid diseases has been accompanied by a relatively high risk of transplant-related mortality. This relates to the older age profile of these patients and to the extensive therapy many patients receive before evaluation for stem cell transplantation.

Transplants for Solid Tumours

Because of the poor response of many solid tumours to conventional doses of chemotherapy, investigators have explored the use of high dose chemotherapy with or without TBI followed by autologous transplant. Studies that used PBSC have predominated in recent years, and the simplicity and reduced morbidity of PBSC transplants have encouraged these studies. By far the largest number of transplants have been performed for breast cancer. In patients with advanced metastatic malignancy, the results have been poor. The best results have been found for transplants performed for diseases that are usually responsive to conventional dose chemotherapy, e.g. breast cancer, ovarian cancer, and at a time when the tumour was still sensitive to such chemotherapy (Bensinger *et al*, 1997). Because of the poor results seen in patients with advanced metastatic disease, high-dose therapies are now being tested as adjuvant therapy for patients with chemosensitive solid tumours at high risk of relapse. Preliminary results of Phase II autografting studies in patients with high risk stage II and III breast cancer suggest that disease-free survivals are extended by this approach and that long-term survivals may be significantly increased. Three-year relapse-free survivals of 60–70% have been reported (Antman et al, 1997; Peters et al, 1993) as compared to 40–50% for patients receiving conventional adjuvant chemotherapy only. The superiority of high-dose therapy, as compared to conventional-dose therapy as a treatment for various stages of breast cancer, still remains to be confirmed by carefully-controlled Phase III studies.

3.2. Transplants for non-malignant disorders

Stem cell transplantation for non-malignant disorders has mostly involved the use of allogeneic transplants from HLA-identical siblings. Initially this mainly involved transplants for aplastic anaemia where allografting cured approximately 50% of patients. However, graft rejection and GVHD were significant problems. Improved conditioning regimens and GVHD prevention with a combination of methotrexate and cyclosporine have led to impressive long-term survival rates of 85–90% in allograft recipients (Fig. 3) (Doney et al, 1997; Storb et al, 1997). Equally impressive have been the results of allografting for the treatment of beta-thalassemia. The Pesaro Group have reported a 75% cure rate for children transplanted with marrow for HLA-identical sibling donors (Lucarelli and Clift, 1994). Preliminary data have indicated that similar results may be achievable for patients with sickle cell disease (Walters et al, 1996). Despite the promising results, allografting remains controversial as a treatment for severe hemoglobinopathies because of the risks of treatment-related mortality in patients who may otherwise survive several decades and who through the use of intensive chelation therapy, can slow iron accumulation and forestall resultant organ damage. Another group of patients for whom allografting has proved successful are children with genetically-determined immunodeficiency syndromes, storage disease, and other metabolic diseases. Allografting, performed with or without

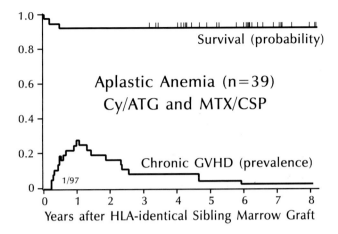

Years after HLA-identical Sibling Marrow Graft

Fig. 3. Survival after allogeneic transplantation from HLA-matched siblings for aplastic anaemia. (A) Improved survivals of patients treated in the last decade were a result of improved conditioning regimens and GVHD prophylaxis. The addition of antithymocyte globulin to cyclophosphamide-based conditioning regimens and use of MTX/CSP have largely eliminated graft rejection and GVHD as causes of treatment failure. The prevalence of chronic GVHD is greatest in the first three years post-transplant and <10% of patients remain on treatment at >3 years.

intensive conditioning regimens, has led to cure of these diseases such as severe combined immune deficiency disease (O'Reilly *et al*, 1994). There has been rising interest over the last several years in the possibility of using stem cell transplantation as treatment for auto-immune diseases (Marmont, 1994). Results of transplants for aplastic anaemia and for a small number of patients who suffered from autoimmune disease concurrent with haematologic diseases have shown that allografting is a highly effective form of controlling these diseases. The results of preclinical studies in rodents have shown that allografting and, to a lesser extent, autografting can control exper-imental autoimmune diseases (Ikehara *et al*, 1985). Initial clinical studies have focussed on the use of high-dose immunosuppressive therapy and autologous stem cell transplant for diseases such as multiple sclerosis, systemic lupus erythematosis and systemic sclerosis. Preliminary results indicate that major disease responses may be achieved with this type of treatment, although longer follow-up will be necessary to determine long-term success. Allografting will no doubt be explored should autologous transplants prove to be ineffective.

3.3. HLA-non-identical stem cell grafts

To increase the available donor pool and thereby offer potentially curative treatment, studies using HLA-non-identical family members and phenotypically HLA-matched unrelated donors have been performed (Anasetti *et al*, 1990; Beatty *et al*, 1991, 1993; Sullivan *et al*, 1986). A high incidence of acute and chronic GVHD and an increased risk of graft rejection have been observed. Despite the increased risk of these complications as compared to the use of HLA-matched family donors, the use of HLA-matched unrelated donors has produced acceptable results. Studies using molecular typing methods have shown that disparities at HLA-DRB1, HLA-DQ and HLA-C are important in determining risk of GVHD and graft rejection (Petersdorf *et al*, 1997, 1995). A requirement for matching at these loci can improve outcomes after unrelated donor transplants, but unfortunately also substantially reduces the potential donor pool for many patients. In patients with early chronic phase CML who underwent unrelated donor marrow transplantation in Seattle, an impressive 70% three-year disease-free survival has been achieved (Servida *et al*, 1996). However, while these results are overall similar to those after transplants from HLA-identical sibling donors, survivors of unrelated donor transplants experience more complications associated with therapy, including for many patients the need for prolonged immunosuppressive treatment as treatment for chronic GVHD.

4. Complications of Transplant

The main factors predicting outcome of transplant include patient age, type of transplant (autograft versus allograft), type of donor (related versus unrelated), disease type and stage, and pre-existing medical problems. The principal complications that lead to treatment failure are toxicity of conditioning regimens, immune deficiencies leading to infection, poor graft function, GVHD, and relapse of disease.

4.1. Regimen-related toxicities of transplant preparative regimens

To achieve maximum anti-tumour effects, regimens have been intensified to a level where significant non-haematopoietic toxicities are seen (Table 5). The principal life-threatening toxicities of these regimens are veno-occlusive disease (VOD) of the liver, mucositis, diarrhoea, pancytopenia, and interstitial pneumonitis. Severe pancytopenia is seen in every patient and is usually promptly corrected by haematopoiesis derived from the transplant. Serious VOD is seen in 15–28% of patients (McDonald *et al*, 1986) and severe

Table 5. Toxicities caused by high-dose conditioning regimens.

Early	Late
Mucositis[a]	Infertility[a]
Nausea/vomiting[a]	Endocrine insufficiencies
Severe pancytopenia[a]	Secondary malignancy
Enterocolitis	Cataracts
Acute mycocarditis	Leukoencephalopathy
Veno-occlusive disease of the liver	Restrictive lung disease
Interstitial pneumonia	Myelodysplastic syndromes[b]
Leukoencephalopathy	
Haemorrhagic cystitis	
Acute renal failure	
Erythroderma	
Alopecia[a]	

[a]Invariable side effects of conditioning regimens currently used for treatment of malignancy.
[b]Associated with autologous transplants and may be due to pre-transplant therapies.

idiopathic pneumonia in approximately 3% (Kantrow *et al*, 1997; Meyers *et al*, 1982). Gastrointestinal toxicity is common, including nausea and vomiting, painful mucositis and diarrhoea (McDonald *et al*, 1986). Long-term side effects include endocrine dysfunction, infertility, cataracts, and in children impaired growth, impaired sexual function and, in some instances, reduced intellectual function (Deeg *et al*, 1984; Sullivan *et al*, 1991). The risk of second malignancies after transplant is greater than the risk of primary malignancies occurring in the general population (Curtis *et al*, 1997). Autologous transplantation can be complicated by the development of bone marrow malignancy in the form of myelodysplasia or AML, unrelated to the original malignancy. This complication has been reported to occur in up to 20% of patients with lymphoma, but most likely occurs in considerably less than 10% of autograft recipients. The only curative treatment for this complication is a haematopoietic stem cell transplant from a donor, but the toxicities of such treatment are prohibitive and this approach is rarely successful.

4.2. Haematologic and immune recovery
(reviewed in Lum, 1987; Parkman, 1994)

Granulocyte and platelet recovery are usually complete by 40–50 days post-transplant. However, variations in the counts after transplant are common and often precipitated by intercurrent infections, GVHD, or drug therapy. Recovery of natural killer (NK) cell function, monocytes and macrophages occurs early post-transplant. Defects in the function of T and B cells, including defective chemotaxis, may persist for many months. Lymphocyte dysfunction is often prolonged and characterised by diminished humoral- and cell-mediated responses. Peripheral blood B-cell numbers and B-cell function are depressed, CD4+ T cells are depressed, and there is increased CD8 suppressor activity associated with an inverted CD4:CD8 ratio. Reconstitution of immunity is often complete at one year post-transplant, but in patients with chronic GVHD, clinical and laboratory evidence of immune deficiency persists. In patients without ongoing GVHD or immunosuppressive therapy vaccinations are usually given after one year post-transplant in an attempt to restore immunity to childhood pathogens, although it is unclear whether this is really required. With or without vaccinations, re-emergence of childhood diseases has been the exception in transplanted patients, except for the varizella-zoster virus.

4.3. Infections

Severe pancytopenia lasts for approximately two to three weeks after the conditioning therapy. Although bacterial sepsis is frequent during this period, the availability of potent broad spectrum antibiotics means that death from this complication is uncommon. Viral and fungal infections occurring after transplant are serious problems because they are more difficult to treat due to the limited efficacy of the currently available treatments (Bowden and Meyers, 1985; Weiner *et al*, 1986; Winston *et al*, 1984). These infections usually occur at greater than one month post-transplant and after granulocyte recovery has occurred. Cytomegalovirus (CMV) infections have been a particularly frequent and serious complication. Reactivation of CMV from host or transfused cells in the early post-transplant months can cause life-threatening pneumonia, previously fatal in approximately 15% of patients who had allografts for malignancy. Advances in preventative measures have included the use of CMV sero-negative blood products in CMV sero-negative transplant recipients (Bowden *et al*, 1991), and more recently prophylaxis with ganciclovir (Goodrich *et al*, 1991; Reed *et al*, 1988). While ganciclovir suppresses the development of CMV infections, treatment-related neutropenia and the development of delayed CMV infection have somewhat diminished the overall effectiveness of ganciclovir prophylaxis. Fungal infections due to *Candida* or aspergillosis are increasingly seen, often in patients with protracted GVHD who receive extensive corticosteroid therapy. Also, patients with pre-transplant fungal infections or extended periods of neutropenia prior to transplant may experience fulminating fungal infection early after treatment. These infections are often resistant to drug therapy and are associated with a high mortality. Fluconazole has become routinely administered as prophylaxis against Candida infections and has been effective in this regard. Herpes simplex infections are common after transplant and effectively prevented with acyclovir. Varicella zoster reactivation occurs in about 40% of transplant recipients and usually responds well to treatment with acyclovir. *Pneumocystis carinii* infection, which previously was a cause of post-transplant pneumonias (3% of patients), is readily prevented with trimethoprim-sulfametoxazole. In general, autograft recipients are at much lower risk of serious infections than allograft recipients because posttransplant immunosuppressive therapy is not required.

4.4. Graft-versus-host disease

(reviewed in Glucksberg *et al*, 1974; Sale and Shulman, 1984; Santos *et al*, 1985; Storb, 1986; Storb and Thomas, 1985; van Bekkum and Löwenberg, 1985)

Acute and chronic GVHD are major causes of morbidity and mortality after allografting. GVHD is caused by allo-reactive T cells directed at non-major histocompatibility complex (MHC) antigens recognised on host antigen presenting cells, and also against MHC antigens when donor-recipient MHC disparity exists. Acute GVHD, defined as GVHD occurring within the first 100 days after transplant, primarily affects the skin, liver and gastrointestinal tract. The principal risk factors for development of GVHD are summarised in Table 6. 15–50% of patients receiving HLA-identical sibling donor transplants develop significant acute GVHD, and this is associated with an increased risk of transplant-related mortality (Storb *et al*, 1989), primarily as the result of infectious complications. A complex series of cellular interactions generates a cascade of cytokine release the role of which in the pathogenesis of GVHD is controversial (Jadus and Websic, 1992). If cytokines were responsible for some of the GVHD manifestations, relevant cytokines could be targeted to develop treatment strategies. Initial studies have commenced to evaluate targeting cytokines such as tumour necrosis factor alpha and interleukin 1 receptor in the treatment of GVHD.

Table 6. Risk factors for the development of acute and chronic GVHD.

Acute GVHD	Chronic GVHD
M HLA-disparity	HLA-disparity
Unrelated donor	Unrelated donor
Advanced malignancy	Preceding acute GVHD
Sex-mismatched donor/recipient pair	Increasing patient age
Parous female donor	Corticosteroids
(Increasing patient/donor age)	PBSC transplants
TBI dose > 1200 cGy	

Table 7. Agents used or under evaluation for prophylaxis and treatment of GVHD.[a]

	Prophylaxis	Treatment
Methotrexate	+	
Cyclosporine	+	+
Corticosteroids	+	+
T-cell depletion	+	
FK506	+	+
Antithymocyte globulin	+	+
Anti-T cell monoclonal antibodies	+	+
Mycophenolate mofetil[b]	+	+
Rapamycin[b]	+	+
15-deoxyspergualin[b]		+
CTLA4-Ig[b]	+	+
Cytokine antagonists, e.g. anti-TNF-alpha antibody[b]	+	+
Azathioprine[c]		+
Thalidomide[c]		+
Psoralen ultraviolet A range (PUVA) therapy		+
Topical corticosteroids (skin, gastrointestinal tract)		+

CTLA4-Ig = cytotoxic T lymphocyte antigen 4 -immunoglobulin fusion molecule.
[a]Combination therapy is commonly given for prevention of acute GVHD.
[b]Phase I or preclinical studies currently being performed.
[c]Mainly used for treatment of chronic GVHD.

The most effective prevention and treatment strategies for GVHD to date have targetted the T cells. Usually this involves the administration of immunosuppressive agents after transplant that are given alone or in combination (Table 7). The most commonly used are cyclosporine, FK506, methotrexate (MTX) and corticosteroids. In contrast to solid organ transplants, indefinite immunosuppression is usually not required, and transplant tolerance may develop as early as three to six months post-transplant. A combination of cyclosporine and MTX has given better GVHD prophylaxis than seen with either agent alone, and has led to improved survival in patients with less advanced malignancy (Fig. 4) (Storb et al, 1989) and non-malignant disorders (Fig. 3) (Storb et al, 1991, 1987). With advanced malignancy, improved GVHD control is associated with improved early post-transplant survival but also with an increased risk of relapse, suggesting a loss of an important graft-derived anti-tumor effect. To a limited extent, this dilemma has been resolved by better anti-leukaemic conditioning programmes administered before transplant. Currently, a number of newer agents are being evaluated for their ability to prevent GVHD. These include mycophenolate mofetil (MMF), CTLA4-Ig, rapamycin, a variety of anti-T-cell monoclonal antibodies, and cytokine antagonists such as a monoclonal antibody to TNF-α.

An alternative and highly-effective approach to the prevention of GVHD involves the removal of T cells from the graft (Marmont et al, 1991; Martin et al, 1986). However, although severe GVHD is uncommon in recipients of T-cell depleted allografts, this benefit is offset by the increased risks of graft rejection, relapse of malignancy, and post-transplant immunodeficiency as compared to non-T-cell depleted allografts (Apperley et al, 1986; Marmont et al, 1991). To date, a survival advantage has not been demonstrated from the use of this technique, although more sophisticated approaches to T-cell depletion that involve more precise manipulation of the T-cell dose and T-cell subsets (Champlin et al, 1990; Soiffer et al, 1992) in the graft appear superior to those used in earlier studies which employed extensive T-cell removal from the graft.

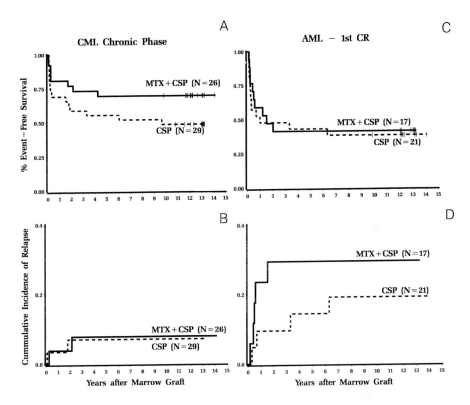

Fig. 4. Effect of GVHD prophylaxis on survival and relapse after allogeneic BMT using HLA-identical family donors in good risk leukaemia (CML in chronic phase and AML in first complete remission). In CML (panels A and B) survival is better with MTX/CSP than with CSP alone and risk of relapse is similar. In AML, survival is not increased by use of MTX/CSP due to an increased risk of relapse (panel D). See the data (Storb *et al*, 1989) updated as of 1997.

Treatment of acute GVHD usually involves the administration of corticosteroids as front-line therapy. Failure to respond to such therapy usually portends a poor prognosis in terms of outcome from GVHD (Martin *et al*, 1990). Second-line agents include antithymocyte globulin (ATG), cyclosporine, and, increasingly, the other agents listed in Table 7.

Chronic GVHD, defined as GVHD occurring after 100 days post-transplant, clinically resembles autoimmune diseases such as scleroderma, Sjogren's syndrome and primary biliary cirrhosis (reviewed in Atkinson, 1990; Atkinson et al, 1990; Glucksberg et al, 1974; Storb, 1986). A major problem is persistent severe immune deficiency, and 25% of affected patients may die from infectious complications. Significant chronic GVHD occurs in 30–50% of patients receiving HLA-matched sibling marrow transplants and usually within two years of transplant. The most effective therapy involves the use of prednisone ± cyclosporine. However, for many patients this approach is not satisfactory, and other drugs under study include FK506, thalidomide and MMF. In patients who survive, treatment can usually be discontinued after several years (Fig. 3).

4.5. Graft-versus-tumour effects of allografting

The anti-leukaemia effect of allogeneic marrow was first demonstrated in murine transplant studies. The term graft-versus-leukaemia (GVL) was later used to distinguish anti-tumour activity of the graft from GVHD, although in a human transplant setting, distinguishing between the two has not been possible. The GVL effect was first suggested in humans by observations that acute and chronic GVHD were associated with a lowered risk of leukaemic relapse (Weiden et al, 1981), and confirmed by observations that recipients of syngeneic or T cell-depleted grafts experienced a two-fold greater risk of relapse than recipients of unmodified allografts (Horowitz et al, 1990; Marmont et al, 1991). These observations suggested that, in an MHC-matched setting, GVL was mediated by T cells that recognised minor histo-compatibility antigens. Although the development of GVHD after allografting reduces the likelihood of relapse, it does not necessarily lead to improved patient survival because of the associated mortality. However, for patients with advanced leukaemia for whom the prognosis is poor, the development of GVHD and associated reduced risk of relapse does lead to improved long-term survival as compared to patients who do not develop GVHD. In practice, it has not been possible to control GVHD with the precision required to exploit the benefit of the GVL effect during the transplant process, and in earlier attempts to boost anti-tumour effects through transplantation of additional donor peripheral blood buffy coat cells, reduced survival was observed due to excess GVHD (Sullivan *et al*, 1989). Newer studies will seek to define the optimal timing and dosing of such cell boosts. Important observations as to the anti-leukaemia effect of donor cells have been made in recent studies in which donor lymphocyte infusions (DLI) were given to treat relapsed malignancy after allografting. It appears possible, particularly in patients with CML, to induce complete remissions of leukemia and possible cure. Approximately 80% of patients with relapsed CML who undergo DLI achieve complete cytogenetic remissions and these patients usually also achieve molecular remissions as determined by polymerase chain reaction (PCR) analysis to detect bcr/abl transcripts (Collins, Jr. *et al*, 1997; Kolb *et al*, 1995). DLI are not without risk, and severe myelosuppression and/ or GVHD have occurred in a majority of patients.

4.6. Graft failure

Poor graft function is common after transplant but often resolves after contributing factors such as infection and drugs are dealt with. Persistence of poor graft function is associated with a high mortality, and the use of recombinant haematopoietic growth factors may have improved survival (Nemunaitis *et al*, 1990). True immunologic graft rejection is rare after the use of TBI-based regimens except when HLA-mismatched donors are used and/or the graft is T cell-depleted. The use of additional host immunosuppression with ATG or anti-T cell antibodies given pre-transplant may reduce the risk of graft rejection under these circumstances. True graft rejection in patients with aplastic anaemia can often be successfully treated by a second transplant (Storb *et al*, 1987), and more recently monoclonal antibody-based transplant regimens have also been described for patients with malignant diseases (Stucki *et al*, 1997).

4.7. Recurrence of malignancy

Relapse is a major cause of treatment failure after allografting or autografting for most types of malignancy. Factors that affect the risk of relapse include the disease type, disease stage, and the type of transplant. High relapse rates are common after transplants for advanced leukaemia, multiple myeloma, and disseminated solid tumours. Autologous transplant recipients are at a higher risk of relapse when compared to allograft recipients due to the lack of a GVL effect, and in some cases due to the infusion of tumour cells with the graft. Except for CML, relapse of malignancy is usually very difficult to treat effectively. Occasionally, Epstein-Barr virus (EBV) positive B-cell lymphomas develop in donor cells, primarily after the use of mismatched or T cell-depleted allografts (Deeg *et al*, 1984; Martin *et al*, 1987). These lymphomas can be effectively treated by infusion of donor T cells or EBV-specific donor T cell clones.

Second allografts have been associated with a high rate of regimen-related mortality and rarely control disease, except in a subgroup of young patients who develop GVHD (Radich *et al*, 1993). For most patients the most logical approach to the treatment of relapsed disease appears to be the infusion of donor leukocytes. Although success has been primarily seen in treating CML, methods to increase the alloreactivity of the donor cells using agents such as IL-2 and IL-12 may enhance results, particularly if GVHD can be controlled. The use of T cells transduced *in vitro* with a suicide gene may make this possible (Bonini *et al*, 1997).

Future attempts at reducing the risk of relapse after transplant will depend on two main approaches. The first involves developing more effective and more tumour-specific regimens that lead to greater tumour kill without increased complications (Matthews *et al*, 1995). The second relates to the use of immune cells that have more specificity and activity against malignant cells without increasing the risk of developing GVHD, and thereby constituting an improvement on the current approaches to DLI (also discussed under "Graft-versus-Tumour Effects of Allografting" and in the following section).

5. Future Directions of Stem Cell Transplantation

Despite significant advances in bone marrow transplantation, the main challenges facing clinicians have remained much the same, i.e. relapse of disease, regimen-related toxicities, GVHD, and a lack of donors for many patients. The development of highly-effective preparative regimens has the potential to deal with these problems. More effective regimens could reduce the risk of relapse and graft rejection simultaneously and thereby allow the increased use of T cell-depleted allografts. If the use of HLA-haploidentical transplants can be made more tolerable, almost all patients would have a family member who could act as a donor. Because the currently used agents such as TBI, cyclophosphamide, busulfan, etc, cannot be readily intensified above their current levels without prohibitive toxicity, the addition of monoclonal antibodies or other agents directed specifically at haematopoietic and/or immune cells is essential for future progress. Preliminary studies have shown that the use of radio-labelled monoclonal antibodies directed at either CD45 for leukaemia (Matthews *et al*, 1995) or CD20 for lymphoma (Press *et al*, 1987) can allow delivery of more intensive therapy to sites of disease without increasing toxicity to vital organs such as the liver or lungs.

A novel alternative approach to conventional allografting involves the use of low-dose conditioning regimens with the goal of establishing mixed donor-recipient haematopoietic chimerism. Establishing a proportion, e.g. 30–50%, of stable haematopoiesis from normal donor cells may be an effective therapy for genetic diseases such as thalassemia and sickle cell disease as well as for patients with aplastic anaemia. For treating malignant diseases this would establish host tolerance against donor cells, allowing donor lymphocytes to be given later to attack malignant cells. One may therefore avoid the use of toxic high-dose conditioning regimens and most of the side effects listed in Table 5. We have demonstrated the feasibility of this approach in a canine preclinical model (Storb *et al*, 1997). Using low-dose non-myeloablative TBI (200 cGy) and potent post-transplant immunosuppression for 35 days after marrow grafting from MHC-compatible littermate donors, stable substantial mixed chimerism could be established as

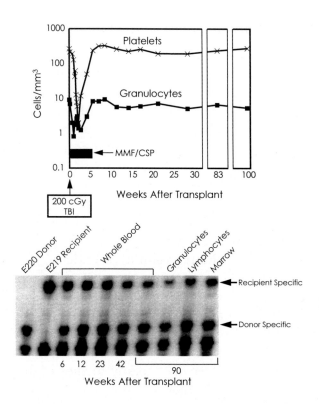

Fig. 5. Granulocyte and platelet counts in a dog after conditioning with a non-myeloablative dose of 200 cGy TBI and given a marrow graft from a DLA-identical littermate on day 0, followed by post-grafting immunosuppression with mycophenolate mofetil/cyclosporine (MMF/CSP) for no more than 35 days. The bottom panel shows the results of testing for $(CA)_n$ dinucleotide repeats of donor and recipient cells before transplantation (lanes 1 and 2) and recipient cells after marrow transplantation (lanes 3 to 10). Stable mixed chimerism is evident by the persistence of donor haematopoiesis for at least 90 weeks post-transplant.

shown in Fig. 5. Based on these studies, we have initiated clinical studies in patients with haematologic malignancy who are poor candidates for conventional high-dose allografting regimens to test the feasibility of establishing mixed chimerism to provide a platform for the subsequent infusion of donor immune cells.

The use of donor immune cells to kill malignant cells rather than high-dose regimens has the potential to improve outcomes through reducing transplant complications related to the preparative regimens. However, for safety purposes more specificity in controlling lymphocyte activity is required for using these cells as therapeutic tools for achieving engraftment and treating malignancy. Progress in terms of reducing toxicity of so-called "adoptive immunotherapy" may come from the use of careful dosing of T cells or T cell subsets, through the use of cytolytic T cell clones directed against tumour cells, or through the use of T cell populations transduced with "suicide" genes such as the herpes simplex virus thymidine kinase gene. The latter may allow for selective killing by ganciclovir of cells that may cause GVHD after T cell infusions. The use of T cell clones against CMV for prophylaxis against infection (Riddell *et al*, 1992) and against EBV as prophylaxis against lymphoma (Heslop *et al*, 1996) have already demonstrated the principles of adoptive immunotherapy using cloned lymphocytes. Eventually, cloned T cells with activity against tumour cell antigens or lineage-specific antigens and against infectious pathogens may be a routine part of allogeneic transplantation.

An increasing array of available recombinant molecules has prompted extensive studies into the *in vitro* manipulation of haematopoietic progenitors. The use of *ex vivo* progenitor cell expansion may facilitate even more rapid engraftment, tumour cell purging from autografts and also the application of gene therapy for the treatment of malignant and non-malignant diseases. The technology for isolating stem cells from the peripheral blood or marrow using antibodies against the CD34 antigen is increasingly used to facilitate graft manipulation and thereby the prevention of GVHD after transplantation. Recent transplant studies using blood from the umbilical cord have shown that the use of this source of stem cells is feasible in children, although its successful application to transplants in adults remains to be demonstrated. *In vitro* expansion of the cord blood products may ultimately increase their utility through overcoming cell dose limitations.

Finally, the developments in molecular biology and immuno-cytochemistry allow for extremely sensitive techniques to detect the presence of tumour cells in the marrow or blood after transplant. The use of this technology to detect persistence of minimal residual tumour or early signs of relapse will ultimately help to determine the need for additional "pre-emptive" post-transplant therapies, which could include the use of donor leukocyte administration or administration of immunostimulatory cytokines such as IL-2 or IL-12.

6. Acknowledgements

The authors thank Bonnie Larson, Harriet Childs and Gary Schoch for their assistance in the preparation of this manuscript.

7. References

ANASETTI, C., BEATTY, P.G., STORB, R., MARTIN, P.J., MORI, M., SANDERS, J.E., THOMAS, E.D. and HANSEN, J.A. (1990). Effect of HLA incompatibility on graft-versus-host disease, relapse, and survival after marrow transplantation for patients with leukemia or lymphoma, *Hum. Immunol.* **29**, 79–91.

ANASETTI, C., ANDERSON, G., APPELBAUM, F.R., BUCKNER, C. D., MARTIN, P.J., NEMUNAITIS, J., SINGER, J., STORB, R., SULLIVAN, K.M., THOMAS, E.D. and HANSEN, J.A. (1993). Phase III study of rhGM-CSF in allogeneic marrow transplantation from unrelated donors, *Blood* **82** (Suppl 1), 454a (Abstract).

ANDERSON, J.E., APPELBAUM, F.R., FISHER, L.D., SCHOCH, G., SHULMAN, H., ANASETTI, C., BENSINGER, W.I., BRYANT, E., BUCKNER, C.D., DONEY, K., MARTIN, P.J., SANDERS, J.E., SULLIVAN, K.M., THOMAS, E.D., WITHERSPOON, R.P., HANSEN, J.A. and STORB, R. (1993). Allogeneic bone marrow transplantation for 93 patients with myelodysplastic syndrome, *Blood* **82**, 677–681.

ANDERSON, J.E., APPELBAUM, F.R., SCHOCH, G., GOOLEY, T., ANASETTI, C., BENSINGER, W.I., BRYANT, E., BUCKNER, C.D., CHAUNCEY, T.R., CLIFT, R.A., DONEY, K., FLOWERS, M., HANSEN, J.A., MARTIN, P.J., MATTHEWS, D.C., SANDERS, J.E., SHULMAN, H., SULLIVAN, K.M., WITHERSPOON, R.P. and STORB, R. (1996). Allogeneic marrow transplantation for refractory anemia: A comparison of two preparative regimens and analysis of prognostic factors, *Blood* **87**, 51–58.

ANDERSON, J.E., APPELBAUM, F.R., SCHOCH, G., GOOLEY, T., ANASETTI, C., BENSINGER, W.I., BRYANT, E., BUCKNER, C.D., CHAUNCEY, T., CLIFT, R.A., DEEG, H.J., DONEY, K., FLOWERS, M., HANSEN, J.A., MARTIN, P.J., MATTHEWS, D.C., NASH, R.A., SANDERS, J.E., SHULMAN, H., SULLIVAN, K.M., WITHERSPOON, R.P. and STORB, R. (1996). Allogeneic marrow transplantation for myelodysplastic syndrome with advanced disease morphology: A phase II study of busulfan, cyclophosphamide, and total-body irradiation and analysis of prognostic factors, *J. Clin. Oncol.* **14**, 220–226.

ANTMAN, K.H., ROWLINGS, P.A., VAUGHAN, W.P., PELZ, C.J., FAY, J.W., FIELDS, K.K., FREYTES, C.O., GALE, R.P., HILLNER, B.E., HOLLAND, H.K., KENNEDY, M.J., KLEIN, J.P., LAZARUS, H.M., MCCARTHY, P.L., JR., SAEZ, R., SPITZER, G., STADTMAUER, E.A., WILLIAMS, S.F., WOLFF, S., SOBOCINSKI, K.A., ARMITAGE, J.O. and HOROWITZ, M.M. (1997). High-dose chemotherapy with autologous hematopoietic stem-cell support for breast cancer in North America, *J. Clin. Oncol.* **15**, 1870–1879.

APPELBAUM, F.R., DAHLBERG, S., THOMAS, E.D., BUCKNER, C.D., CHEEVER, M.A., CLIFT, R.A., CROWLEY, J., DEEG, H.J., FEFER, A., GREENBERG, P., KADIN, M., SMITH, W., STEWART, P., SULLIVAN, K., STORB, R. and WEIDEN, P. (1984). Bone marrow transplantation or chemotherapy after remission induction for adults with acute nonlymphoblastic leukemia — A prospective comparison, *Ann. Intern. Med.* **101**, 581–588.

APPERLEY, J.F., JONES, L., HALE, G., WALDMANN, H., HOWS, J., ROMBOS, Y., TSATALAS, C., MARCUS, R.E., GOOLDEN, A.W.G., GORDON-SMITH, E.C., CATOVSKY, D., GALTON, D.A.G. and GOLDMAN, J.M. (1986). Bone marrow transplantation for patients with chronic myeloid leukaemia: T-cell depletion with Campath-1 reduces the incidence of graft-versus-host disease but may increase the risk of leukaemic relapse, *Bone Marrow Transplantation* **1**, 53–66.

ATKINSON, K. (1990). Chronic graft-versus-host disease, *Bone Marrow Transplantation* **5**, 69–82.

ATKINSON, K., HOROWITZ, M.M., GALE, R.P., VAN BEKKUM, D.W., GLUCKMAN, E., GOOD, R.A., JACOBSEN, N., KOLB, H., RIMM, A.A., RINGDÉN, O., ROZMAN, C., SOBOCINSKI, K.A., ZWAAN, F.E. and BORTIN, M.M. (1990). Risk factors for chronic graft-versus-host disease after HLA-identical sibling bone marrow transplantation, *Blood* **75**, 2459–2464.

ATTAL, M., HAROUSSEAU, J.-L., STOPPA, A.-M., SOTTO, J.-J., FUZIBET, J.-G., ROSSI, J.-F., CASASSUS, P., MAISONNEUVE, H., FACON, T., IFRAH, N., PAYEN, C., BATAILLE, R. and FOR THE INTERGROUPE FRANÇAIS DU MYÉLOME. (1996). A prospective, randomized trial of autologous bone marrow transplantation and chemotherapy in multiple myeloma, *N. Engl. J. Med.* **335**, 91–97.

BEATTY, P.G., HANSEN, J.A., LONGTON, G.M., THOMAS, E.D., SANDERS, J.E., MARTIN, P.J., BEARMAN, S.I., ANASETTI, C., PETERSDORF, E.W., MICKELSON, E.M., PEPE, M.S., APPELBAUM, F.R., BUCKNER, C.D., CLIFT, R.A., PETERSEN, F.B., STEWART, P.S., STORB, R.F., SULLIVAN, K.M., TESLER, M.C. and WITHERSPOON, R.P. (1991). Marrow transplantation from HLA-matched unrelated donors for treatment of hematologic malignancies, *Transplantation* **51**, 443–447.

BEATTY, P.G., ANASETTI, C., HANSEN, J.A., LONGTON, G.M., SANDERS, J.E., MARTIN, P.J., MICKELSON, E.M., CHOO, S.Y., PETERSDORF, E.W., PEPE, M.S., APPELBAUM, F.R., BEARMAN, S.I., BUCKNER, C.D., CLIFT, R.A., PETERSEN, F.B., SINGER, J., STEWART, P.S., STORB, R.F., SULLIVAN, K.M., TESLER, M.C., WITHERSPOON, R.P. and THOMAS, E.D. (1993). Marrow transplantation from unrelated donors for treatment of hematologic malignancies: Effect of mismatching for one HLA locus, *Blood* **81**, 249–253.

BENSINGER, W.I., BUCKNER, C.D., ANASETTI, C., CLIFT, R., STORB, R., BARNETT, T., CHAUNCEY, T., SHULMAN, H. and APPELBAUM, F.R. (1996). Allogeneic marrow transplantation for multiple myeloma: An analysis of risk factors on outcome, *Blood* **88**, 2787–2793.

BENSINGER, W.I., BUCKNER, C.D., SHANNON-DORCY, K., ROWLEY, S., APPELBAUM, F.R., BENYUNES, M., CLIFT, R., MARTIN, P., DEMIRER, T., STORB, R., LEE, M. and SCHILLER, G. (1996). Transplantation of allogeneic CD34+ peripheral blood stem cells in patients with advanced hematologic malignancy, *Blood* **88**, 4132–4138.

BENSINGER, W.I., ROWLEY, S.D., DEMIRER, T., LILLEBY, K., SCHIFFMAN, K., CLIFT, R.A., APPELBAUM, F.R., FEFER, A., BARNETT, T., STORB, R., CHAUNCEY, T., MAZIARZ, R.T., KLARNET, J., MCSWEENEY, P., HOLMBERG, L., MALONEY, D.G., WEAVER, C.H. and BUCKNER, C.D. (1996). High-dose therapy followed by autologous hematopoietic stem-cell infusion for patients with multiple myeloma, *J. Clin. Oncol.* **14**, 1447–1456.

BENSINGER, W.I., BUCKNER, C.D. and GAHRTON, G. (1997). Allogeneic stem cell transplantation for multiple myeloma, *Hematol./Oncol. Clin. N. Am.* **11**, 147–157.

BENSINGER, W.I., SCHIFFMAN, K.S., HOLMBERG, L., APPELBAUM, F.R., MAZIARZ, R., MONTGOMERY, P., ELLIS, E., RIVKIN, S., WEIDEN, P., LILLEBY, K., ROWLEY, S., PETERSDORF, S., KLARNET, J.P., NICHOLS, W., HERTLER, A., MCCROSKEY, R., WEAVER, C.H. and BUCKNER, C.D. (1997). High-dose busulfan, melphalan, thiotepa and peripheral blood stem cell infusion for the treatment of metastatic breast cancer, *Bone Marrow Transplantation* **19**, 1183–1189.

BIGGS, J.C., HOROWITZ, M.M., GALE, R.P., ASH, R.C., ATKINSON, K., HELBIG, W., JACOBSEN, N., PHILLIPS, G.L., RIMM, A.A., RINGDEN, O., ROZMAN, C., SOBOCINSKI, K., ZEUM, J. and BORTIN, M. (1992). Bone marrow transplants may cure patients with acute leukemia never achieving remission with chemotherapy, *Blood* **80**(4), 1090.

BONINI, C., FERRARI, G., VERZELETTI, S., SERVIDA, P., ZAPPONE, E., RUGGIERI, L., PONZONI, M., ROSSINI, S., MAVILIO, F., TRAVERSARI, C. and BORDIGNON, C. (1997). HSV-TK gene transfer into donor lymphocytes for control of allogeneic graft-versus-leukemia, *Science* **276**, 1719–1724.

BORTIN, M.M., HOROWITZ, M.M. and RIMM, A.A. (1992). Progress report from the International Bone Marrow Transplant Registry, *Bone Marrow Transplantation* **10**, 113–122.

BOSLY, A., COIFFIER, B., GISSELBRECHT, C., TILLY, H., AUZANNEAU, G., ANDRIEN, F., HERBRECHT, R., LEGROS, M., DEVAUX, Y., JAUBERT, J., PIGNON, B., MICHAUX, J., HUMBLET, Y., DUPRIEZ, B., THYSS, A. and LEDERLIN, P. (1992). Bone marrow transplantation prolongs survival after relapse in aggressive-lymphoma patients treated with the LNH-84 regimen, *J. Clin. Oncol.* **10**, 1615–1623.

BOWDEN, R.A. and MEYERS, J.D. (1985). Infectious complications following marrow transplantation. In *Plasma Therapy and Transfusion Technology*, pp 285–302.

BOWDEN, R.A., SLICHTER, S.J., SAYERS, M.H., MORI, M., CAYS, M.J. and MEYERS, J.D. (1991). Use of leukocyte-depleted platelets and cytomegalovirus-seronegative red blood cells for prevention of primary cytomegalovirus infection after marrow transplant, *Blood* **78**, 246–250.

CHAMPLIN, R. FOR THE ADVISORY COMMITTEE OF THE INTERNATIONAL BONE MARROW TRANSPLANT REGISTRY. (1987). Bone marrow transplantation for acute leukemia: A preliminary report from the International Bone Marrow Transplant Registry, *Transplant Proc.* **19**, 2626–2628.

CHAMPLIN, R., HO, W., GAJEWSKI, J., FEIG, S., BURNISON, M., HOLLEY, G., GREENBERG, P., LEE, K., SCHMID, I., GIORGI, J., YAM, P., PETZ, L., WINSTON, D., WARNER, N. and REICHERT, T. (1990). Selective depletion of CD8+ T lymphocytes for prevention of graft-versus-host disease after allogeneic bone marrow transplantation, *Blood* **76**, 418-423.

CHOPRA, R., GOLDSTONE, A.H., PEARCE, R., PHILIP, T., PETERSEN, F., APPELBAUM, F., DE VOL, E. and ERNST, P. (1992). Autologous versus allogeneic bone marrow transplantation for non-Hodgkin's lymphoma: A case-controlled analysis of the European bone marrow transplant group registry data, *J. Clin. Oncol.* **10**, 1690–1695.

CIVIN, C.I., STRAUSS, L.C., BROVALL, C., FACKLER, M.J., SCHWARTZ, J.F. and SHAPER, J.H. (1984). Antigenic analysis of hematopoiesis. III. A hematopoietic progenitor cell surface antigen defined by a monoclonal antibody raised against KG-1a cells, *J. Immunol.* **133**, 157–165.

CLIFT, R.A., BUCKNER, C.D., THOMAS, E.D., KOPECKY, K.J., APPELBAUM, F.R., TALLMAN, M., STORB, R., SANDERS, J., SULLIVAN, K., BANAJI, M., BEATTY, P.S., BENSINGER, W., CHEEVER, M., DEEG, J., DONEY, K., FEFER, A., GREENBERG, P., HANSEN, J.A., HACKMAN, R., HILL, R., MARTIN, P.,

MEYERS, J., MCGUFFIN, R., NEIMAN, P., SALE, G., SHULMAN, H., SINGER, J., STEWART, P., WEIDEN, P. and WITHERSPOON, R. (1987). The treatment of acute non-lymphoblastic leukemia by allogeneic marrow transplantation, *Bone Marrow Transplantation* **2**, 243–258.

CLIFT, R.A., BUCKNER, C.D., APPELBAUM, F.R., BRYANT, E., BEARMAN, S.I., PETERSEN, F.B., FISHER, L.D., ANASETTI, C., BEATTY, P., BENSINGER, W.I., DONEY, K., HILL, R.S., MCDONALD, G.B., MARTIN, P., MEYERS, J., SANDERS, J., SINGER, J., STEWART, P., SULLIVAN, K.M., WITHERSPOON, R., STORB, R., HANSEN, J.A. and THOMAS, E.D. (1991). Allogeneic marrow transplantation in patients with chronic myeloid leukemia in the chronic phase: A randomized trial of two irradiation regimens, *Blood* **77**, 1660–1665.

CLIFT, R.A., BUCKNER, C.D., THOMAS, E.D., BENSINGER, W.I., BOWDEN, R., BRYANT, E., DEEG, H.J., DONEY, K.C., FISHER, L.D., HANSEN, J.A., MARTIN, P., MCDONALD, G.B., SANDERS, J.E., SCHOCH, G., SINGER, J., STORB, R., SULLIVAN, K.M., WITHERSPOON, R.P. and APPELBAUM, F.R. (1994). Marrow transplantation for chronic myeloid leukemia: A randomized study comparing cyclophosphamide and total body irradiation with busulfan and cyclophosphamide, *Blood* **84**, 2036–2043.

COLLINS, R.H., JR., SHPILBERG, O., DROBYSKI, W.R., PORTER, D.L., GIRALT, S., CHAMPLIN, R., GOODMAN, S.A., WOLFF, S.N., HU, W., VERFAILLIE, C., LIST, A., DALTON, W., OGNOSKIE, N., CHETRIT, A., ANTIN, J.H. and NEMUNAITIS, J. (1997). Donor leukocyte infusions in 140 patients with relapsed malignancy after allogeneic bone marrow transplantation, *J. Clin. Oncol.* **15**, 433–444.

CURTIS, R.E., ROWLINGS, P.A., DEEG, H.J., SHRINER, D.A., SOCIÉ, G., TRAVIS, L.B., HOROWITZ, M.M., WITHERSPOON, R.P., HOOVER, R.N., SOBOCINSKI, K.A., FRAUMENI, J.F., JR., BOICE, J.D., JR., SCHOCH, H.G., SALE, G.E., STORB, R., TRAVIS,

W.D., KOLB, H.-J., GALE, R.P. and PASSWEG, J.R. (1997). Solid cancers after bone marrow transplantation, *N. Engl. J. Med.* **336**, 897–904.

DEEG, H.J., STORB, R. and THOMAS, E.D. (1984). Bone marrow transplantation: A review of delayed complications. (Review). *Br. J. Haematol.* **57**, 185–208.

DONEY, K., LEISENRING, W., STORB, R., APPELBAUM, F.R. and FOR THE SEATTLE BONE MARROW TRANSPLANT TEAM. (1997). Primary treatment of acquired aplastic anemia: Outcomes with bone marrow transplantation and immunosuppressive therapy, *Ann. Intern. Med.* **126**, 107–115.

DURRANT, I.J., PRENTICE, H.G., RICHARDS, S.M. and FOR THE MEDICAL RESEARCH COUNCIL WORKING PARTY ON LEUKEMIA IN ADULTS. (1997). Intensification of treatment for adults with acute lymphoblastic leukaemia: Results of the UK medical research council randomized trial UKALL XA, *Br. J. Haematol.* **99**, 84–92.

FERRANT, A., LABOPIN, M., FRASSONI, F., PRENTICE, H. G., CAHN, J.Y., BLAISE, D., REIFFERS, J., VISANI, G., SANZ, M.A., BOOGAERTS, M.A., LOWENBERG, B. and GORIN, N.C. (1997). Karyotype in acute myeloblastic leukemia — prognostic significance for bone marrow transplantation in first remission. A European Group for Blood and Marrow Transplantation Study, *Blood* **90**, 2931–2938.

GALE, R.P. and HOELZER, D. (1989). Acute lymphoblastic leukemia: Current controversies, future directions (news), *Leukemia* **3**, 681–686.

GALE, R.P., HOROWITZ, M.M., WEINER, R.S., ASH, R.C., ATKINSON, K., BABU, R., DICKE, K.A., KLEIN, J.P., LOWENBERG, B., REIFFERS, J., RIMM, A.A., ROWLINGS, P.A., SANDBERG, A.A., SOBOCINSKI, K.A., VEUM-STONE, J.

and BORTIN, M.M. (1995). Impact of cytogenetic abnormalities on outcome of bone marrow transplants in acute myelogenous leukemia in first remission, *Bone Marrow Transplantation* **16**, 203–208.

GLUCKSBERG, H., STORB, R., FEFER, A., BUCKNER, C. D., NEIMAN, P.E., CLIFT, R.A., LERNER, K.G. and THOMAS, E.D. (1974). Clinical manifestations of graft-versus-host disease in human recipients of marrow from HL-A-matched sibling donors, *Transplantation* **18**, 295–304.

GOODRICH, J.M., MORI, M., GLEAVES, C.A., DU MOND, C., CAYS, M., EBELING, D.F., BUHLES, W.C., DEARMOND, B. and MEYERS, J.D. (1991). Early treatment with ganciclovir to prevent cytomegalovirus disease after allogeneic bone marrow transplantation, *N. Engl. J. Med.* **325**, 1601–1607.

HERRERA, C., GARCIA-PEREZ, M.J., RAMIREZ, R., MARTIN, C., ALVAREZ, M.A., MARTINEZ, F., GOMEZ, P., GARCIA-CASTELLANO, J.M. and TORRES, A. (1997). Lymphokine-activated killer (LAK) cell generation from peripheral blood stem cells by *in vitro* incubation with low-dose interleukin-2 plus granulocyte-macrophage colony-stimulating factor, *Bone Marrow Transplantation* **19**, 545–551.

HESLOP, H.E., SMITH, C.A., NG, C., LOFTIN, S.K., SIXBEY, J., KRANCE, R.A., BRENNER, M.K. and ROONEY, C.M. (1996). Efficacy of adoptively transferred virus specific cytotoxic T lymphocytes for prophylaxis and treatment of EBV lymphoma, *Blood* **88**, 681a, #2713 (Abstract).

HOROWITZ, M.M., GALE, R.P., SONDEL, P.M., GOLDMAN, J.M., KERSEY, J., KOLB, H., RIMM, A.A., RINGDEN, O., ROZMAN, C., SPECK, B., TRUITT, R.L., ZWAAN, F.E. and BORTIN, M.M. (1990). Graft-versus-leukemia reactions after bone marrow transplantation, *Blood* **75**, 555–562.

IKEHARA, S., GOOD, R.A., NAKAMURA, T., SEKITA, K., INOUE, S., OO, M.M., MUSO, E., OGAWA, K. and HAMASHIMA, Y. (1985). Rationale for bone marrow transplantation in the treatment of autoimmune diseases, *Proc. Natl. Acad. Sci. USA* **82**, 2483–2487.

JADUS, M.R. and WEBSIC, H.T. (1992). The role of cytokines in graft-versus-host reactions and disease, *Bone Marrow Transplantation* **10**, 1–14.

JONES, R.J., AMBINDER, R.F., PIANTADOSI, S. and SANTOS, G.W. (1991). Evidence of graft-versus-lymphoma effect associated with allogeneic bone marrow transplantation, *Blood* **77**, 649–653.

KANTROW, S.P., HACKMAN, R.C., BOECKH, M., MYERSON, D. and CRAWFORD, S.W. (1997). Idiopathic pneumonia syndrome: Changing spectrum of lung injury after marrow transplantation, *Transplantation* **63**, 1079–1086.

KHOURI, I.F., KEATING, M.J., VRIESENDORP, H.M., READING, C.L., PRZEPIORKA, D., HUH, Y.O., ANDERSSON, B.S., VAN BESIEN, K.W., MEHRA, R.C., GIRALT, S.A., IPPOLITI, C., MARSHALL, M., THOMAS, M.W., O'BRIEN, S., ROBERTSON, L.E., DEISSEROTH, A.B. and CHAMPLIN, R.E. (1994). Autologous and allogeniec bone marrow transplantation for chronic lymphocytic leukemia: Preliminary results, *J. Clin. Oncol.* **12**, 748–758.

KOLB, H.J., SCHATTENBERG, A., GOLDMAN, J.M., HERTENSTEIN, B., JACOBSEN, N., ARCESE, W., LJUNGMAN, P., FERRANT, A., VERDONCK, L., NIEDERWIESER, D., VAN RHEE, F., MITTERMUELLER, J., DE WITTE, T., HOLLER, E. and ANSARI, H. (1995). Graft-versus-leukemia effect of donor lymphocyte transfusions in marrow grafted patients. European Group for Blood and Marrow Transplantation Working Party Chronic Leukemia, *Blood* **86**, 2041–2050.

KRAUSE, D.S., FACKLER, M.J., CIVIN, C.I. and MAY, W.S. (1996). CD34: Structure, biology, and clinical unity, *Blood* **87**, 1–13.

LANGENMAYER, I., WEAVER, C., BUCKNER, C.D., LILLEBY, K., APPELBAUM, F.R., LONGIN, K., ROWLEY, S., STORB, R., SINGER, J. and BENSINGER, W.I. (1995). Engraftment of patients with lymphoid malignancies transplanted with autologous bone marrow, peripheral blood stem cells or both, *Bone Marrow Transplantation* **15**, 241–246.

LUCARELLI, G. and CLIFT, R.A. (1994). Bone marrow transplantation in Thalassemia. In: *Bone Marrow Transplantation*, S.J. Forman, K.G. Blume and E.D. Thomas, eds., Blackwell Scientific Publications, Boston, MA, pp 829–839.

LUM, L.G. (1987). A Review: The kinetics of immune reconstitution after human marrow transplantation, *Blood* **69**, 369–380.

MARMONT, A.M. (1994). Immune ablation followed by allogeneic or autologous bone marrow transplantation: A new treatment for severe autoimmune diseases, *Stem Cells* **12**, 125–135.

MARMONT, A.M., HOROWITZ, M.M., GALE, R.P., SOBOCINSKI, K., ASH, R.C., VAN BEKKUM, D.W., CHAMPLIN, R.E., DICKE, K.A., GOLDMAN, J.M., GOOD, R.A., HERZIG, R.H., HONG, R., MASAOKA, T., RIMM, A.A., RINGDEN, O., SPECK, B., WEINER, R.S. and BORTIN, M.M. (1991). T-cell depletion of HLA-identical transplants in leukemia, *Blood* **78**, 2120–2130.

MARTIN, P.J., HANSEN, J., STORB, R. and THOMAS, E.D. (1987). Human marrow transplantation: An immunological perspective. In: *Advances in Immunology*, F.J. Dixon, K.F. Austen, L.E. Hood and J.W. Uhr, eds., Academic Press, Orlando, Florida, pp 379–438.

MARTIN, P.J., HANSEN, J.A., STORB, R. and THOMAS, E.D. (1986). Applications of monoclonal antibodies for prevention of graft-versus-host disease. In: *Monoclonal Antibodies in Haematopathology*, F. Grignani, M.F. Mantelli and D.Y. Mason, eds., Raven Press, New York, pp 139–148.

MARTIN, P.J., SCHOCH, G., FISHER, L., BYERS, V., ANASETTI, C., APPELBAUM, F.R., BEATTY, P.G., DONEY, K., MCDONALD, G. B., SANDERS, J.E., SULLIVAN, K.M., STORB, R., THOMAS, E.D., WITHERSPOON, R.P., LOMEN, P., HANNIGAN, J. and HANSEN, J.A. (1990). A retrospective analysis of therapy for acute graft-versus-host disease: Initial treatment, *Blood* **76**, 1464–1472.

MATTHEWS, D.C., APPELBAUM, F.R., EARY, J.F., FISHER, D.R., DURACK, L.D., BUSH, S.A., HUI, T.E., MARTIN, P.J., MITCHELL, D., PRESS, O.W., BADGER, C.C., STORB, R., NELP, W.B. and BERNSTEIN, I.D. (1995). Development of a marrow transplant regimen for acute leukemia using targeted hematopoietic irradiation delivered by ^{131}I-labeled anti-CD45 antibody, combined with cyclophosphamide and total body irradiation, *Blood* **85**, 1122–1131.

McDONALD, G.B., SHULMAN, H.M., SULLIVAN, K.M. and SPENCER, G.D. (1986). Intestinal and hepatic complications of human bone marrow transplantation, *Gastroenterology* **90**, 460–477, 770–784.

MEYERS, J.D., FLOURNOY, N. and THOMAS, E.D. (1982). Nonbacterial pneumonia after allogeneic marrow transplantation: A review of ten years' experience, *Rev. Infect. Dis.* **4**, 1119–1132.

MICHALLET, M., ARCHIMBAUD, E., BANDINI, G., ROWLINGS, P.A., DEEG, H.J., GAHRTON, G., MONTSERRAT, E., ROZMAN, C., GRATWOHL, A. and GALE, R.P. (1996). HLA-Identical sibling bone marrow transplantation in younger patients with chronic lymphocytic leukemia, *Ann. Intern. Med.* **124**, 311–315.

NEMUNAITIS, J., SINGER, J.W., BUCKNER, C.D., DURNAM, D., EPSTEIN, C., HILL, R., STORB, R., THOMAS, E.D. and APPELBAUM, F.R. (1990). Use of recombinant human granulocyte-macrophage colony-stimulating factor in graft failure after bone marrow transplantation, *Blood* **76**, 245–253.

O'REILLY, R.J., FRIEDRICH, W. and SMALL, T.N. (1994). Transplantation approaches for severe combined immunodeficiency disease, Wiskott-Aldrich syndrome, and other lethal genetic, combined immunodeficiency disorders. In: *Bone Marrow Transplantation*, S.J. Forman, K.G. Blume and E.D. Thomas, eds., Blackwell Scientific Publications, Boston, MA, pp 849–873.

PARKMAN, R. (1994). Immunological reconstitution following bone marrow transplantation. In: *Bone Marrow Transplantation*, S.J. Forman, K.G. Blume and E.D. Thomas, eds., Blackwell Scientific Publications, Boston, MA, pp 504–512.

PETERS, W.P., ROSS, M., VREDENBURGH, J.J., MEISENBERG, B., MARKS, L.B., WINER, E., KURTZBERG, J., BAST, R.C., JR., JONES, R., SHPALL, E., WU, K., ROSNER, G., GILBERT, C., MATHIAS, B., CONIGLIO, D., PETROS, W., HENDERSON, I.C., NORTON, L., WEISS, R.B., BUDMAN, D. and HURD, D. (1993). High-dose chemotherapy and autologous bone marrow support as consolidation after standard-dose adjuvant therapy for high-risk primary breast cancer, *J. Clin. Oncol.* **11**, 1132–1143.

PETERSDORF, E.W., LONGTON, G.M., ANASETTI, C., MARTIN, P.J., MICKELSON, E.M., SMITH, A.G. and HANSEN, J.A. (1995). The significance of HLA-DRB1 matching on clinical outcome after HLA-A, B, DR identical unrelated donor marrow transplantation, *Blood* **86**, 1606–1613.

PETERSDORF, E.W., LONGTON, G.M., ANASETTI, C., MICKELSON, E.M., MCKINNEY, S.K., SMITH, A.G., MARTIN, P.J. and HANSEN, J.A. (1997). Association of HLA-C disparity with graft failure after marrow transplantation from unrelated donors, *Blood* **89**, 1818–1823.

PHILIP, T., GUGLIELMI, C., HAGENBEEK, A., SOMERS, R., VAN DER LELIE, H., BRON, D., SONNEVELD, P., GISSELBRECHT, CAHN, J., HAROUSSEAU, J., COIFFIER, B., BIRON, P., MANDELL, F. and CHAUVIN, F. (1995). Autologous bone marrow transplantation as compared with salvage chemotherapy in relapses of chemotherapy-sensitive non-Hodgkin's lymphoma, *N. Engl. J. Med.* **333**, 1540–1545.

PRESS, O.W., APPELBAUM, F., LEDBETTER, J.A., MARTIN, P.J., ZARLING, J., KIDD, P. and THOMAS, E.D. (1987). Monoclonal antibody 1F5 (anti-CD20) serotherapy of human B cell lymphomas, *Blood* **69**, 584–591.

RABINOWE, S.N., SOIFFER, R.J., GRIBBEN, J.G., DALEY, H., FREEDMAN, A.S., DALEY, J., PESEK, K., NEUBERG, D., PINKUS, G., LEAVITT, P.R., SPECTOR, N.A., GROSSBARD, M.L., ANDERSON, K., ROBERTSON, M.J., MAUCH, P., CHAYT-MARCUS, K., RITZ, J. and NADLER, L.M. (1993). Autologous and allogeneic bone marrow transplantation for poor prognosis patients with B-cell chronic lymphocytic leukemia, *Blood* **82**, 1366–1376.

RADICH, J.P., SANDERS, J.E., BUCKNER, C.D., MARTIN, P.J., PETERSON, F.B., BENSINGER, W., MCDONALD, G.B., MORI, M., SCHOCH, G. and HANSEN, J.A. (1993). Second allogeneic marrow transplantation for patients with recurrent leukemia after initial transplant with total-body irradiation-containing regimens, *J. Clin. Oncol.* **11**, 304–313.

REED, E.C., BOWDEN, R.A., DANDLIKER, P.S., LILLEBY, K.E. and MEYERS, J.D. (1988). Treatment of cytomegalovirus pneumonia with ganciclovir and intravenous cytomegalovirus immunoglobulin in patients with bone marrow transplants, *Ann. Intern. Med.* **109**, 783–788.

RIDDELL, S.R., WATANABE, K.S., GOODRICH, J.M., LI, C.R., AGHA, M.E. and GREENBERG, P.D. (1992). Restoration of viral immunity in immunodeficient humans by the adoptive transfer of T cell clones, *Science* **257**, 238–241.

SALE, G.E. and SHULMAN, H.M. (1984). *The Pathology of Bone Marrow Transplantation*, Masson, Inc., New York.

SANTOS, G.W., HESS, A.D. and VOGELSANG, G.B. (1985). Graft-versus-host reactions and disease. (Review). *Immunol Rev* **88**, 169–192.

SCHILLER, G., VESCIO, R., FREYTES, C., SPITZER, G., SAHEBI, F., LEE, M., WU, C.H., CAO, J., LEE, J.C., HONG, C.H., LICHTENSTEIN, A., LILL, M., HALL, J., BERENSON, R. and BERENSON, J. (1995). Transplantation of CD34+ peripheral blood progenitor cells after high-dose chemotherapy for patients with advanced multiple myeloma, *Blood* **86**, 390–397.

SEBBAN, C., LEPAGE, E., VERNANT, J.-P., GLUCKMAN, E., ATTAL, M., REIFFERS, J., SUTTON, L., RACADOT, E., MICHALLET, M., MARANINCHI, D., DREYFUS, F. and FIERE, D. (1994). Allogeneic bone marrow transplantation in adult acute lymphoblastic leukemia in first complete remission: A comparative study, *J. Clin. Oncol.* **12**, 2580–2587.

SERVIDA, P., GOOLEY, T., HANSEN, J.A., BJERKE, J., MARTIN, P.J., PETERSDORF, E.W. and ANASETTI, C. (1996). Improved survival of haploidentical related donor marrow transplants mismatched for HLA-A or B versus HLA-DR, *Blood* **88**, 484a, #1925 (Abstract).

SIMMONS, P.J., PRZEPIORKA, D., THOMAS, E.D. and TOROK-STORB, B. (1987). Host origin of marrow stromal cells following allogeneic bone marrow transplantation, *Nature* **328**, 429–432.

SOIFFER, R.J., MURRAY, C., MAUCH, P., ANDERSON, K.C., FREEDMAN, A.S., RABINOWE, S.N., TAKVORIAN, T., ROBERTSON, M.J., SPECTOR, N. and GONIN, R. (1992). Prevention of graft-versus-host disease by selective depletion of CD6-positive T lymphocytes from donor bone marrow, *J. Clin. Oncol.* **10**, 1191–1200.

STORB, R. (1986). Graft-versus-host disease after marrow transplantation. In: *Transplantation: Approaches to Graft Rejection*, H.T. Meryman, ed., Alan R. Liss, Inc., New York, pp 139–157.

STORB, R., ANASETTI, C., APPELBAUM, F., BENSINGER, W., BUCKNER, C.D., CLIFT, R., DEEG, H.J., DONEY, K., HANSEN, J., LOUGHRAN, T., MARTIN, P., PEPE, M., PETERSEN, F., SANDERS, J., SINGER, J., STEWART, P., SULLIVAN, K.M., WITHERSPOON, R. and THOMAS, E.D. (1991). Marrow transplantation for severe aplastic anemia and thalassemia major, *Semin. Hematol.* **28**, 235–239.

STORB, R., DEEG, H.J., PEPE, M., APPELBAUM, F.R., ANASETTI, C., BEATTY, P., BENSINGER, W., BERENSON, R., BUCKNER, C.D., CLIFT, R., DONEY, K., LONGTON, G., HANSEN, J., HILL, R., LOUGHRAN, T., JR., MARTIN, P., SINGER, J., SANDERS, J., STEWART, P., SULLIVAN, K., WITHERSPOON, R. and THOMAS, E.D. (1989). Methotrexate and cyclosporine versus cyclosporine alone for prophylaxis of graft-versus-host disease in patients given HLA-identical marrow grafts for leukemia: Long-term follow-up of a controlled trial, *Blood* **73**, 1729–1734.

STORB, R., DEEG, H.J., WHITEHEAD, J., FAREWELL, V., APPELBAUM, F.R., BEATTY, P., BENSINGER, W., BUCKNER, C.D., CLIFT, R., DONEY, K., HANSEN, J., HILL, R., LUM, L.G., MARTIN, P., MCGUFFIN, R., SANDERS, J.E., SINGER, J., STEWART, P., SULLIVAN, K.M., WITHERSPOON, R.P. and THOMAS, E.D. (1987). Marrow transplantation for leukemia and aplastic anemia: Two controlled trials of a combination of methotrexate and cyclosporine versus cyclosporine alone or methotrexate alone for prophylaxis of acute graft-versus-host disease, *Transplant Proc.* **19**, 2608–2613.

STORB, R., LEISENRING, W., ANASETTI, C., APPELBAUM, F.R., BUCKNER, C.D., BENSINGER, W.I., CHAUNCEY, T., CLIFT, R.A., DEEG, H.J., DONEY, K.C., FLOWERS, M.E.D., HANSEN, J.A., MARTIN, P.J., SANDERS, J.E., SULLIVAN, K.M. and WITHERSPOON, R.P. (1997). Long-term follow-up of allogeneic marrow transplants in patients with aplastic anemia conditioned by cyclophosphamide combined with antithymocyte globulin (Letter to the Editor), *Blood* **89**, 3890–3891.

STORB, R., PRENTICE, R.L., SULLIVAN, K.M., SHULMAN, H.M., DEEG, H.J., DONEY, K.C., BUCKNER, C.D., CLIFT, R.A., WITHERSPOON, R.P., APPELBAUM, F.R., SANDERS, J.E., STEWART, P.S. and THOMAS, E.D. (1983). Predictive factors in chronic graft-versus-host disease in patients with aplastic anemia treated by marrow transplantation from HLA-identical siblings, *Ann. Intern. Med.* **98**, 461–466.

STORB, R. and THOMAS, E.D. (1985). Graft-versus-host disease in dog and man: The Seattle Experience. In: *Immunological Reviews No. 88*, G. Möller, ed., Munksgaard, Copenhagen, pp 215–238.

STORB, R., WEIDEN, P.L., SULLIVAN, K.M., APPELBAUM, F.R., BEATTY, P., BUCKNER, C.D., CLIFT, R.A., DONEY, K.C., HANSEN, J., MARTIN, P.J., SANDERS, J.E., STEWART, P., WITHERSPOON, R.P. and THOMAS, E.D. (1987). Second marrow transplants in patients with aplastic anemia rejecting the first graft: Use of a conditioning regimen including cyclophosphamide and antithymocyte globulin, *Blood* **70**, 116–121.

STORB, R., YU, C., WAGNER, J.L., DEEG, H.J., NASH, R.A., KIEM, H.-P., LEISENRING, W. and SHULMAN, H. (1997). Stable mixed hematopoietic chimerism in DLA-identical littermate dogs given sublethal total body irradiation before and pharmacological immunosuppression after marrow transplantation, *Blood* **89**, 3048–3054.

STOREK, J., GOOLEY, T., SIADAK, M., BENSINGER, W.I., MALONEY, D.G., CHAUNCEY, T.R., FLOWERS, M., SULLIVAN, K.M., WITHERSPOON, R.P., ROWLEY, S.D., HANSEN, J.A., STORB, R. and APPELBAUM, F.R. (1997). Allogeneic peripheral blood stem cell transplantation may be associated with a high risk of chronic graft-versus-host disease. *Blood* **90**, 4705–4709.

STUCKI, A., LEISENRING, W., SANDMAIER, B.M., SANDERS, J., ANASETTI, C. and STORB, R. (1997). Increasing survival for severe aplastic anemia patients who undergo a second marrow transplant after rejection of the first graft, *Blood* **90**(Suppl 1), 550a (Abstract #2450).

SULLIVAN, K.M., AGURA, E., ANASETTI, C., APPELBAUM, F.R., BADGER, C., BEARMAN, S., ERICKSON, K., FLOWERS, M., HANSEN, J.A., LOUGHRAN, T., MARTIN, P., MATTHEWS, D., PETERSDORF, E., RADICH, J., RIDDELL, S., ROVIRA, D., SANDERS, J., SCHUENING, F., SIADAK, M., STORB, R. and WITHERSPOON, R.P. (1991). Chronic graft-versus-host disease and other late complications of bone marrow transplantation, *Semin. Hematol.* **28**, 250–259.

SULLIVAN, K.M., APPELBAUM, F.R., HORNING, S.J., ROSENBERG, S.A. and THOMAS, E.D. (1986). Selection of patients with Hodgkin's disease and non-Hodgkin's lymphoma for bone marrow transplantation, *Int. J. Cell Cloning* **4**, 94–106.

SULLIVAN, K.M., STORB, R., BUCKNER, C.D., FEFER, A., FISHER, L., WEIDEN, P.L., WITHERSPOON, R.P., APPELBAUM, F.R., BANAJI, M., HANSEN, J., MARTIN, P., SANDERS, J.E., SINGER, J. and THOMAS, E.D. (1989). Graft-versus-host disease as adoptive immunotherapy in patients with advanced hematologic neoplasms, *N. Engl. J. Med.* **320**, 828–834.

THOMAS, E.D., BUCKNER, C.D., BANAJI, M., CLIFT, R.A., FEFER, A., FLOURNOY, N., GOODELL, B.W., HICKMAN, R.O., LERNER, K.G., NEIMAN, P.E., SALE, G.E., SANDERS, J.E., SINGER, J., STEVENS, M., STORB, R. and WEIDEN, P.L. (1977). One hundred patients with acute leukemia treated by chemotherapy, total body irradiation, and allogeneic marrow transplantation, *Blood* **49**, 511–533.

THOMAS, E.D. and STORB, R. (1970). Technique for human marrow grafting, *Blood* **36**, 507–515.

THOMAS, E.D., STORB, R., CLIFT, R.A., FEFER, A., JOHNSON, F.L., NEIMAN, P.E., LERNER, K.G., GLUCKSBERG, H. and BUCKNER, C.D. (1975). Bone-marrow transplantation, *N. Engl. J. Med.* **292**, 832–843, 895–902.

VAN BEKKUM, D.W. and LÖWENBERG, B. (1985). *Bone Marrow Transplantation. Biological Mechanisms and Clinical Practice.* Marcel Dekker, Inc., New York & Basel.

WALTERS, M.C., PATIENCE, M., LEISENRING, W., ECKMAN, J.R., SCOTT, J.P., MENTZER, W.C., DAVIES, S.C., OHENE-FREMPONG, K., BERNAUDIN, F., MATTHEWS, D.C., STORB, R. and SULLIVAN, K.M. (1996). Bone marrow transplantation for sickle cell disease, *N. Engl. J. Med.* **335**, 369–376.

WEIDEN, P.L., SULLIVAN, K.M., FLOURNOY, N., STORB, R., THOMAS, E.D. and THE SEATTLE MARROW TRANSPLANT TEAM. (1981). Antileukemic effect of chronic graft-versus-host disease. Contribution to improved survival after allogeneic marrow transplantation, *N. Engl. J. Med.* **304**, 1529–1533.

WEINER, R.S., BORTIN, M.M., GALE, R.P., GLUCKMAN, E., KAY, H.E.M., KOLB, H., HARTZ, A.J. and RIMM, A.A. (1986). Interstitial pneumonitis after bone marrow transplantation, *Ann. Intern. Med.* **104**, 168–175.

WINSTON, D.J., HO, W.G., CHAMPLIN, R.E. and GALE, R.P. (1984). Infectious complications of bone marrow transplantation, *Exp. Hematol.* **12**, 205–215.

Chapter 3

IMMUNOLOGICAL DEVELOPMENTS IN SUPPORT OF ORTHOPAEDIC SURGERY

3.1 Cardiac Myocytes as Rare Targets of Cell-Mediated Immune Responses
J.B. Sundstrom and A.A. Ansari (*Emory University School of Medicine, Atlanta, USA*)

3.2 Immunology of Bone Allografts: Current Knowledge
G.E. Friedlaender *et al* (*Yale University School of Medicine, New Haven, USA*)

Upon his return from England and after pursuing his Ph.D., Dr. Sell brought with him a profound interest in establishing immunology as it applies to a variety of specialties. He became prominent in attracting scientists to the field of transplantation immunology at the Navy. Several scientists were assigned to the responsibility of developing immunosuppressive therapy through generation of anti-thymocyte globulin. The report in chapter 1 by Dr. Contreras attests to the success of this approach and the continuing contributions of investigators at the Navy to this field. Dr. Sell was also instrumental in facilitating the development of histocompatibility testing during this time and was one of the contributors to the establishment of the American Society of Histocompatibility and Immunogenetics (ASHI). Many immunological techniques were also developed for monitoring patients undergoing transplantation. Dr. Sundstrom reports in this chapter on modern technology now being investigated using cardiac myocytes for monitoring immunological events and understanding the role of cells undergoing immunological attack. The application of immunological principles was also a major undertaking for the field of musculoskeletal tissue transplantation. Dr. Friedlaender reports on immunological principles as they relate to bone transplantation in both experimental and clinical settings.

D.M.S.

3.1 CARDIAC MYOCYTES AS RARE TARGETS OF CELL-MEDIATED IMMUNE RESPONSES

J.B. SUNDSTROM & A.A. ANSARI

Department of Pathology and Laboratory Medicine
Emory University School of Medicine
Atlanta, Georgia, USA

1. Introduction

Immune-mediated injury of cardiac tissues has been associated with a variety of clinical and experimental conditions of heart disease ranging from viral (Guthrie *et al*, 1984; Liu *et al*, 1996) and auto-immune myocarditis (Rose and Hill, 1996; Penninger *et al*, 1997), dilated cardiomyopathies (Goldman and McKenna, 1995), hyperacute and chronic cardiac allograft rejection (Duquesnoy and Demetris, 1995) as well as transplantation-associated atherosclerosis (Ewel and Foegh, 1993). Although the exact mechanisms of immune-mediated cardiac myocyte injury are varied and remain ill-defined, they fall into two general categories: those which cause tissue damage by directly targeting antigens expressed or presented uniquely by the cardiac myocytes and those which damage cardiac myocytes indirectly as a result of an inflammation triggered by other (non-muscle) cardiac tissues. Examples of the latter are myocyte damage that may occur during TH1 inflammatory responses initiated during viral myocarditis. These immune events lead to the recruitment of activated macrophages which release potent antimicrobial agents (e.g. oxygen radicals, nitric oxide (NO), tumour necrosis factor alpha (TNF-α)) into the cardiac tissues which indirectly and non-specifically injure myocytes (Matsumori, 1997). Also, indirect injury leading to necrosis of cardiac myocytes may occur due to a failure in the supply of oxygen which results when the microvasculature is destroyed in transplantation-associated atherosclerosis (Hosenpud, 1993). Examples of the former are cardiomyocyte damage (or dysfunction) caused by the specific actions of complement fixing antibodies that have been reported for both viral and autoimmune cardiomyopathies (Neumann et al, 1994, 1990). Also, CD8[+] or CD4[+] T cells have been shown to directly target virally-infected cardiomyocytes in murine models of viral myocarditis (Van Houten and Huber, 1989; Huber et al, 1988) or uniquely expressed cardiac myocyte antigens in experimental models of autoimmune myocarditis (Pummerer et al, 1996; Hanawa et al, 1996).

In an attempt to gain a clearer understanding of the cellular mechanisms involved in immune-mediated damage of human cardiac myocytes, our laboratory has focussed our research on investigating the ability of human cardiac myocytes to trigger proliferative responses in primed antigen specific CD4[+] T cells or to present specific antigen and serve as targets for armed effector CD8[+] T cells. Both of these cell-mediated immune responses rely on an intimate cognate interaction between the T cell receptor (TCR) and processed antigen, stably presented by major histocompatibility complex (MHC) Class I/II displayed on the myocyte. The ability to process and present antigen to primed CD4[+] or CD8[+] T cells has been documented for various types of non-professional antigen presenting cells (Sundstrom and Ansari, 1995). However, human cardiac myocytes have not been considered even as facultative antigen presenting cells (APCs) and their intrinsic ability to process and present antigens has not been formally studied. In this report we describe our findings which suggest that human cardiac myocytes are rarely direct targeted cell-mediated immune events due to their intrinsic limitations in antigen processing and presentation.

2. T Cell Recognition of Antigenic Determinants on Non-Antigen Presenting Cells

The process by which T cells respond to specific antigen and become activated involves at least two signals: one antigen specific and one antigen non-specific. The T cell's recognition of linear oligomeric peptides presented by MHC molecules displayed on the surface of the antigen presenting cell is mediated by its clonally rearranged TCR, which is specific for the peptide-MHC complex. Endogenous peptides are processed for presentation by MHC Class I to CD8+ restricted T cells, whereas exogenous peptides are processed for presentation by MHC Class II to CD4+ restricted T cells. A brief summary of the two main pathways for antigen processing for MHC Class I or Class II is depicted in Fig. 1. The cognate interactions between TCRs and MHC-peptide complexes induce a (first) signal which is transduced by the CD3 complex associated with the TCR through a network of second messengers to the T cell nucleus. The simultaneous interactions between cellular adhesion molecules (CAMs) and costimulatory molecules (CSMs) and their specific ligands expressed on the surfaces of T cells and APCs help to stabilise TCR-peptide-MHC interactions as well as supply (second) signals which act synergistically with TCR-mediated (first) signals in "switching on" gene activation programmes within the nucleus of the T cell. An in-depth review of T cell activation and antigen recognition has been presented elsewhere (Janeway and Bottomly, 1994; Robey and Allison, 1995).

Professional APCs display a quantity and quality of MHC-peptide complexes and CSMs able to induce naive T cells to become armed or activated. However, many highly-differentiated cells of non-lymphoid lineage (e.g. cardiac myocytes) lack the constitutive expression of MHC-peptide complexes or CSMs sufficient to induce such primary responses in naive or resting T cells. Nevertheless, many such "non-antigen presenting cells" are able to present antigen and serve as specific targets to primed T cells, which are less dependent on second signals for coactivation (Croft, 1994). Furthermore, cytokines

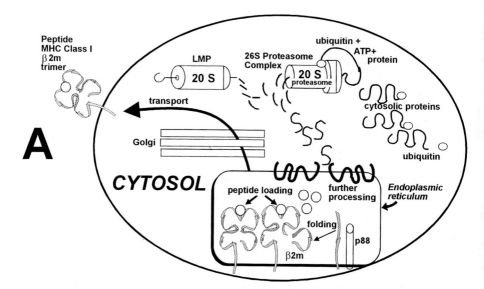

Fig. 1. (A) **MHC Class I processing**. Processing of endogenous antigens for presentation by MHC Class I begins in the cytosol with the proteolytic degradation of ubiquitin-tagged proteins by the multicatalytic proteasome (LMP). The Transporter of Antigenic Peptides (TAP) delivers size-selected processed oligomeric peptides from the cytosol into the ER where they may undergo further processing. Inside the ER, nascent MHC Class I associates with chaperone proteins (e.g. p88) which facilitate proper folding of the molecule into its α1, α2, and α3 domains. Then, as properly-processed peptides (8–11 residues in length) bind to the peptide loading groove (defined by the α1 and α2 domains) a heavy chain/peptide/β2-microglobulin complex forms and the protein chaperone(s) disassociates. The stable MHC Class I/peptide trimer is then transported through the golgi and expressed on the cell surface.

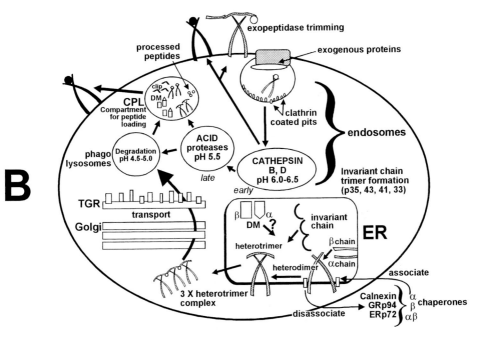

Fig. 1. (B) **MHC Class II processing**. Processing of extracellular antigens occurs as exogenous proteins are internalised via phagocytosis, pinocytosis, or receptor-mediated endocytosis in clathrin coated pits and shuttled into an endocytic route from early to late endosomes and eventually to phagolysosomes with concomitant proteolytic degradation by acid proteases (e.g. cathepsins). MHC Class II assembly occurs independently of endocytic antigen processing. Nascent MHC Class II, synthesised in the ER, associates with chaperone proteins which facilitate proper folding of the MHC Class II α and β heavy chains and retards egress of MHC Class II from the ER until they are properly configured and associated in a trimeric complex with the invariant chain (Ii). The peptide antigen binding groove formed by the MHC Class II heterodimer binds to a conserved region of the invariant chain referred to as the Class II invariant peptide (CLIP). The MHCαβ-Ii heterotrimer (nonameric complex) dissociates from the calnexin chaperone and is transported through the golgi and transgolgi reticulum (TGR) to a late endosomal compartment for peptide loading (CPL) where the DM facilitates the replacement of CLIP with processed antigenic peptide. Once loaded with peptide the MHC Class II-peptide complex is transported to and expressed on the cell surface.

associated with inflammation, e.g. interferon gamma (IFN-γ), are able to up-regulate expression of MHC antigens and certain CAM/CSMs, which in turn restores or augments the ability of non-antigen presenting cells to induce allo-responses and to present nominal antigen.

3. T Cell Responses to Allo-Antigen Versus Nominal Antigen

Given that T cell responses to allo-antigen are significantly stronger than to nominal antigen, our laboratory first examined the cellular basis for immune-mediated injury to cardiac myocytes in the context of chronic cardiac allograft rejection. To study these mechanisms *in vitro*, we developed the surrogate SV40-transformed foetal human cardiac myocyte (FHCM) cell line, W-1. This cell line which was derived from an enriched population of FHCMs from a single donor, as previously described (Wang *et al*, 1991), constitutively expresses MHC Class I, ICAM-1, and LFA-3. Treatment of W-1s with IFN-γ induces the expression of stable MHC II-peptide complexes and causes an up-regulation of expression of MHC Class I and ICAM-1 (Ansari *et al*, 1994). Nevertheless, *in vitro* neither W-1s nor FHCMs are able to induce allo-proliferative responses or anergy in unfractionated peripheral blood mononuclear cells (PBMCs) or in T cells (Chang and Flavell, 1995). Furthermore, reconstitution of W-1s with glycosyl phosphatidylinositol-anchored B7-1 does not restore their ability to induce allo-responses (manuscript in preparation).

In view of new insights into the molecular basis of allo-recognition, we reasoned that these results might be explained in terms of the intrinsic abilities of W-1 to process and present self-antigens. There is growing acceptance of the view that individual T cell clones recognising multiple allogeneic determinants, formed by single processed oligomeric peptides complexed with MHC Class I/II molecules and displayed on the surface of the APC, determines the high precursor frequency of allo-reactive T cells (Sundstrom and Ansari, 1995). The requirement of peptide plus MHC for allo-recognition implies that the diversity of peptides associated with

MHC Class I/II antigens governs the characteristic allo-antigenic diversity of cells of different tissue lineages. In the context of these findings, we reasoned that an alternative hypothesis for the observed lack of allogenicity of the W-1 cell line could be that cardiac myocytes possess a limited ability to process and present antigenic peptides for presentation by MHC, thus resulting in the display of a number of allotopes insufficient to surpass a threshold leading to allo-activation or anergy that could be measured by conventional techniques. To test this hypothesis, we measured the ability of W-1s to process and present immunogenic peptides for presentation to antigen primed $CD8^+$ or $CD4^+$ restricted T cells.

4. Ability of Cardiac Myocytes to Process and Present Nominal Antigen

The observation that cardiac myocytes are so weakly immunogenic that they appear to be unable to induce allo-responses in T cells raises a question as to whether they are still able to serve as direct targets of cellular immune responses. Our approach was to divide this question into two parts: (1) can MHC Class I or Class II expressing cardiac myocytes present synthetic antigenic peptides to $CD8^+$ or $CD4^+$ T cells? and (2) can they process endogenous or exogenous antigens for presentation to primed $CD8^+$ or $CD4^+$ T cells which recognise specific oligomeric peptides associated with MHC Class I or II, respectively?

To address these issues, we first evaluated the ability of HLA-A*0201 W-1s to process and present antigenic peptides for MHC Class I restricted presentation to $CD8^+$ CTLs specific for the influenza M1 58-66 peptide derived from the influenza A matrix protein. In standard 6 H CTL assays the percent specific lysis of W-1 targets increases proportionately with increasing pulsing concentrations of exogenous M1 58-66 peptide. However, even with peptide concentrations as high as 10 µM, W-1 targets are lysed with only 50% efficiency as peptide-pulsed HLA-A*0201 EBV-PBL control target cells. Pretreatment of W-1 targets with IFN-γ improves their efficiency in presenting flu peptides to HLA-A2 restricted $CD8^+$ CTLs, although their net specific lysis remains significantly less than that seen with peptide-pulsed HLA-A*0201 Epstein-Barr virus peripheral blood lymphocyte (EBV-PBL) control target cells (unpublished observations).

We examined the ability of W-1s to process endogenous antigen by infecting W-1s with vaccinia constructs containing the full length influenza A matrix 1 protein. We observed that although W-1s constitutively express MHC Class I, they are unable to process and present antigenic peptides to CD8+ CTLs specific for the influenza M1 58-66 peptide. However, pretreatment with IFN-γ restored their ability to process and present the M1 58-66 peptide, although with only 50% of the efficiency as HLA-A*0201 EBV-PBL control target cells (unpublished observations).

Similar experiments to study the processing and presentation of exogenous antigens by MHC Class II on HLA-DR β1*0301 W-1s were conducted using the TT 830-843 peptide (P2), derived from Tetanus toxin (TT), in standard five-day proliferation assays with TT-primed HLA-DR β1*0301 T cells. Although pretreatment of W-1s with IFN-γ induces the expression of stable MHC Class II-peptide complexes, IFN-γ pretreated W-1s were unable to process or present the TT 830-843 peptide to TT-primed T cells whereas HLA-DR β1*0301 EBV-PBL controls were. The induced expression of MHC Class II is only 10% of that constitutively expressed on EBV-PBLs. However, peptide binding studies confirmed that the P2 peptide was able to bind to HLA-DR β1*0301 expressing W-1s, although P2 peptide binding to HLA-DR β1*0301 W-1s was only 0.5% of that seen with HLA-DR β1*0301 EBV-PBLs. These observations led us to consider whether the intransigence of MHC Class II expressing W-1s to P2 peptide binding or TT antigen processing might be due to slow MHC-peptide turnover rates or expression of genes involved in antigen processing relative to EBV-PBL controls.

5. Constitutive and Induced Expression of Genes Associated with Antigen Processing and Presentation in Cardiac Myocytes

Within the MHC Class II locus, located on the short arm of human chromosome 6 are the genes which encode the MHC Class I heavy chain, the Class II α and β chains, and critical cellular components for the Class I and Class II antigen processing pathways. Two subunits of the 20s proteasome, encoded by LMP-2 and LMP-7, and the transporters of antigenic peptides, encoded by TAP-1 and TAP-2, together process and transport endogenous antigens into the endoplasmic reticulum (ER) where they associate with nascent MHC Class I molecules, which are subsequently transported to and expressed on the cell surface (Lehner and Cresswell, 1996; York and Rock, 1996). Though the role of DMA and DMB continues to be elucidated, DM has recently been shown to be involved in the exchange of processed antigenic peptides for processed invariant chain peptide (CLIP) on nascent MHC Class II molecules within the compartment for peptide loading (CPL) (Weber *et al*, 1996; Denzin and Cresswell, 1995; Sloan *et al*, 1995). Regulation of MHC Class II gene expression is coordinated by the Class II transactivator (CIITA) which is also located within the MHC Class II gene locus (Chang and Flavell, 1995). Although it is located on a separate chromosome, the gene encoding Ii is co-regulated with the expression of the MHC Class II genes due to shared promoter/enhancer elements (Nordeng and Bakke, 1994). Deficient expression of any of these genes has been shown to result in defective or absence of antigen presentation by MHC antigens (Mach *et al*, 1996). Therefore, in order to assess antigen processing and presentation defects of the W-1 cell line from the perspective of gene expression, mRNA levels for each of these genes were determined by semi-quantitative RT-PCR and then normalised relative to constitutive levels of gene expression measured in EBV-PBL controls (for genes associated with MHC Class II antigen processing pathway) or measured in primary or SV40 transformed microvascular endothelial cells as well as EBV-PBLs (for genes associated with MHC Class I antigen processing pathway).

For the MHC Class II antigen processing pathway, the relative levels of gene expression for CIITA, MHC II, Ii and DMA/B were determined only in IFN-γ pretreated W-1s, since constitutive levels of expression were undetectable. We determined that the (IFN-γ) induced expression of genes encoding DMA/B, Ii and CIITA ranged from 50–90% of those measured in EBV-PBLs. However, the gene expression for MHC Class II was only 10–20% of that seen in EBV-PBLs, which is consistent with the relative surface expression for MHC Class II as measured by flow microfluorometry. These data suggest that although IFN-γ can up-regulate the transcription of multiple genes critical to the Class II processing pathway, the markedly weak level of expression of MHC Class II mRNA most likely has the strongest influence (at the transcriptional level) in limiting the ability of W-1s to process and present antigenic peptides for MHC Class II.

For MHC Class I antigen processing pathway, the levels of constitutive gene expression for LMP-2/7, TAP-1/2 and MHC Class I were significantly lower than corresponding levels measured in EBV-PBLs. However, the (IFN-γ) induced levels of gene expression in W-1s were comparable to constitutive levels measured in EBV-PBLs as well as in representative (non-antigen presenting) human lung or dermal microvascular endothelial cell lines. Therefore, at the level of gene expression, antigen processing and presentation for MHC Class I can be restored (*in vitro*) by pre-treatment with high concentrations of recombinant IFN-γ.

6. Pulse-Chase Studies

To complement our transcriptional profile of gene expression, the levels of expression and turnover rates of the gene translation products for MHC Class I/II, Ii, DMA/B, LMP-2/7 and TAP-1/2 for W-1s were compared with corresponding values obtained with EBV-PBLs. The levels of [^{35}S]-labelled immuno-precipitates from (IFN-γ) induced W-1s were significantly lower relative to EBV-PBLs. Furthermore, the half-lives of all [^{35}S]-labelled immuno-precipitates measured were 200% greater than corresponding levels from EBV-PBLs. Thus, the low levels of expression together with the slow turnover rates for the translation products of genes associated with antigen processing and presentation support the concept of a lethargic pace of antigen processing within the (IFN-γ) induced W-1 cell line and are consistent with the observed functional defects in antigen presentation by W-1s.

7. Summary

Although the immunopathogenesis associated with many cardiomyopathies leads to myocyte drop-out, there is little evidence that cardiac myocytes are the direct targets of immune-mediated injury. For most part, cardiac myocytes remain antigenically silent and immunologically inert. Our research with the human foetal cardiac myocyte cell line, W-1, supports these conclusions. We have been able to demonstrate that W-1s can be destroyed *in vitro* by antigen-specific CD8+ CTLs, but only after pretreatment with supra-physiologic levels of IFN-γ or pulsing with relatively high molar concentrations of synthetic peptide. Therefore, we have been able to show that cardiac myocytes can serve as targets of direct immune-mediated injury but only under experimental conditions that favour such outcomes. We suggest that three possible reasons for such a lack of immune recognition are that cardiac myocytes (1) are unable to process and display a threshold number of antigenic peptide-MHC complexes to trigger requisite TCR-mediated signals, (2) are unable to display a threshold number or variety of critical CAMs/CSMs capable of delivering requisite second signals, or (3) display unique surface antigen(s) which deliver cognate signals to effector T cells that inhibit their activation.

Targets of cytolytic T cells are usually destroyed by apoptosis. Armed effector CD8+ T cells destroy their targets by the combined actions of granzymes and perforin. Alternate apoptotic pathways are mediated through interactions of FAS expressed on the surface of the target cell and FAS ligand expressed on activated effector CD4+ or CD8+ T cells. FAS is constitutively expressed on W-1s and can be up-regulated with IFN-γ. However, it is not known if FAS-mediated apoptosis can be induced in cardiac myocytes. Nevertheless, there are reports of apoptosis of cardiac myocytes in cardiomyopathies related to ischaemia/reperfusion and myocardial infarction (Olivetti et al, 1996; MacLellan and Schneider, 1997; Bromme and Holtz, 1996). However, these apoptotic events are usually not immune-mediated. More recent reports of apoptosis in myocytes found in cardiac allografts undergoing rejection remain controversial (Laguens et al, 1996; Jollow et al, 1997; Larsen et al, 1995). We conclude that cardiac myocytes are rarely the direct targets of cell-mediated immune responses and that myocyte injury mainly occurs indirectly and is a consequence of immunopathogenesis directed towards other lineages of cardiac tissues.

8. References

ANSARI, A.A., SUNDSTROM, J.B., RUNNELS, H., JENSEN, P., KANTER, K., MAYNE, A. and HERSKOWITZ, A. (1994). The absence of constitutive and induced expression of critical cell-adhesion molecules on human cardiac myocytes. Its role in transplant rejection, *Transplantation 1994* **57**, 942–949.

BROMME, H.J. and HOLTZ, J. (1996). Apoptosis in the heart: When and why? *Molecular & Cellular Biochemistry*, 261–275.

CHANG, C.H. and FLAVELL, R.A. (1995). Class II transactivator regulates the expression of multiple genes involved in antigen presentation, *J. Exp. Med.* **181**(2), 765–767.

CROFT, M. (1994). Activation of naive, memory and effector T cells, *Current Opinion in Immunology* **6**(3), 431–437.

DENZIN, L.K. and CRESSWELL, P. (1995). HLA-DM induces CLIP dissociation from MHC class II alpha beta dimers and facilitates peptide loading, *Cell* **82**, 155–165.

DUQUESNOY, R.J. and DEMETRIS, A.J. (1995). Immunopathology of cardiac transplant rejection, *Current Opinion in Cardiology* **10**, 193–206.

EWEL, C.H. and FOEGH, M.L. (1993). Chronic graft rejection: Accelerated transplant arteriosclerosis, *Immunological Reviews* **134**, 21–31.

GOLDMAN, J.H. and McKENNA, W.J. (1995). Immunopathogenesis of dilated cardiomyopathies, *Current Opinion in Cardiology* **10**, 306–311.

GUTHRIE, M., LODGE, P.A. and HUBER, S.A. (1984). Cardiac injury in myocarditis induced by Coxsackievirus group B, type 3 in Balb/c mice is mediated by Lyt 2+ cytolytic lymphocytes, *Cellular Immunology* **88**(2), 558–567.

HANAWA, H., INOMATA, T., SEKIKAWA, H., ABO, T., KODAMA, M., IZUMI, T. and SHIBATA, A. (1996). Analysis of heart-infiltrating T-cell clonotypes in experimental autoimmune myocarditis in rats, *Circulation Research* **78**, 118–125.

HOSENPUD, J.D. (1993). Immune mechanisms of cardiac allograft vasculopathy: An update, *Transplant Immunology* **1**, 237–249.

HUBER, S.A., HEINTZ, N. and TRACY, R. (1988). Coxsackievirus B-3-induced myocarditis: Virus and actinomycin D treatment of myocytes induces novel antigens recognized by cytolytic T lymphocytes, *J. Immunol.* **141**(9), 3214–3219.

JANEWAY, C.A.J. and BOTTOMLY, K. (1994). Signals and signs for lymphocyte responses, *Cell* **76**, 275–285.

JOLLOW, K.C., SUNDSTROM, J.B., GRAVANIS, M.B., KANTER, K., HERSKOWITZ, A. and ANSARI, A.A. (1997). Apoptosis of mononuclear cell infiltrates in cardiac allograft biopsy specimens questions studies of biopsy-cultured cells, *Transplantation* **63**, 1482–1489.

LAGUENS, R.P., MECKERT, P.M., MARTINO, J.S., PERRONE, S. and FAVALORO, R. (1996). Identification of programmed cell death (apoptosis) *in situ* by means of specific labeling of nuclear DNA fragments in heart biopsy samples during acute rejection episodes, *J. Heart & Lung Transpl.* **15**, 911–918.

LARSEN, C.P., ALEXANDER, D.Z., HENDRIX, R., RITCHIE, S.C. and PEARSON, T.C. (1995). Fas-mediated cytotoxicity. An immunoeffector or immunoregulatory pathway in T cell-mediated immune responses? *Transplantation* **60**, 221–224.

LEHNER, P.J. and CRESSWELL, P. (1996). Processing and delivery of peptides presented by MHC class I molecules, *Current Opinion in Immunology* **8**, 59–67.

LIU, P., MARTINO, T., OPAVSKY, M.A. and PENNINGER, J. (1996). Viral myocarditis: Balance between viral infection and immune response, *Can. J. Cardiol.* **12**, 935–943.

MACH, B., STEIMLE, V., MARTINEZ-SORIA, E. and REITH, W. (1996). Regulation of MHC class II genes: Lessons from a disease, *Ann. Rev. Immunol.* **14**, 301–331.

MacLELLAN, W.R. and SCHNEIDER, M.D. (1997). Death by design. Programmed cell death in cardiovascular biology and disease, *Circulation Research* **81**, 137–144.

MATSUMORI, A. (1997). Molecular and immune mechanisms in the pathogenesis of cardiomyopathy — role of viruses, cytokines, and nitric oxide, *Japanese Circulation Journal* **61**, 275–291.

NEUMANN, D.A., BUREK, C.L., BAUGHMAN, K.L., ROSE, N.R. and HERSKOWITZ, A. (1990) Circulating heart-reactive antibodies in patients with myocarditis or cardiomyopathy, *J. Am. Coll. Cardio.* **16**, 839–846.

NEUMANN, D.A., ROSE, N.R., ANSARI, A.A. and HERSKOWITZ, A. (1994). Induction of multiple heart autoantibodies in mice with coxsackievirus B3- and cardiac myosin-induced autoimmune myocarditis, *J. Immunol.* **152**, 343–350.

NORDENG, T.W. and BAKKE, O. (1994). The biological role of invariant chain (Ii) in MHC class II antigen presentation, *Immunol. Lett.* **43**, 47–55.

OLIVETTI, G., QUAINI, F., SALA, R., LAGRASTA, C., CORRADI, D., BONACINA, E., GAMBERT, S.R., CIGOLA, E. and ANVERSA, P. (1996). Acute myocardial infarction in humans is associated with activation of programmed myocyte cell death in the surviving portion of the heart, *J. Mol. & Cell. Cardio.* **28**, 2005–2016.

PENNINGER, J.M., PUMMERER, C., LIU, P., NEU, N. and BACHMAIER, K. (1997). Cellular and molecular mechanisms of murine autoimmune myocarditis, *APMIS* **105**, 1–13.

PUMMERER, C.L., LUZE, K., GRASSL, G., BACHMAIER, K., OFFNER, F., BURRELL, S.K., LENZ, D.M., ZAMBORELLI, T.J., PENNINGER, J.M. and NEU, N. (1996). Identification of cardiac myosin peptides capable of inducing autoimmune myocarditis in BALB/c mice, *J. Clinical Investigation* **97**, 2057–2062.

ROBEY, E. and ALLISON, J.P. (1995). T-cell activation: Integration of signals from the antigen receptor and costimulatory molecules, *Immunology Today* **16**, 306–310.

ROSE, N.R. and HILL, S.L. (1996). Autoimmune myocarditis, *Int. J. Cardiol.* **54**, 171–175.

SLOAN, V.S., CAMERON, P., PORTER, G., GAMMON, M., AMAYA, M., MELLINS, E. and ZALLER, D.M. (1995). Mediation by HLA-DM of dissociation of peptides from HLA-DR, *Nature* **375**, 802–806.

SUNDSTROM, J.B. and ANSARI, A.A. (1995). Comparative study of the role of professional versus semiprofessional or nonprofessional antigen presenting cells in the rejection of vascularized organ allografts, *Transpl. Immunol.* **3**(4), 273–289.

VAN HOUTEN, N. and HUBER, S.A. (1989). Role of cytotoxic T cells in experimental myocarditis, *Springer Seminars in Immunopathology* 11(1), 61–68.

WANG, Y.C., NECKELMANN, N., MAYNE, A., HERSKOWITZ, A., SRINIVASAN, A., SELL, K.W. and AHMED-ANSARI, A. (1991). Establishment of a human fetal cardiac myocyte cell line, *In Vitro Cellular & Developmental Biology* 27(1), 63–74.

WEBER, D.A., EVAVOLD, B.D. and JENSEN, P.E. (1996). Enhanced dissociation of HLA-DR-bound peptides in the presence of HLA- DM, *Science* 274, 618–620.

YORK, I.A. and ROCK, K.L. (1996). Antigen processing and presentation by the class I major histocompatibility complex, *Ann. Rev. Immunol.* 14, 369–396.

3.2 IMMUNOLOGY OF BONE ALLOGRAFTS: CURRENT KNOWLEDGE

G.E. FRIEDLAENDER

Department of Orthopaedics and Rehabilitation
Yale University School of Medicine
P.O. Box 208071
New Haven, CT 06520-8071, USA

D.M. STRONG

Puget Sound Blood Center/Northwest Tissue Center
921 Terry Avenue
Seattle, WA 98108, USA

H.J. MANKIN

The Orthopaedic Oncology Unit and Bone Bank
Orthopaedic Service, Massachusetts General Hospital
55 Fruit Street
Boston, MA 02114-2696, USA

1. Introduction

The transplantation of tissues and organs represents one of the most fascinating strategies to repair or replace diseased anatomical structures. Indeed, references to the use of allogeneic and xenogeneic bone have appeared frequently over the past hundred years (Friedlaender et al, 1983; Macewen, 1881) and sporadically for centuries (Bick, 1968). However, these approaches present considerable challenges in terms of understanding and controlling the nature and consequences of immune responses directed against these tissues. This circumstance is particularly important since the clinical behaviour of bone allografts, including some associated complications, most certainly reflects the biology of incorporation, and this, in turn, may be influenced by immunological events (Friedlaender, 1991; Horowitz and Friedlaender, 1991b).

Bone, by its character, differs substantially from solid organ and immediately revascularised tissue with respect to transplantation. Bone regenerates, and does so with autogenous resources including cells, cytokines and blood vessels, regardless of the source of graft material. Bone also shares, with other transplantable organs and tissues, the ability to induce a variety of immunological responses reflecting its allogeneic or xenogeneic nature (Friedlaender, 1987). The understanding and reconciliation of these two sets of circumstances, particularly in humans, remains unresolved and controversial. This manuscript will review our current knowledge pertaining to immune responses induced by bone allografts in animal models and humans, and their apparent consequences on graft biology and clinical function.

2. Bone Biology

The process of bone regeneration is common to skeletal homeostasis, the repair of fractures and the incorporation of bone grafts, and the cascading sequence of biologic events common to this wide spectrum of regenerative activity is often described as the remodelling cycle. Cell populations are activated and become committed to resorption of pre-existing bone matrix (osteoclasts) followed by the accretion of new mineralised tissue (osteoblasts) (Burchardt, 1983; Friedlaender, 1987; Heiple, 1963). These events require a blood supply as well as a system of humoral factors (cytokines) that integrate and regulate these events. This circular sequence, or continuum of cellular and molecular events, is in large measure regulated by soluble factors, cytokines, that facilitate cell-cell interactions and modulate their activities in an autocrine or, more frequently, paracrine fashion (Goldring, 1996; Mundy, 1996).

Cytokine families include interleukins (e.g. IL-1, IL-6), tumour necrosis factors (TNF), growth factors [insulin-like growth factor (IGF)] and particularly members of the transforming growth factor-beta (TGF-β) superfamily, e.g. bone morphogenetic proteins (BMPs) and colony stimulating factors [e.g. monocyte-colony stimulating factor (M-CSF)], and granulocyte macrophage colony stimulating factor (GM-CSF). Many of these factors have multiple and overlapping activities, and have been found to be produced by and influential in more than one biological system. For example, IL-1 was first identified as a product of immunocompetent mononuclear cells that influenced the activity of other immune cells. This cytokine is now known to be produced by connective tissue cells and stimulates bone resorption (Goldring, 1996). Several members of the TGF-β super-family have been shown to cause the recruitment of mesenchymal stem cells and their differentiation into chondrogenic and osteogenic populations (Mundy,1996). Osteogenic protein-1 (OP-1 or BMP-7) and BMP-2 have been particularly well-characterised and produced by recombinant DNA techniques (Cook, 1996; Riley, 1996). Pending experience with ongoing animal investigations and clinical trials, these factors will be available commercially for the promotion of osteo-inductive activity, including bone graft enhancement or substitution.

3. Immune Responses

3.1. In general

Potential sources of immunogenicity related to bone grafts include collagen, a weak antigen in most systems, and non-collagenous matrix molecules. For example, xenogeneic proteoglycans injected into the knee joint of rabbits will induce a systemic response (Friedlaender *et al*, 1983). It is generally agreed, however, that the major source of alloantigens presented by bone grafts are cell-surface glycoproteins of the major histocompatibility complex (MHC), or HLA in humans. These antigens can be further categorised as Class I, found on virtually all nucleated cells including osteoblasts and platelets, and Class II, more restricted in their distribution and found on macrophages, B cells and other antigen presenting cells. In solid organ transplantation, antibodies to Class I antigens are clearly detrimental to graft success, while the presence of anti-Class II activity is less well correlated with graft outcome (Horowitz and Friedlaender, 1987, 1991b).

3.2. Animal-derived data

Numerous animal investigations over the years, using a variety of assay techniques, have demonstrated the ability of fresh allogeneic bone to induce humoral and cell-mediated responses in rats, cats, dogs, sheep and other investigational models (Burwell, 1976; Friedlaender, 1983; Friedlaender and Horowitz, 1992; Friedlaender *et al*, 1996; Stevenson and Horowitz, 1992; Stevenson *et al*, 1991). These responses include histologic evidence of inflammation, accelerated skin graft rejection patterns, blast transformation in regional lymph nodes, and the appearance of cytotoxic humoral antibodies and/or activated lymphocytes. More recently, in a well-characterised rat model, fresh allogeneic bone, with marrow depleted by washing, was associated with the activation of T cells of the killer/suppressor phenotype (Horowitz and Friedlaender, 1991a; Horowitz *et al*, 1994).

It has been further demonstrated in animals that immune responses to bone allografts can be reduced by freezing these transplants and further diminished, often to undetectable levels, by freeze drying tissues prior to transplantation (Friedlaender *et al*, 1976). Stevenson and colleagues, working with both rat and dog models, demonstrated a reduction in the magnitude of anti-Class I responses with matching at the MHC loci, and suggestions of improved incorporation with either histocompatibility matching or the use of immunosuppressive agents (Cyclosporin) was observed (Stevenson *et al*, 1989, 1991, 1997). Survival of vascular allografts in a canine model could only be accomplished with the use of immunosuppression, analogous to circumstances with solid organ transplantation. Ultimately, the ability of a bone graft to incorporate depends on revascularisation. Circumstances that interfere with graft vascularity include preservation techniques (freezing or freeze drying), histocompatibility mismatches, irradiation of the recipient bed and systemic chemotherapy.

3.3. Human-derived information

Information related to immune responses in humans is relatively limited compared with animal-related investigations, but results in humans generally parallel animal-derived data. Fresh allografts elicit humoral responses (Langer *et al*, 1978). These responses exist but are diminished in intensity and frequency with deep-freezing of the grafts, and are reduced further by freeze drying (Rodrigo *et al*, 1976; Friedlaender *et al*, 1984). Clinical experience with large osteochondral allografts, while satisfactory, is still fraught with a substantial complication rate, primarily during the first two to three years (Mankin *et al*, 1996). Infection, failure of incorporation at the graft-host junction and fracture through the substance of the allograft each occur in approximately 10–15% of patients. It is tempting to ascribe at least some of these biologically-compromised behaviours to immunological events (Friedlaender, 1991). While some support for this relationship between immune responses and graft success has been derived from animal investigations, this scenario remains speculative. In humans, evidence is even more tenuous, but at least two clinical series have provided some support.

Muscolo and co-workers have reported their experiences with 46 patients receiving frozen bone allografts (Muscolo *et al*, 1996). A trend (not statistically significant) towards improved radiographic scores was observed if one or two Class I antigens were matched in contrast to no matches. In a smaller group with retrieved specimens available, five of 16 patients with histologic evidence of inflammation also had reduced scores for clinical success. The correlation, however, was tenuous, perhaps reflecting the diversity of immune responses capable of being generated over a spectrum from acute "rejection" to the induction of tolerance. In this study, matching for Class II HLA specificities did not appear to influence radiologic scores.

Strong and colleagues have demonstrated patterns of sensitisation in a group of 84 recipients of massive frozen osteochondral allografts (Strong *et al*, 1996). More than one-third (39%) were pre-sensitised to either Class I or II antigens, perhaps related to a high rate of prior blood transfusions and pregnancies (28 of 44 females in this series). Following transplantation, 67% demonstrated antibodies to Class I and/or Class II specificities, 49 of 88 (58%) to Class I, and 46 of 84 (55%) to Class II antigens. While follow-up has been lengthy (more than five years), the subjectivity of plain X-ray has limited the ability to define with sufficient accuracy the biological status of these grafts. In a related study of 74 patients, time to union, frequency of union and functional status, in general, were best in non-sensitised individuals (91% judged good or excellent compared with 65% good or excellent in the sensitised group, $p = 0.024$, see Table 1) (Friedlaender *et al*, 1998). Of the 42 female patients in this series, there was a significant improvement in clinical function in the 28 women who experienced pregnancy at some point prior to receiving their allograft compared with the 14 who had never been pregnant (Table 2). Regardless of sensitisation, the majority of patients in this series had satisfactory clinical results (54 of 74 patients, 73%), emphasising our incomplete

Table 1. Relationship of clinical outcome to sensitisation.

Patient Group (n)	Excellent-Good Outcome (n)	Fair-Poor Outcome (n)
Non-sensitised (22)*	91% (20)	9% (2)
Sensitised (52)*	65% (34)	35% (18)
Total	73% (54)	27% (20)

n = number of patients
* = p = 0.024

Table 2. Relationship of pregnancy to clinical outcome.

Prior Pregnancy (n)	Excellent-Good Outcome (n)	Fair-Poor Outcome (n)
Yes (28)*	89% (25)	11% (3)
No (14)*	36% (5)	64% (9)

n = number of patients
* = p = 0.001

understanding of both the nature of immune responses following bone allograft implantation and the relationship of these responses to the biological fate of these grafts.

4. Conclusions

Burchardt and co-investigators demonstrated, in a canine fibula model, three distinct patterns of graft incorporation based upon radiographic and histologic evaluation (Burchardt *et al*, 1978). Type 1 repair reflected the normal successful sequence of events; Type 3 repair was characterised by overt failure of union at the graft-host junction and often unopposed resorption of the graft; Type 2 repair was intermediate, with delayed union and fracture of the graft common. These investigators speculated that Type 1 repair was characteristic of autografts (histocompatible), while the Type 2 pattern reflected minor MHC mismatches, and Type 3 repair was the consequence of major histoincompatibility. In their model, fresh autografts proceeded to a Type 1 repair 80% of the time and the remaining 20% of animals healed by a Type 2 pattern. Allografts demonstrated Type 2 repairs in 60% of dogs, with 20% each associated with Type 1 and Type 3 patterns. Thus, these studies reflected the notion that a relationship existed between graft biology and histocompatibility; but the correlation, using rather crude measures of both biology and immunologic responses, was not clearly established.

More recently, Horowitz and co-workers have emphasised important relationships, in general, between the immune response and the bone (skeletal) remodelling system (Horowitz and Friedlaender, 1991). In addition to sharing cells with common bone marrow ancestry, cytokines generated by immunocompetent cells (TGF-β, IL-2, IL-6, etc) play significant roles in the regulation of bone remodelling, particularly during homeostasis but, presumably, fracture repair and graft incorporation as well. If this hypothesis is confirmed using more sophisticated and quantitative measures of graft biology and immunologic events, then regulation of immune responses, either through the manipulation of graft-related antigens or modification of effector responses (including immunosuppressive agents) may improve the reliability of bone graft incorporation and decrease some of the most perplexing complications associated with their use.

5. References

BICK, E.M. (1968). *Source Book of Orthopaedics.* Hafner, New York, p 243.

BURCHARDT, H. (1983). The biology of bone graft repair, *Clin. Orthop.* **174**, 28–42.

BURCHARDT, H., JONES, H., GLOWCZEWSKIE, F., RUDNER, C. and ENNEKING, W.F. (1978). Freeze-dried allogeneic segmental cortical-bone grafts in dogs, *J. Bone Joint Surg.* **60A**, 1082–1090.

BURWELL, R.G. (1976). The fate of bone grafts. In: *Recent Advances in Orthopaedics.* A.G. Apley. ed., William and Wilkins, Baltimore, pp 115–207.

COOK, S.D. and RUEGER, D.C. (1996). Osteogenic protein-1: Biology and applications, *Clin. Orthop.* **324**, 29–38.

FRIEDLAENDER, G.E. (1983). Immune responses to osteochondral allografts. Current knowledge and future directions, *Clin. Orthop.* **174**, 58–68.

FRIEDLAENDER, G.E. (1987). Bone Grafts. The basic science rationale for clinical applications, *J. Bone Joint Surg.* **69A**, 786–790.

FRIEDLAENDER, G.E. (1991). Bone allografts: The biological consequences of immunological events, *J. Bone Joint Surg.* **73A**, 1119–1122.

FRIEDLAENDER, G.E. and HOROWITZ, M.C. (1992). Immune responses to osteochondral allografts: Nature and significance, *Orthopedics* **15**, 1171–1175.

FRIEDLAENDER, G.E., LADENBAUER-BELLIS, I.M. and CHRISMAN, O.D. (1983). Immunogenicity of xenogeneic cartilage matrix components in a rat model, *Yale J. Biol. Med.* **56**, 211–217.

FRIEDLAENDER, G.E., MANKIN, H.J. and SELL, K.W. (1983). *Osteochondral Allograft: Biology, Banking and Clinical Applications.* Little, Brown & Co., Boston.

FRIEDLAENDER, G.E., STRONG, D.M. and MANKIN, H.J. (Unpublished data).

FRIEDLAENDER, G.E., STRONG, D.M. and SELL, K.W. (1976). Studies on the antigenicity of bone. I. Freeze-dried and deep-frozen bone allografts in rabbits, *J. Bone Joint Surg.* **58A**, 854–858.

FRIEDLAENDER, G.E., STRONG, D.M. and SELL, K.W. (1984). Studies on the antigenicity of bone. II. Donor-specific anti-HLA antibodies in human recipients of freeze-dried bone allografts, *J. Bone Joint Surg.* **66A**, 107–112.

GOLDRING, S.R. and GOLDRING, M.B. (1996). Cytokines and skeletal physiology, *Clin. Orthop.* **324**, 13–23.

HEIPLE, K.G., CHASE, S.W. and HERNDON, C.H. (1963). A comparative study of the healing process following different types of bone transplantation, *J. Bone Joint Surg.* **45A**, 1593–1612.

HOROWITZ, M.C. and FRIEDLAENDER, G.E. (1987). Immunologic aspects of bone transplantation. A rationale for future studies, *Orthop. Clin. North Am.* **18**, 227–233.

HOROWITZ, M.C. and FRIEDLAENDER, G.E. (1991a). Induction of specific T-cell responsiveness to allogeneic bone, *J. Bone Joint Surg.* **73A**, 1157–1168.

HOROWITZ, M.C. and FRIEDLAENDER, G.E. (1991b). The immune response to bone grafts. In: *Bone and Cartilage Allografts.* G. E. Friedlaender and V.M. Goldberg, eds., American Academy of Orthopaedic Surgeons, Park Ridge, IL, pp 85–101.

HOROWITZ, M.C., FRIEDLAENDER, G.E. and QIAN, H-Y. (1994). T-cell activation and the immune response to bone allograft, *Transact. Orthop. Res. Soc.* **19**, 180.

LANGER, F., GROSS, A.E., WEST, M. and UROVITZ, E.P. (1978). The immunogenicity of allograft knee joint transplants, *Clin. Orthop.* **132**, 155–162.

MACEWEN, W. (1881). Observations concerning transplantation of bone. Illustrated by a case of inter-human osseous transplantation, whereby over two-thirds of the shaft of a humerus was restored, *Proc. R. Soc. Lond.* **32**, 232–234.

MANKIN, H.J., GEBHARDT, M.C., JENNINGS, L.C., SPRINGFIELD, D.S. and TOMFORD, W.W. (1996). Long-term results of allograft replacement in the management of bone tumors, *Clin. Orthop.* **324**, 86–97.

MUNDY, G.R. (1996). Regulation of bone formation by bone morphogenetic proteins and other growth factors, *Clin. Orthop.* **324**, 24–28.

MUSCOLO, D.L., AYERZA, M.A., CALABRESE, M.E., REDAL, M.A. and ARAUJO, E.S. (1996). Human leukocyte antigen matching, radiographic score, and histologic findings in massive frozen bone allografts, *Clin. Orthop.* **326**, 115–126.

RILEY, E.H., LANE, J.M., URIST, M.R., LYONS, K.M. and LIEBERMAN, J.R. (1996). Bone morphogenetic protein-2: Biology and applications, *Clin. Orthop.* **324**, 39–46.

RODRIGO, J.J., FULLER, T.C. and MANKIN, H.J. (1976). Cytotoxic HLA antibodies in patients with bone and cartilage allografts, *Trans. Orthop. Res. Soc.* **1**, 131.

STEVENSON, S., GOLDBERG, V.M., SHAFFER, J., FIELD, G., DAVY, D. and KLEIN, L. (1989). Interactions among immuno-suppression, immune response and histomorphometry in canine fibular vascularised and nonvascularised segmental allografts. *Transact. Orthop. Res. Soc.* **14**, 272.

STEVENSON, S. and HOROWITZ, M.C. (1992). Current concepts review: The response to bone allografts, *J. Bone Joint Surg.* **74A**, 939–950.

STEVENSON, S., Li, X.Q., DAVY, D.T., KLEIN, L. and GOLDBERG, V.M. (1997). Critical biological determinants of incorporation of non-vascularised cortical bone grafts. Quantification of a complex process and structure, *J. Bone Joint Surg.* **79A**, 1–16.

STEVENSON, S., Li, X.Q. and MARTIN, B. (1991). The fate of cancellous and cortical bone after transplantation of fresh and frozen tissue-antigenmatched and mismatched osteochondral allografts in dogs, *J. Bone Joint Surg.* **73A**, 1143–1156.

STEVENSON, S., SHAFFER, J.W., DAVY, D., LI, X.Q., KLEIN, L., FIELD, G. and GOLDBERG, V.M. (1991). Tissue antigen matching enhances the patency and internal remodeling in vascularised fibular allografts, *Transact. Orthop. Res. Soc.* **16**, 458.

STRONG, D.M., FRIEDLAENDER, G.E., TOMFORD, W.W., SPRINGFIELD, D.S., BURCHARDT, H.C., ENNEKING, W.F. and MANKIN, H.J. (1996). Immunological responses in human recipients of osseous and osteochondral allografts, *Clin. Orthop.* **326**, 107–114.

Chapter 4

CRYOPRESERVATION OF
ORGANS AND TISSUE

4.1 Surgical Reconstruction by Allograft: Cryopreservation of
Tissues and Organs
H.T. Meryman (*Naval Medical Research Institute, Bethesda, USA*)

4.2 A Twenty-Year Experience with Hypothermic Pulsatile
Perfusion as the Primary Mode of Renal Preservation
R.S. Filo (*Organ Transplant Center, University Hospital,
Indianapolis, USA*)

4.3 Preservation of Chondrocyte Viability During Long-Term
Refrigerated Storage of Osteochondral Allografts
L. Csönge (*West Hungarian Regional Tissue Bank, Hungary*) and
H. Newman-Gage *et al* (*Northwest Tissue Center/Puget Sound
Blood Center, Seattle, USA*)

4.4 The Effects of Cryopreservation and Irradiation on Human
Patellar Tendon Allografts
S. Rezaiamiri *et al* (*Harborview Medical Center and University of
Washington, Seattle, USA*) and
D.M. Strong (*Puget Sound Blood Center/Northwest Tissue Center,
USA*)

Dr. Sell's growing interest in clinical transplantation during the
1960s led to additional applications in organ and tissue preservation
technology based at the Navy Tissue Bank. Various protocols were

developed for the cryopreservation and storage of tissues such as bone marrow, tendons, kidneys, hearts, and heart valves. For example, scientists at the Navy became leaders in the field of organ perfusion preservation. Dr. Ronald Filo, who has contributed to this chapter, was one of the leaders of the group developing perfusion preservation of kidneys. At that time tissue bank technicians were trained not only in tissue recovery and processing, but also in organ retrieval and perfusion preservation. The increased interest led this group along with other Navy scientists to participate in the establishment of yet another society called the Society for Cryobiology.

Dr. Sell had recognised very early in his training in England the connection between interests in transplantation and the banking of organs and tissues. During this period, Dr. Sell worked with Dr. R. Stevenson, Dr. V. Perry, Dr. T.I. Malinin, and Dr. H. Meryman in investigating various cryopreservation protocols. Drs. Stevenson, Malinin and Meryman all participated in the 1997 Symposium honouring Dr. Sell. Dr. Meryman provides his insights into the present and future application of cryopreservation of tissues and organs. These concepts have been extended and are reported here by Dr. Csönge in the preservation of chondrocyte viability as well as Dr. Rezaiamiri in the effects of cryopreservation on human patellar tendon allografts.

D.M.S.

4.1 SURGICAL RECONSTRUCTION BY ALLOGRAFT: CRYOPRESERVATION OF TISSUES AND ORGANS

H.T. MERYMAN

Transfusion and Cryopreservation Research Program
Naval Medical Research Institute
NMRI Bldg. 29, 8901 Wisconsin Avenue
Bethesda, MD 20889-5607
USA

1. Introduction

None of us, I dare say, will live to see our dreams fulfilled. Ken Sell was no exception. Not because he was taken from us prematurely — which he was. Not because his dreams were unrealistic — which they never were. And not because he failed to exert all of his energy and talent to their fulfillment — which would have been totally out of character. It was because they were big dreams — dreams that even a big man could not bring to pass single-handedly. One of those big dreams concerned tissue banking. It was a dream we both shared and I would now like to offer a progress report.

In these still early days of tissue banking, except for skin, heart valves and corneas, which are special cases, we deal only in dead tissues — bone, fascia, tendon and dura — tissues that can easily be frozen or lyophilised because they are already dead and that can be transplanted because they are less immunogenic. Viable skin grafts can be stored frozen but can only provide transient covering for burns because they are subsequently rejected. Penetrating corneal allografts are in a special category because the eye is an immunologically privileged site. Heart valves which reside in a high blood flow environment are perhaps less prone to immunologic assault. But other than these three exceptions, we do not bank living tissues. In fact, except for the major organs, we do not transplant any living tissues since immuno-suppression, the only current way to prevent rejection, is too dangerous to use unless the alternative is death. But even if rejection were not an obstacle, we do not, at present, have any way to preserve — and therefore to bank — living tissues.

Allograft rejection is under attack in many laboratories around the world and there are many promising approaches under study. Antibodies against the accessory signals that are essential for the activation of CD4 cells by antigen presenting cells (APCs) have enabled the retention of baboon kidney allografts without immuno-suppression. The establishment of a chimeric state between recipient and donor has been shown to provide lifelong allograft acceptance. We can look forward with some confidence to safe, practical methods for preventing rejection that will make it no longer necessary to limit transplants to those that are life-saving.

If living tissue allografts can be safely transplanted without rejection, will they also need to be banked? Many tissues will need to be matched for size and, where skin is present, for color as well. Testing for viral and bacterial contamination is mandatory. The few days of storage available through refrigeration or perfusion will be inadequate. Freeze drying is incompatible with the survival of nucleated cells and cryopreservation appears to be essential.

2. Freezing Injures Cells and Tissues in Four Ways

2.1. Extracellular ice

The growth of extracellular ice concentrates the extracellular solution, leading to osmotic dehydration of the cells. Since living cells do not appear to contain nuclei for ice formation, extracellular freezing and the resulting cell dehydration is the most common cause of freezing injury. Cryoprotectants such as glycerol and dimethylsulfoxide (Me_2SO) can prevent dehydration injury by reducing the amount of ice formed on a purely colligative basis (Meryman, 1974). Any solute with sufficient solubility in water can be a colligative anti-freeze but, in order to be useful for tissues, they must be non-toxic at high concentration and, in order not to dehydrate the cells on an osmotic basis, they must freely penetrate the plasma membrane — two requirements that severely limit the choices.

2.2. Intracellular ice

It is possible to freeze so rapidly that there is insufficient time for water to leave the cells and dehydration injury can be prevented. Polymers such as polyvinylpyrrolidone, hydroxyethyl starch and dextran exert their cryoprotective effects by reducing the rate of water loss from the cells (Takahashi *et al*, 1988). Aqueous solutions of these compounds are highly viscous. As extracellular ice concentrates the polymer solution and the temperature falls, the solution rapidly becomes so viscous that water can no longer diffuse to the ice crystals and extracellular freezing ceases. However, although cells contain no intracellular ice nuclei, at about $-40°C$ or below, depending on concentration, aqueous solutions become self-nucleating and although ice may not grow at this temperature, it will form rapidly during rewarming. Intracellular crystals of ice in excess of about 200 nm in diameter are mechanically destructive to intracellular structures. The addition of penetrating cryoprotectants such as Me_2SO can alleviate this problem somewhat by lowering the nucleation temperature and the melting point of the intracellular solution and increasing its viscosity. Intracellular ice can still form during thawing and rapid rewarming is mandatory for such preparations. In theory, one might store the tissue at a temperature above the freezing point of the cell interior. Unfortunately, for this strategy, there are other nucleating forces such as vibration, radiation and random fluctuations of molecules that can initiate intracellular freezing and cause progressive destruction of cells during storage.

2.3. Mechanical injury

The third cause of freezing injury to tissues is mechanical. In a suspension of glycerolised red cells in which dehydration injury is prevented by reducing the amount of ice formed, the presence of extracellular ice is inconsequential. In a tissue, however, extracellular ice ruptures intercellular structures and can rupture capillaries and small vessels. The presence of extracellular, interstitial ice is incompatible with tissue survival.

2.4. Cold denaturation of proteins

The fourth source of freezing injury, cold denaturation of proteins, has only recently been identified (Tsonev et al, submitted 1997). The recent development of techniques for quantitating protein unfolding at physiological concentrations and pH have revealed a rapid and continuous unfolding at temperatures near 0°C. Of particular importance is the observation that these structural changes do not reverse on return to higher temperature, indicating that the native conformation is not, as generally believed, the global free energy minimum. From the standpoint of cryopreservation, this suggests that refrigerated storage and storage at modest sub-freezing temperatures may be limited in duration by protein denaturation even if the adverse effects of ice and dehydration are avoided. Temperatures in the range −60°C to −80°C are low enough to avoid cold denaturation, placing an upper limit on the temperatures necessary for prolonged storage of viable tissues.

3. Discussion

If storage must be at temperatures below −60°C, it is clear that both extracellular and intracellular freezing will be major obstacles to the development of a successful cryopreservation regimen. The only really satisfactory solution will be to avoid the formation of ice altogether.

Figure 1 provides a clue as to how this might be accomplished. The curve T_M shows the relationship between melting temperature and the concentration of an aqueous solution. Although this is also the nominal freezing point curve, in fact, freezing almost always occurs at a lower temperature. The initiation of freezing requires the presence of an ice nucleus. Ice nuclei can be on the surface of the container, on a dust particle, or even an array of hydrophilic sites on a molecule that approximate the positions of oxygen atoms in an ice lattice. Different nuclei will nucleate at different temperatures depending on their size, and a solution will supercool until a nucleus initiates freezing. Samples of water carefully treated to remove all particulate sources of nucleation can be supercooled to nearly −20°C.

As temperature falls, the critical size for an ice nucleus becomes smaller and at about −40°C random aggregations of water molecules can nucleate ice. The curve T_H shows the relationship between solute concentration and this homogeneous nucleation temperature where spontaneous self-nucleation occurs. This temperature also falls as solute

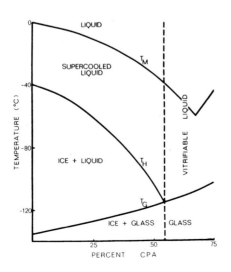

Fig. 1. Phase diagram for a model aqueous solution at temperatures below 0°C.

concentration increases. The bottom curve illustrates the relationship between solute concentration and the glass transition temperature T_G, where the solution has become so viscous that the translational movement of water molecules no longer takes place at a discernible rate. Below T_G whatever solution that has not already been frozen becomes a glass and no further physical events will take place. To cryopreserve tissues without ice formation, the goal, then, is to reduce specimen temperature to T_G, i.e. to vitrify it, without the initiation of freezing. Figure 1 shows the way to do this.

If one follows the T_H curve down to the right, it eventually intersects the T_G curve. In other words, if the aqueous solution has a concentration equal to or higher than that at the intersection of T_H and T_G, spontaneous freezing will not take place before the temperature falls below T_G and a safe storage condition has been achieved.

There are two obstacles to this strategy. First, heterogeneous nucleation, which can occur at temperatures anywhere between the melting point and T_H, can initiate freezing before T_G has been reached. Fortunately, at the very high solute concentrations required to reach T_G without freezing, heterogeneous nucleation appears to be largely suppressed. The second obstacle is the high solute concentration, of the order of 55%, that is required for vitrification.

Our studies of this system have focussed on two aspects of the perfusion of high concentrations of cryoprotectant solutions: the osmotic effects and the toxic effects. The osmolality of a 55% solution will be very high. Only if the majority of the solutes penetrate the cells can lethal cell dehydration be avoided. However, since most penetrating solutes cross the cell membrane more slowly than water, there can be a transient osmotic imbalance that will dehydrate the cells. During removal of the perfusate, the opposite is true and the cells will swell. The rate of introduction and removal and the concentration of the cryoprotectant must therefore be carefully controlled to prevent excessive shrinking or swelling. To some extent the process can be accelerated by making the base (non-penetrating) solution hypo- or hypertonic to counteract these transient osmotic imbalances during loading and unloading. The loading and unloading protocols are further complicated by the fact that the viscosity of the perfusate increases with both increase in concentration and temperature reduction, and permeation slows.

Toxicity is an ill-defined term based more on evidence of damage than on any specific mechanism. At high cryoprotectant concentrations, injury increases with the duration of exposure and decreases at lower temperature. The fact that toxicity is best minimised by rapid loading and unloading and by carrying this out at low temperature conflicts with the fact that osmotic stresses are exacerbated by these same measures, thereby making optimum loading and unloading protocols difficult to design. It is a tribute to Dr. Greg Fahy, who has directed our organ and tissue cryopreservation programme for many years that it is now possible to load a rabbit kidney with a 55% cryoprotective solution, remove it and have the majority of kidneys support life after reimplantation and contra-lateral nephrectomy (Fahy *et al*, 1984). Such kidneys can be vitrified and techniques for rapid rewarming by radio-frequency heating are under development.

The rabbit kidney has been used as a particularly demanding model with a definitive assay. Clearly what can be accomplished with a kidney can be applied to tissues and, in many cases, more easily because tissues have smaller size, more tolerance for osmotic stresses and more ability to heal.

This vitrification programme has been underway for over 20 years and there are still obstacles to overcome, primarily those related to rewarming. However, we are more confident of eventual success than ever before and can even begin to hope that, when allograft rejection has at last been satisfactorily conquered, the technology for cryopreservation will be there too, making it possible at last to bank living human tissues for the reconstruction of body parts lost through trauma or surgery. It is a dream worthy of Ken Sell.

4. Acknowledgement

This work was supported by NMRDC Work Unit No. 1462. The opinions and assertions contained herein are the private ones of the author and should not be construed as official or as representing those of the Department of Defense or the US Navy.

5. References

FAHY, G.M., MACFARLANE, D.R., ANGELL, C.A. and MERYMAN, H.T. (1984). Vitrification as an approach to cryopreservation, *Cryobiology* **21**, 407–426.

MERYMAN, H.T. (1974). Freezing injury and its prevention in living cells. In: *Ann. Rev. Biophysics and Bioengineering.* Vol. 3, pp 341–363.

TAKAHASHI, T.S., HIRSH, A., ERBE, E. and WILLIAMS, R.J. (1988). Mechanisms of cryoprotection by extracellular polymeric solutes, *Biophysical J.* **54**, 509–518.

TSONEV, L.I., HIRSH, A.G., MEHL, P.M. and LITVINOVITCH, S. (1997). Evidence that cold denaturation of proteins near 0°C is a general phenomenon, *Biophysical J.* (submitted).

4.2 A TWENTY-YEAR EXPERIENCE WITH HYPOTHERMIC PULSATILE PERFUSION AS THE PRIMARY MODE OF RENAL PRESERVATION

R.S. FILO

Division of Organ Transplantation
Indiana University Medical Center
Indianapolis, IN, USA

1. Introduction

Currently, although simple flush and cold storage is used by over 95% of the transplant centres throughout the world, the debate as to the relative merits of the two forms of *ex vivo* renal preservation, i.e. hypothermic machine perfusion (MP) versus simple cold storage (CS), has persisted for most of the past 20 years (Belzer and Southard, 1980; McClelland and Cecka, 1987). The complexity of MP preservation demands proper formal training or extensive laboratory experience if one is to become proficient with the technique. While pulsatile perfusion has initially accepted as the best method for short-term renal preservation, during the late 1970s, many transplant centres with a paucity of experience and limited access to adequate training in hypothermic MP were achieving less than optimal results. An increasing number of reports implicating this mode of preservation as a possible cause of renal injury as well as the intrinsic simplicity of the CS technique led most transplant centres to switch to the CS method of renal preservation. Initially Collin's, modified Collin's, or Sach's solution were employed as the flush and storage media. Later, Belzer and Southard (1980) introduced UW solution and it has become the most commonly used cold storage solution for all organs in this country. By the mid 1980s only about 10% of the cadaveric kidneys that were transplanted in the USA were preserved by MP preservation performed at just a handful of the 250 centres performing renal transplantation (Koyama *et al*, 1993).

Numerous studies have documented a clear superiority of MP over simple CS with regard to the incidence of delayed graft function (DGF), particularly with preservation times of more than 24 hrs (Henry *et al*, 1988; Koyama *et al*, 1993; Kumar *et al*, 1991). The concept of a detrimental effect of DGF, i.e. defined as the need for dialysis in the first week after transplantation, on cadaveric renal allograft survival was initially suggested in the early 1980s (Sanfilippo *et al*, 1984). It has since become a well established dogma. However, despite a persistent 10–20% higher incidence of DGF seen with the use of simple CS, it continues to be employed as the most common form of renal preservation by a large margin. These facts can only be reconciled by the ongoing perception prevalent in the transplant community that any advantage confirmed by MP with regard to better early renal function has not always translated into measurably improved long-term allograft survival rates (Koyama *et al*, 1993). In other words, although there is convincing evidence supporting the contention that MP kidneys have a lower incidence of DGF than simple CS and that recipients with DGF have poorer allograft survival rates, there appears to be insufficient data showing that pumped kidneys have sufficiently superior allograft survival rates to convince practitioners to alter their behaviour.

Today, there are only a few transplant centres, such as our own at Indiana University, that have remained steadfast disciples of the Belzer MP technique for renal preservation. Over the past 20 years, those programmes using MP almost exclusively for renal preservation have repeatedly reported their incidence of DGF to be 5–15% of their cadaveric recipients, while analysis of United Network for Organ

Sharing (UNOS) and other data has shown the incidence of DGF for simple CS at most centres to ranged between 20–40% depending on the duration of preservation (Koyama *et al*, 1993). The most recent national data from UNOS shows a mean incidence for DGF of 20.7% for all centres (UNOS, 1997).

As noted above, although most transplant centres have yet to be convinced of achieving superior results with pumped kidneys, the additional costs incurred by the requirement for dialysis in their recipients of cadaveric kidneys with DGF has led some centres to reconsider the MP method of renal preservation. Furthermore, the increasingly severe shortage of cadaveric organs has led to the expansion of the organ donor pool by consideration of older and physiologically less-than-ideal kidneys, as well as kidneys from non-heart-beating cadaver donors. The necessity of considering increased utilisation of kidneys from this "expanded" donor population has rekindled a new interest and reappraisal of the role of hypothermic machine perfusion for renal preservation (Burdick *et al*, 1997). It is to serve this purpose that I relate our extensive experience with *ex vivo* renal preservation by hypothermic machine perfusion over the past 20 years.

2. Background

The early 1970s saw the evolution of renal transplantation into a legitimate treatment of end-stage renal disease. During those very early days of transplantation, Captain Ken Sell (MC) USN, a pioneer in tissue banking and one of the founding fathers of the American Association of Tissue Banks, foresaw a need for *ex vivo* long-term viable storage of solid organs for transplantation. To that end he encouraged a group of us at the Naval Medical Research Institute (NMRI) to systematically begin looking at problems and possible solutions to the freezing of complex solid organs such as the kidney.

In 1970, the first report appeared pointing out the merits of cadaveric kidney preservation by continuous hypothermic pulsatile perfusion with cryoprecipitate plasma (CPP) for their storage prior to transplantation (Belzer and Kountz, 1970). While several studies had demonstrated that dog kidneys could be viably maintained for up to 72 hours with MP, clinically machine perfusion enabled predictable preservation of life sustaining kidney function for a maximum of about 48 hours. Thus, it was obvious that if organ preservation was desirable for more than a few days it would require the development of a new technique likely involving the viable freezing and thawing of the entire kidney. During the early animal experimental studies on the feasibility of solid organ freezing, our group was able to demonstrate, in literally scores of kidneys, the clear superiority of the "Belzer-type" hypothermic machine perfusion over simple flush and ice storage in the preparation of kidneys for viable freezing. Machine perfusion provided better homogeneity of tissue perfusion (Small *et al*, 1973), more uniform introduction, dispersion, and removal of cryoprotectants like dimethylsulfoxide or glycerol necessary to maintain cell viability during

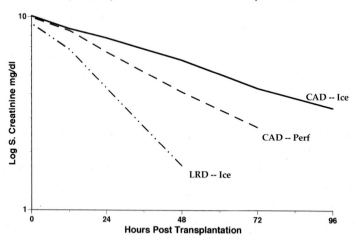

Fig. 1. A comparison of the log rate decrease in serum creatinine as a measure of early recovery of post-renal transplant function. LRD — Ice ≈ 1 hr of CS; CAD — Ice = 20.6 hrs of CS; CAD — Perf. = 24.8 hrs of MP. n = 20 consecutive kidneys for each group. LRD = Living Related Donor; CS = Simple Cold Storage; CAD = Cadaveric Donor; MP = Hypothermic Machine Perfusion.

freezing (Filo *et al*, 1976), and a more rapid recovery of renal function after reimplantation (Small *et al*, 1977). It is likely that it is these very properties of perfusion preservation which are important in preserving organ integrity and renal function better than could be achieved with CS for periods from 24 to 48 hours. Figure 1 shows the differences in the rate of recovery of early renal function after transplantation of cadaveric kidneys undergoing either 20 hours of CS or 24 hours of MP, compared with HLA identical living related donor (LRD) kidneys having less than one hour of cold ischaemia.

Initially at NMRI and later at Indiana, we generated an abundance of data supporting Belzer's original work on the merits and superiority of hypothermic perfusion over simple cold storage. We also discovered and reported certain mechanisms of renal "perfusion injury". In these studies we demonstrated that the CPP perfusate itself could cause both immunologic and mechanical injury to the perfused kidney either by specific antibody-mediated reactions (Filo *et al*, 1974) or the ongoing precipitation of cold unstable cryoprecipitates, i.e. fibrinogen, cryoglobulins and immune complexes, in the kidney vasculature (Filo *et al*, 1978). As we would later learn, even albumin, which has been denatured through improper preparation or handling, can precipitate in the renal vasculature during cold perfusion (Southard *et al*, 1981). Other reports began appearing in the literature on the significant role of perfusion injury in the clinical setting (Light *et al*, 1975; Hill *et al*, 1976; Spector *et al*, 1976). While our own studies clearly indicated the CPP perfusate as a major source of renal perfusion injury, we learned of other possible mechanisms of "perfusion injury" which could be prevented through the use of on-line filters and proper perfusion technique. Furthermore, we were able to confirm the value of mannitol and renal capsulotomy to reduce the reperfusion injury and parenchymal edema promulgated by David Hume in the early days of renal transplantation. Figure 2 shows the results of a previously unpublished study carried out in our lab in the early 1980s in the canine model. It demonstrates the positive effect of renal capsulotomy on the recovery of early renal function after 24 hours of MP and reimplantation. One can equate renal capsulotomy with fasciotomy which is done to

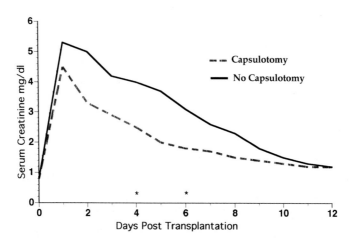

Fig. 2. The effect of renal capsulotomy on recovery of kidney function after 24 hrs of machine perfusion preservation and autotransplantation. n = 6 for both groups. (*) Denotes $p < 0.05$ between treatment groups at timepoint.

improve circulation to skeletal muscle after ischaemic injury. In both cases the release of the strong connective tissue binding of the tissue/organ permits it to swell due to reperfusion injury and still maintain adequate haemo-perfusion.

Our own experience both clinically and in the laboratory have convinced us of the intrinsic superiority of properly performed hypothermic MP preservation over simple CS for renal preservation. This has led us to develop and clinically test a synthetic 5% albumin plasma-like (SAP) solution as the our new perfusate for renal perfusion preservation. In 1977, we reported our findings from a controlled clinical trial of machine perfusion with either 5% SAP or CPP perfusate. This trial showed comparable or better results in the SAP group with regard to recovery of early renal function and allograft survival rates (Filo *et al*, 1977). Furthermore, SAP was devoid of the major problems associated with the use of CPP perfusate in that it was easier to prepare, more stable at cold temperatures, and was free of risk from causing viral or other transmittable infections.

Based on these studies, we converted from CPP to the albumin-based perfusate for all clinical renal perfusion preservation at Indiana University Medical Center. Our renal preservation technique consisted of an initial short cold storage period of up to six hours in Sachs, Euro-Collins, or UW solution while transporting the organs from the donor hospital to the perfusion lab, followed by the basic "Belzer-technique" of hypothermic pulsatile perfusion on a Waters machine using 5% albumin plasma-like perfusate until transplantation. This technique of renal preservation has been used consistently at our centre for the past 20 years. Although we have been very satisfied with the clinical results of MP using our 5% albumin perfusate, we have shown that this mode of preservation has its limitations in preventing the glomerular endothelial injury as well as a specific time course associated with perfusion preservation (Evan *et al*, 1983; Gattone *et al*, 1985).

3. Analysis

What follows is a retrospective analysis of our 20-year experience using MP renal preservation. Over the years, it has been readily apparent to those of us at our transplant centre that the level of early renal function we had come to expect as the norm from our MP cadaveric kidneys was not the experience of our colleagues at many other centres. The presentation of this data is not intended as proof that MP is superior to cold storage for clinical renal preservation since that is beyond the capability of this type of analysis. However, there is value in reviewing a carefully chronicled and hopefully unbiased experience over a 20-year span. Nonetheless, it is entirely appropriate to raise a word of caution regarding the limitations and possible, though unintended, bias inherent in the retrospective treatment of such data.

We have preserved over 2000 cadaveric kidneys by the technique described above. While the method of renal preservation at our centre has gone essentially unchanged, other parameters which can affect early renal function have changed significantly over the years. On-site donor management has been relatively standardised and is performed primarily by Organ Procurement Organization coordinators. The mean donor age has increased from 24.8 ± 11 years in 1985 to nearly 35 years by 1995. Today, nearly 20% of the organ donors are over 55 years of age as opposed to almost nil 20 years ago. There are an ever-increasing number of organ donors dying from some form of cerebral vascular accident, replacing motor vehicle accidents and closed head injury as the most common cause of brain death throughout the decade of 1970s and in the first half of 1980s. Today, like most centres, over three quarters of our kidneys are procured from multi-organ donors, an uncommon event until the mid 1980s. Although it has yet to be shown to adversely affect early renal function when properly performed, the procurement of multiple organs from a single donor can increase both warm and uncontrolled cold ischaemic times for kidneys. Finally, there have been multiple changes in the immunosuppressive regimens used to treat patients over the past 20 years. Since 1985, most recipients of cadaveric kidneys underwent induction with either anti-thymocyte (ATGAM), anti-lymphocyte globulin (MALG), or monoclonal anti-T cell antibody (OKT3). Due to their inherent nephrotoxicity, typically, we have delayed the initiation of cyclosporine A or tacrolimus therapy until after good renal function has been established, i.e. a mean of 3.5 days after transplantation. Throughout the 90s most of our cadaveric recipients have been treated under one of the many drug research protocols.

Fifty-five percent, or 1108 of the 2000 kidneys were transplanted at our own transplant centre and these recipients have provided the bulk of the data for this analysis. Of the remaining kidneys, 14% (281) were shared at the local OPO level and transplanted within our service area, 27% (529) were shared either regionally or nationally via the Southeastern Organ Procurement Foundation (SEOPF) or UNOS and subsequently transplanted, and 4% (82) were not transplanted. Although adequate follow-up has been achieved in only about 60% of the distantly shared kidneys, the incidence of DGF has stayed fairly constant at about 20% or twice the rate of locally transplanted kidneys. This DGF rate of shared kidneys has been increasing since

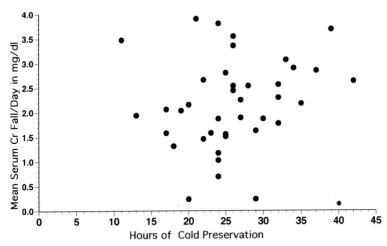

Fig. 3. Scattergram of the slope of recovery of renal function as measured by daily decrease in the serum creatinine (mg/dl) plotted against the kidneys total preservation time in hours (n = 50).

we discontinued shipping kidneys on MP in 1990 because so few centres were capable of perfusion preservation.

In 1985, we analysed the results of our first 1000 MP kidneys. Prior to that analysis our prejudice was that all forms of preservation, including MP, resulted in some linear deterioration of renal function. Therefore, all kidney transplants at our centre were performed as emergent operations, more often than not in the middle of the night, in order to minimise renal preservation times. Figure 3 is a scattergram plot of preservation times versus the rate of renal function recovery and shows that from four to 40 hours of MP, there was no correlation between the duration of preservation and the level of early renal function. Based on these data, cadaveric transplant operations at our institution were subsequently scheduled and performed as semi-elective cases whenever the mode of preservation was MP. This capacity for semi-elective scheduling of renal transplant procedures

Mean and Range of Renal Preservation Times By Decades

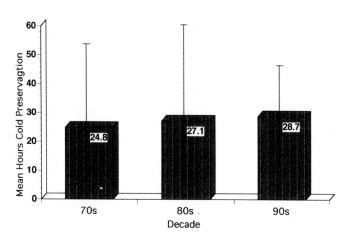

Fig. 4. Total mean and range bars for renal preservation times (ice + pump) of kidneys that were transplanted at Indiana University over the past three decades. n = 166 for 1970s; n = 489 for 1980s; n = 553 for the 1990s. Difference between 1970s–1990s, p < 0.05.

provides more flexibility in the scheduling of the operating rooms and helps to reduce the impact and stress on operating room personnel when multiple organs must be transplanted, i.e. heart, liver, lungs, pancreas, etc, in a fairly short time frame. Therefore, as shown in Fig. 4, our mean total preservation times, i.e. ice + pump times, have increased significantly from 24.8 ± 7 to 28 ± 8 hours (p ≤ 0.5) over the past two decades without any negative effect on early renal function or need for dialysis.

Figure 5 depicts the incidence of DGF along with yearly activity for the past ten years. Recipients of all locally transplanted cadaveric (CAD) kidneys have a mean incidence of DGF of 10.6% per year for the entire 20-year span. However, when the data are segregated by decade there is a significant fall in the mean incidence of DGF from 14.6% observed during the first decade and 7.6% seen over the last ten years (p ≤ 0.5). Closer analysis of the data provided no ready explanation for this reduction in the incidence of DGF between decades.

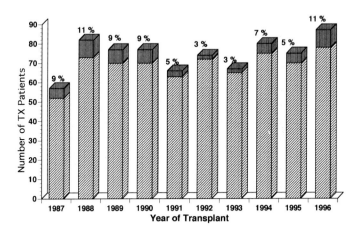

Fig. 5. Incidence of delayed graft function (DGF) as a function of yearly cadaveric transplant activity. None of the differences between years are significant.

Both parameters we found to adversely affect the incidence of DGF in our initial analysis in 1985, i.e. multiple transplant status and high preformed reactive antibody (PRA) ≥ 80%, were not significantly different in our transplant population between the two decades and thus could not account for the reduced rate of DGF seen in the last decade.

Figures 6 and 7 show the significant increase we found in the incidence of DGF with the known immune risks factors of retransplantation and a high PRA. Recipients in the multi-transplant (Multi-Tx) status or have a high PRA ≥ 80% were over two times more likely to experience DGF than patients undergoing their first renal transplant or those whose PRA was less than 80% for all preservation intervals. These data suggest that perhaps not all DGF are of the same ilk. Other immunologic factors such as unrecognised humoral renal injury or allograft rejection could account for up to half of the cases of DGF in these high-risk group of patients. It may well be this group of patients, who are undergoing early immune attack which account

Incidence of Delayed Graft Function Based on Preservation Times

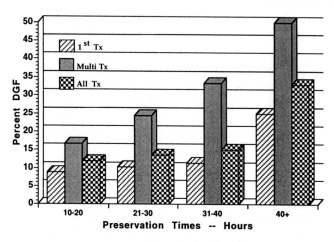

Fig. 6. Incidence of delayed graft function (DGF) based on the duration of preservation time for first and multiple cadaveric transplants. Note that not until preservation times of greater than 40 hrs did the incidence of DGF for pumped kidneys (hypothermic machine perfused) increase significantly, $p < 0.05$.

Incidence of Delayed Graft Function Based on % PRA

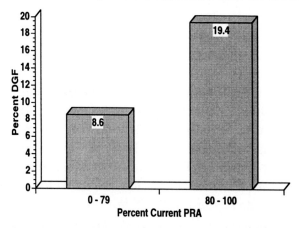

Fig. 7. Incidence of delayed graft function (DGF) is adversely affected by the very high levels of preformed reactive antibody (PRA) in cadaveric renal transplant recipients. PRA levels of $\geq 80\%$ were associated with a two-fold greater probability of DGF, $p < 0.05$.

for the bulk of allograft losses seen in patients experiencing DGF and not due simply to acute tubular necrosis (ATN) from cold ischaemia or drug-induced nephrotoxicity. Our data in Fig. 6 confirm the findings of other studies in that the incidence of DGF for MP kidneys, especially for recipients of first cadaveric (CAD) transplants, does not significantly increase with perfusion preservation times from ten to 40 hours which does not appear to be the case for CS of kidneys.

As noted previously, there were several changes in our immuno-suppressive management between the first and second decade which might have accounted for the significant decrease in the incidence of DGF, particularly if there was some fraction of DGF caused by an early immune injury and not ATN. One factor known to change between the decades was our change to an antibody induction immuno-suppressive protocol for nearly all of our cadaveric recipients during the last ten years. Induction with ATGAM or MALG has been shown to decrease the incidence of rejection at least during the interval that

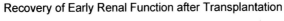

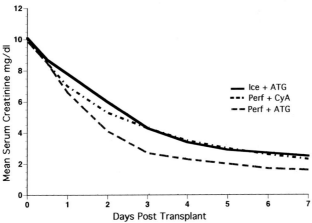

Fig. 8. Effect of immediate treatment with cyclosporine A or ATG induction and the mode of preservation on the recovery of renal function. Mean preservation times were 24.8 hrs for machine perfusion (Perf) groups and 20.1 hrs for the cold storage (Ice) group. n = 20 for each group.

the antibody therapy is being administered, which might provide some reduction in the observed incidence of DGF.

Figure 8 shows the beneficial effect of delaying the administration of cyclosporine on the recovery of renal function even in MP-preserved kidneys. The nephrotoxic effect of cyclosporine A given too early in the post-transplant course seems to nullify the improved renal function gained by MP preservation. The recovery rate of renal function becomes similar to that seen with ATG induction after 24 hours of CS. Though not statistically significant, the apparent increase DGF rate in 1996 (11%) may be a result of certain study protocols prohibiting antibody induction with the initiation of cyclosporine A at the time of transplant.

4. Conclusion

In summary, one can conclude from this analysis that the MP mode of renal preservation has been highly effective in consistently resulting in a low incidence of DGF under a variety of conditions. We feel comfortable with renal preservation times of 36 to 40 hours in kidneys from physiologically good donors and established renal function prior to initiation of any nephrotoxic drugs. It is our opinion that MP preserves organ integrity and renal function better than any form of CS preservation employed to date; however, we have not observed that MP with SAP is capable of rejuvenating or improving renal function in kidneys from physiologically sub-optimal donors. Furthermore, unless there are gross abnormalities in perfusion parameters, i.e. flow rates, pressures, weight gain, etc., during machine perfusion, we have found that these parameters are not particularly discerning in identifying irreversibly-damaged organs from those that have prompt good function.

5. Acknowledgement

I would like to sincerely thank Mr. Micheal Forney and Mr. Rick Putz. It is due to their unflagging dedication and attention to detail in the performance of their duties at the Organ Preservation Laboratory that has enabled our highly successful machine perfusion mode of preservation and facilitated the preparation of this manuscript.

6. References

BELZER, F.O. and KOUNTZ, S.L. (1970). Preservation and transplantation of human cadaver kidneys: A two-year experience, *Ann. Surgery* **172**, 394–404.

BELZER, F.O. and SOUTHARD, J.H. (1980). The future of kidney preservation, *Transplantation* **30**, 161–165.

BURDICK, J.F., ROSENDALE, J.D., MCBRIDE, M.A., KAUFFMAN, H.M. and BENNETT, L.E. (1997). National impact of pulsatile perfusion on cadaveric kidney transplantation, *Transplantation* **64**(12), 1730–1733.

EVAN, A.P., GATTONE, V.H., FILO, R.S., LEAPMAN, S.B., SMITH E.J. and LUFT, F.C. (1983). Glomerular endothelial injury related to renal perfusion. A scanning electron microscopic study, *Transplantation* **35**(5), 436–441.

FILO, R.S., BELL, R.T., SMALL, A. and SELL, K.W. (1976). Current status of kidney freeze preservation, *Transplant Proc.* **8**(2), 215–220.

FILO, R.S., DICKSON, L.G., SUBA, E.A. and SELL, K.W. (1974). Immunologic injury induced by *ex vivo* perfusion of canine renal autografts, *Surgery* **76**, 88–100.

FILO, R.S., MAINOUS, P.D., KREIGER, D. and SMITH, E.J. (1977). Comparison of synthetic albumin and cryoprecipitated plasma perfusate for clinical renal preservation, *American Society of Transplantation Surgeons Abstracts*, p 3.

FILO, R.S., KREIGER, D., BLOOM, P. and SMITH, E.J. (1978). Perfusion injury due to the formation of immunologically active cryoprecipitates in cryoprecipitated plasma, *Acta Med. Pol.* **19**, 89–104.

GATTONE, V.H., FILO, R.S., EVAN, A.P., LEAPMAN, S.B., SMITH, E.J. and LUFT, F.C. (1985). Time course of glomerular endothelial injury related to pulsatile perfusion preservation, *Transplantation* **39**(4), 396–399.

HENRY, M.L., SOMMER, B.G., and FERGUSON, R.M. (1988). Improved immediate function of renal allografts with Belzer perfusate, *Transplantation* **45**, 73–75.

HILL, G.S., LIGHT, J.A. and PERLOFF, L.J. (1976). Perfusion-related injury in renal transplantation, *Surgery* **79**, 440–447.

KOYAMA, H., CECKA, J.M. and TERASAKI, P.I. (1993). A comparison of cadaver donor kidney storage methods: Pump perfusion and cold storage solutions. In: *Clinical Transplantation*, UCLA Tissue Typing Laboratory, Los Angeles, pp 199–205.

KUMAR, M.S., SAMHAN, M., AL SABAWI, N., AL ABDULLAH, I.H., SILVA, O.S., WHICHE, A.G. and ABOUNA, G.M. (1991). Preservation of cadaveric kidneys longer than 48 hours: Comparison between Euro-Collins solution, UW solution, and machine perfusion, *Transplant Proc.* **23**, 2392–2393.

LIGHT, J.A., ANNABLE, C., PERLOFF, L.J., SULKIN, M.D., HILL, G.S., ETHEREDGE, E.E. and SPEES JR., E.K. (1975). Immune injury from organ preservation. A potential cause of hyperacute rejection in human cadaver kidney transplantation, *Transplantation* **19**(6), 511–516.

McCLELLAND, J. and CECKA, J.M. (1987). Kidney preservation. In: *Clinical Transplantation 1987*, P.I. Terasaki, ed., UCLA Tissue Typing Laboratory, Los Angeles, pp 415.

SANFILIPPO, F., VAUGHN, W.K., SPEES, E. and LUCAS, B.A. (1984). The detrimental effects of delayed graft function in cadaver donor renal transplantation, *Transplantation* **38**, 643–648.

SMALL, A., BELL, R.T., FILO, R.S. and WOODWARD, C.R. (1973). Measurement of intracortical flow distribution in hypothermic isolated perfused kidneys, *Am. J. Physiol.* **225**(5), 1199–1205.

SMALL, A., FEDUSKA, N.J. and FILO, R.S. (1977). Function of autotransplanted kidneys after hypothermic perfusion with dimethylsulfoxide, *Cryobiology* **14**, 23–36.

SOUTHARD, J.H., SENZIG, K.A., HOFFMANN, R. and BELZER, F.O. (1981). Denaturation of albumin: A critical factor in long-term preservation, *J. Surg. Res.* **30**, 80–85.

SPECTOR, D., LIMAS, C., FROST, J.L., ZACHARY, J.B., STERIOFF, S., WILLIAMS, G.M., ROLLEY, R.T. and SADLER, J.H. (1976). Perfusion nephropathy in human transplants, *N. Engl. J. Med.* **295**, 1217–1221.

UNOS (1997). The United Network for Organ Sharing Report of center specific graft and patient survival rates. *Department of Health and Human Services. Kidney* **1**.

4.3 PRESERVATION OF CHONDROCYTE VIABILITY DURING LONG-TERM REFRIGERATED STORAGE OF OSTEOCHONDRAL ALLOGRAFTS

L. CSÖNGE

Hungarian Regional Tissue Bank, Györ, Hungary
and
Fulbright Scholar at the Northwest Tissue Center, USA

H. NEWMAN-GAGE, T. RIGLEY, D. BRAVO,
E. U. CONRAD and D. M. STRONG

Northwest Tissue Center/Puget Sound Blood Center
921 Terry Avenue, Seattle, WA 98104, USA

1. Introduction

Massive, cartilage-bearing articular allografts are commonly transplanted in limb-saving surgeries for patients afflicted by tumours, trauma, or degenerative processes (Mankin *et al*, 1983). Almost certainly, viable chondrocytes are required for long-term maintenance of articular function in these osteochondral transplants (Hagerty *et al*, 1967; McGann *et al*, 1988; Schachar *et al*, 1989). The two options for clinicians and patients requiring osteochondral allografts are fresh or cryopreserved grafts. Each of these has its biological and logistical advantages and disadvantages.

Although fresh osteochondral allografts can undoubtedly ensure a higher proportion of viable chondrocytes in the transplant, attendant with this viability is a greater immunogenicity of the graft. A logistical complication for the use of fresh allografts is that the timing of the transplant surgery must necessarily be dependent upon donor availability. Scheduling surgical time for the transplant procedure must be performed with an alacrity that can be difficult both for patients and hospital personnel.

An advantage of cryopreservation is that accurately-sized banked allografts can be accumulated to create a comprehensive inventory listing in a tissue bank. There is adequate time for complete donor screening, laboratory testing and scheduling of surgical procedures becomes less difficult. Unfortunately, cryopreservation of intact human cartilage has not reached its zenith. Attempts to cryopreserve articular cartilage generally fail, with typical reported viability upon thawing of only 20–40% (Tomford et al, 1982; Schachar et al, 1986; Kawabe et al, 1990; Viviente et al, 1996; Fabbriciani et al, 1997).

Adequacy of donor screening is a significant issue. Because fresh osteochondral allografts are typically transplanted within 48 hours of procurement (Sammarco et al, 1997), there is little time to glean detailed information regarding the donor, and often these tissues must be released for transplant prior to accumulation of all the screening information that is typically required of other bone graft donors. For many donors, it is impossible within this interval to obtain autopsy reports, or accurately evaluate the haemodilution of the blood sample acquired for serology testing. Microbial culture results will not have developed fully due to shortened incubation times, and detailed interviews may not have been conducted with those knowledgeable of the donor's medical and social history details. Although cryopreserved grafts have a lower viability, considerations of this sort commonly preclude tissue banks from providing fresh osteochondral allografts. For some banks, the risks of disease transmission outweigh the benefits of viable cartilage since, in the majority of cases, these are not life-saving surgical procedures and the clinical benefits of viable cartilage have not been substantiated.

We have studied methods of cartilage preservation at 4°C in order to retain viable cartilage, while addressing the issue of donor safety by holding allografts long enough to allow adequate donor screening.

2. Methods

Here, we report on studies in which osteochondral grafts were procured from typical transplant tissue donors and stored at 4°C. The viability of the cartilage was measured frequently over long periods of storage. The talar surfaces of the talo-tibial joint were procured from donors with an age range from 16 to 59. The next-of-kin of these donors had consented for additional research use of the grafts procured. The talus was chosen as a convenient source of joint cartilage that, while exposed during routine tissue bank bone graft procurement, is not normally taken as a transplant graft. In this way, we ensured obtaining samples representative of the typical transplant material in terms of age, health, ischaemic post-mortem intervals, etc., without compromising the availability of transplantable graft material for patients.

Immediately after procurement, the cartilage-bearing talar domes were placed into tissue culture media (X-Vivo 10; BioWhittaker, Walkersville, MD) and refrigerated until delivered to the research laboratory. For the duration of the long-term study, the talar samples were maintained at + 4°C in tissue culture media containing 500 µg/ml Vancocin (Eli Lilly, Indianapolis, IN) and 80 µg/ml gentamicin (Elkins-Sinn, Cherry Hill, NJ). The tissue culture media was replaced by half with fresh media every third day.

The methyl tetrazolium (MTT) viability assay was adapted for use with cartilage samples. The MTT assay has been used as a surrogate marker of cellular viability and to monitor cell activity independently of proliferation in numerous cell types including skin, platelets, tumour cell lines, corneas, heart valve leaflets, hepatocytes, and others (Mossmann, 1983; Gerlier and Thomasset, 1986; Uludag *et al*, 1990; Vistica *et al*, 1991; Hershey *et al*, 1958; Kearney *et al*, 1990; Carney *et al*, 1976, Dushoff *et al*, 1964; Imbert and Cullander, 1997; Lu *et al*, 1997; Fujii *et al*, 1995; Sun *et al*, 1997).

The MTT assay relies on viable cells containing functional mitochondria enzymatically reducing tetrazolium to an intensely-colored pigment. The amount of formazan pigment produced within a given tissue sample is taken to be a meaningful measure of that specimen's viability.

To adapt this assay for use with cartilage, full thickness (from the articulating surface to the subchondral bone) 4 mm diameter punch biopsies of the cartilage were collected and incubated for 1 hour in tetrazolium solutions that ranged in concentration from 0.1–2.0 mg/ml. The concentration that produced the greatest reduction of tetrazolium during that time interval was chosen as the test condition (Fig. 1). In all subsequent experiments, tetrazolium was used at a concentration of 1.0 mg/ml and incubated for 1 hour. After incubation, the formazan pigment produced in the mitrochondrial outer membranes was extracted by an 8–12 hour soak in ethylene glycol monomethyl ether (Methylcellosolve, Sigma). The amount of formazan produced was measured spectrophotometrically and expressed as optical absorbance per milligram of tissue per milliliter of solvent (Abs/mg/ml).

Triplicate biopsies were obtained and tested using the MTT assay from each of ten donors on every third day of storage. Cartilage samples were evaluated over a period of between 30 and 42 days.

In order to demonstrate assay consistency over time, a large number of matched split thickness skin punch biopsies from a typical skin graft donor were cryopreserved by control-rate freezing at 1°C/min (4°C to − 40°C) in tissue culture medium containing 10% dimethylsulfoxide (Me_2SO). These skin samples were thawed and assayed simultaneously and identically with specimens of refrigerator-stored cartilage from a specific donor over a period of many weeks. This control was intended to reveal whether fluctuations in cartilage viability measurements were inherent in the cartilage or had arisen from within the assay system itself. Data were analysed using the F-statistic to evaluate the degree of variability within replicates for each day in comparison to the variability of the viability readings between days.

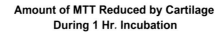

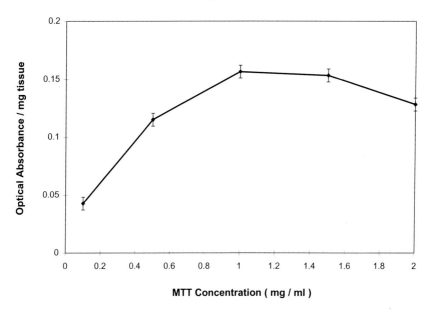

Fig. 1. Graph representative of tests performed using MTT at varying concentrations and incubation intervals. Evaluations of this sort allow for the determination of assay conditions optimised for a particular tissue type and biopsy size.

Fresh cartilage samples of very high viability were collected as surgical discard tissue during amputation procedures from donors (n = 3) whose identities were unknown by the investigators. These samples were assayed using MTT within 1 hour of excision and the mean viability value was defined as 100% viability. Non-viable control specimens, created by desiccation of cartilage biopsies, were used to establish a 0% viability baseline value.

Viability determinations using the tetrazolium method were corroborated by fluorescent dye evaluation of cartilage sections prepared using a vibrating microtome. Sections 20 microns thick of fresh cartilage, cryopreserved cartilage and cartilage that had been stored under our refrigerated test conditions for 45 days, were evaluated using the fluorescent supravital dyes SYTO 16 and propidium iodide (Molecular Probes, Eugene, OR). These fluorescent stains allow simultaneous visualisation of both viable (green) and non-viable (red) cell images.

3. Results

The data presented here show that articular cartilage can be stored for at least 42 days after procurement and still retain a viability much greater than that currently possible with cryopreservation (Fig. 2).

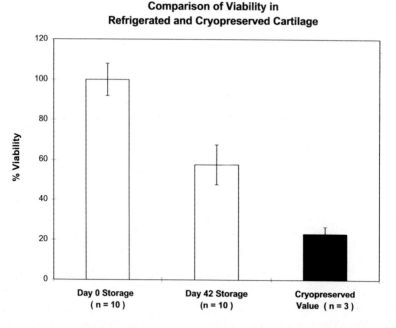

Fig. 2. Values from day 0 measurements were averaged and normalised to 100%. The relative viability of the 42 day 4°C stored cartilage, as well as the mean value for cryopreserved cartilage as reported in the literature (Tomford *et al*, 1982; Schachar *et al*, 1986; Kawabe *et al*, 1990) are also shown. There is a substantial retention in the viability of long-term refrigerator-stored cartilage compared to that of cryopreserved cartilage.

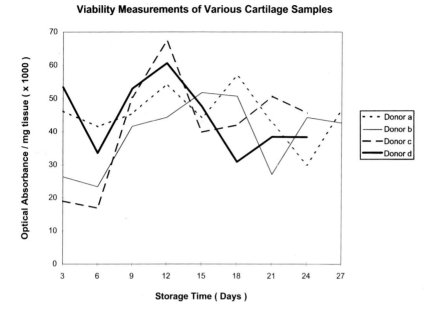

Fig. 3. The inflection points of each line correspond to measurements of MTT reduction by matched cartilage biopsies over time. The averaged values of triplicate measurements are presented without error bars in order to reduce visual clutter and allow the striking range of variability to stand out.

An unexpected finding of this study was the presence of large, recurring fluctuations in the degree of MTT reduction in the cartilage specimens from one day to another over the course of many weeks storage (Fig. 3). This sample of data from four donors is typical of the fluctuations found in every individual cartilage sample measured. Had the cartilage not been examined frequently these fluctuations may have escaped detection. These fluctuations appear to be intrinsic to the cartilage and not a result of variations between replicates according to statistical F-test analysis comparing variations within replicates of each donor to the variability encountered in the measurements across time. Additionally, cryopreserved skin graft samples thawed on each day of MTT assay and simultaneously evaluated using the same reagents and supplies do not show this cyclic MTT reactivity (Fig. 4).

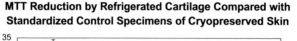

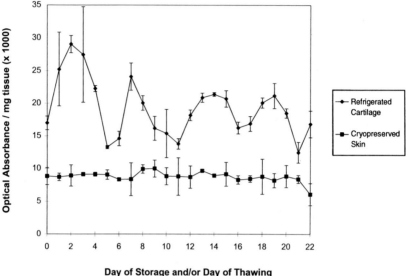

Fig. 4. This chart provides evidence that large fluctuations in the viability of refrigerated articular cartilage observed from day to day result from variations of activity intrinsic to the cartilage itself; when matched cryopreserved skin samples are assayed in tandem with the cartilage, the small degree of variation attributable to the assay becomes apparent. Each data point represents the mean ± the standard error of the mean for n = 3–5 replicates.

Viability observations over time of cartilage specimens from many donors revealed very similar patterns of fluctuation. In order to determine whether the cycling in viability was consistent from donor to donor, the MTT viability values for ten cases were averaged and charted (Fig. 5). The pattern of viability fluctuation over time in 4°C stored cartilage remains evident in this composite data from ten donors. The persistence of this fluctuating pattern following the averaging of many donor's viability assessments indicates a genuine underlying biological phenomenon. The pattern has become less distinct when combined in this way in part because the periodicity

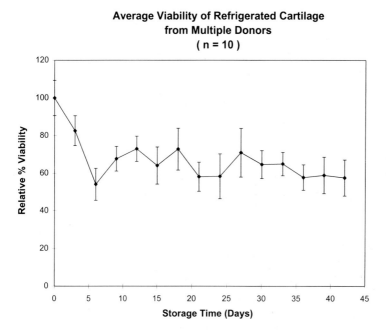

Fig. 5. That a clear appearance of periodic change in apparent viability in this chart has not been lost due to averaging constitutes striking evidence of an underlying biological process common to articular cartilage specimens.

of the fluctuations varies somewhat over time and between donors. Figure 5 also illustrates that even at 42 days of storage the relative percent viability compared to the highest peak observed immediately after processing is 62%.

Fluorescent viability stains (Fig. 6) reveal distinct differences in the proportion of viable cells in fresh cartilage (Fig. 6(a)), cartilage that has been stored for 42 days at refrigerated temperatures (Fig. 6(b)), and cartilage that has been cryopreserved (Fig. 6(c)). These images clearly show the nearly-complete viability of chondrocytes in cadaveric cartilage that has been procured 8 hours after asystole, and stored refrigerated in tissue culture media for 10 hours until evaluated (Fig. 6(a)). Figure 6(b) is from the best example of viability after 42 days of storage. This included continuous slow agitation of the sample

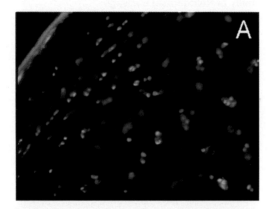

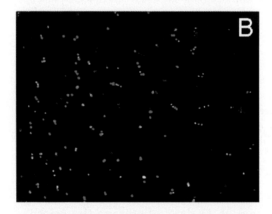

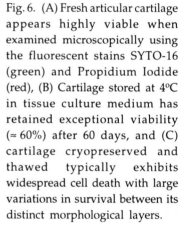

Fig. 6. (A) Fresh articular cartilage appears highly viable when examined microscopically using the fluorescent stains SYTO-16 (green) and Propidium Iodide (red), (B) Cartilage stored at 4°C in tissue culture medium has retained exceptional viability ($\approx$ 60%) after 60 days, and (C) cartilage cryopreserved and thawed typically exhibits widespread cell death with large variations in survival between its distinct morphological layers.

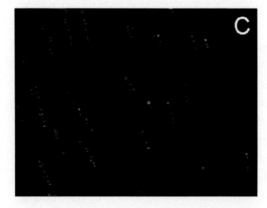

during cold storage. In the cryopreserved specimen (Fig. 6(c)), widespread cell loss is revealed as the majority of cells that admit the propidium iodide dye and thus fluoresce red. Substantial variations in survival between layers was also observed.

4. Discussion

These studies show that it is possible to maintain relatively high levels of viability in articular cartilage with prolonged refrigerated storage. This is important because the longer storage period provides more time to complete donor screening and thereby reduces the risk of disease transmission with fresh osteochondral allografts. Also, refrigerated storage, even up to 42 days, results in the retention of a substantially higher proportion of viable cells than has been achieved with cryopreservation. Although it has not yet been studied, it is interesting to speculate that perhaps longer storage would reduce immunogenicity in large osteochondral allografts while maintaining acceptable numbers of viable chondrocytes. Although a large proportion of chondrocytes survive prolonged storage at 4°C, perhaps the antigen presenting cells contained in the marrow elements and synovial components of cartilage bearing grafts will not withstand this type of storage.

We have observed that the intrinsic activity of mitochondrial enzymes in refrigerated cartilage appears to fluctuate substantially, behaviour not seen in other similarly stored tissues such as skin. Perhaps, because the normal milieu for cartilage is relatively hypoxic, there are intrinsic mechanisms for the conservation of metabolic activity within cartilage.

There are only a few other studies that have examined the effects of long-term refrigerated storage on osteochondral allografts (Bujia *et al*, 1994; Wayne *et al*, 1990). Bujia and colleagues examined the storage of cartilage samples rather than osteochrondral allografts, and assessed the viability using supravital dye and trypan blue exclusion. They examined formaldehyde-fixed as well as refrigerator-stored cartilage. Cartilage exposed to formaldehyde lost 100% of its viability in short order, but cartilage stored in any of three different tissue culture media maintained its viability levels (exceeding 85%) up to beyond 100 days of storage. In contrast, cartilage stored in saline lost viability after 20 days of storage. Wayne and co-workers examined canine osteochondral allografts stored in tissue culture medium for up to 60 days at 4°C. The mechanical and chemical properties they examined, aggregate modulus and apparent permeability, safranin-O binding, glycosaminoglycan content and total collagen concentration, remained normal. Interestingly, they found that chondrocyte viability, as assessed by radio-labelled sulphate uptake, decreased dramatically with time. However, our data, indicating large fluctuations in viability over the period of a few days, suggest that perhaps if additional measurements had been made, the final assessment of viability may have been different.

A recent article evaluates the viability of human cartilage obtained from notch-plasties using the ^{35}S uptake measure. These studies indicate that at 24 hours there is a decrement of 0.8% in ^{35}S uptake and at 48 hours a decrement of 6.4% (Sammarco *et al*, 1997). For comparative purposes, it would have been interesting to repeat these types of measurements over an interval extending beyond the 48 hours. An advantage of the tetrazolium assay over the sulphate uptake measure is that the ease of use facilitates repeated measurements at short intervals over long periods.

With respect to synthesis of glycosaminoglycans, Benya and Nimni (1979) found an eight-fold increase in glycosaminoglycans in collagen at one and three weeks of culture. This gradually declined to a four-fold increase at nine weeks. Others have also noted that storage in refrigerated media stimulates glycosaminoglycan synthesis in bovine articular cartilage and found similar activity peaks on the third day of storage similar to those observed in the present study (Schachar *et al*, 1994).

As a result of finding that a high percentage of viability is retained after prolonged refrigerated storage of osteochondral allografts, we have recently begun a limited trial of transplantation of osteochondral cartilage cores that have been refrigerator-stored for up to 30 days. These have been performed in four instances for localised defects as a result of avascular necrosis in femoral condyles. The average size of the small osteochondral graft was 2.5–3 cm in diameter. The longest follow-up to date is approximately nine months and the recipient maintains excellent function in the affected joint. Similar outcomes are observed for the other three patients with shorter-term follow-up.

These results encourage us to consider that full viability may not be required for the maintenance of long-term functionality in cartilage allografts, and we are hopeful that longer refrigerated storage will reduce the immunogenicity associated with large allograft transplantation. Some caution must be taken, however, due to the increased potential of bacterial contamination in extended 4°C storage. With respect to other tissue banking concerns, prolonged storage provides the opportunity to subject osteochondral allografts to the same rigorous donor screening that is applied to other transplant tissues, thus increasing the safety while maintaining the effectiveness of this type of transplant.

5. References

BENYA, P.D. and NIMNI, M.E. (1979). The stability of the collagen phenotype during stimulated collagen, glycosaminoglycan, and DNA synthesis by articular cartilage organ cultures, *Arch. Biochem. Biophys.* **192**, 327–335.

BUJIA, J., OSETE, J.M., SPREKELSEN, C. and WILMES, E. (1994). Vital preservation of cartilage transplants with tissue culture methods, *Laryngorhinootologie* **73**(5), 249–252.

CARNEY, S.A., HALL, M. and RICKETTS, C.R. (1976). The succinic dehydrogenase and cytochrome c oxidase activities of guinea-pig skin after mild heat damage, *Br. J. Dermatol.* **94**, 295–299.

DUSHOFF, I.M., PAYNE, J., HERSHEY, F.B. and DONALDSON, R.C. (1964). Oxygen uptake and tetrazolium reduction during skin cycle of the mouse, *Am. J. Physiol.* **209**, 231–235.

FABBRICIANI, C., LUCANIA, L., MILANO, G., SCHIAVONE, P.A. and EVANGELISTI, M. (1997). Meniscal allografts: Cryopreservation vs deep-frozen technique. An experimental study in goats, *Knee Surg. Sports Traumatol. Arthrosc.* **5**, 124–134.

FUJII, T., HA, H., YOKOYAMA, H., HAMAMOTO, H., YOON, S.H. and HORI, H. (1995). Applications of MTT assay to primary cultured rat hepatocytes, *Biol. Pharm. Bull.* **18**, 1446–1449.

GERLIER, D. and THOMASSET, N. (1986). Use of MTT colorimetric assay to measure cell activation, *J. Immunol. Methods* **94**, 57–63.

HAGERTY, R.F., BRAID, H.L., BONNER, W.M., JR., HENNIGAR, G.R., LEE, W.H., JR. (1967). Viable and nonviable human cartilage homografts, *Surg. Gynecol. Obstet.* **125**, 485–492

HERSHEY, F.B., CRUICKSHANK, C.N.D. and MULLINS, L.I. (1958). The quantitative reduction of 2,3,5-triphenyl tetrazolium chloride by skin *in vitro, J. Histochem. Cytochem.* **6**, 191–196.

IMBERT, D. and CULLANDER, C. (1997). Assessment of cornea viability by confocal laser scanning microscopy and MTT assay, *Cornea* **16**, 666–674.

KAWABE, N. and YOSHINAO, M. (1990). Cryopreservation of cartilage, *Int. Orthop.* **14**, 231–235.

KEARNEY, J.N., WHELDON, L.A. and GOWLAND, G. (1990). Cryopreservation of skin using a murine model: Validation of a prognostic viability assay, *Cryobiology* **27**, 24–30.

LU, J.H., CHIU, Y.T., SUNG, H.W., HWANG, B., CHONG, C.K., CHEN, S.P., MAO, S.J., YANG, P.Z. and CHANG, Y. (1997). XTT-colorimetric assay as a marker of viability in cryoprocessed cardiac valve, *J. Mol. Cell Cardiol.* **29**, 1189–1194.

MANKIN, H.J., DOPPELT, S., TOMFORD, W. (1983). Clinical experience with allograft implantation. The first ten years, *Clin. Orthop.* **174**, 69–86.

McGANN, L.E., STEVENSON, M., MULDREW, K., and SCHACHAR, N. (1988). Kinetics of osmotic water movement in chondrocytes isolated from articular cartilage and applications to cryopreservation, *J. Orthop. Res.* **6**, 109–115.

MOSSMANN, T. (1983). Rapid colorimetric assay for cellular growth and survival: Application to proliferation and cytotoxicity assays, *J. Immunol. Methods* **65**, 55–63.

SAMMARCO, V.J., GORAB, R., MILLER, R. and BROOKS, P.J. (1997). Human articular cartilage storage in cell culture medium: Guidelines for storage of fresh osteochondral allografts, *Orthopaedics* **20**(6), 497–500.

SCHACHAR, N.S., CUCHERAN, D.J., McGANN, L.E., NOVAK, K.A. and FRANK, C.B. (1994). Metabolic activity of bovine articular cartilage during refrigerated storage, *J. Orthop. Res.* **12**, 15–20.

SCHACHAR, N.S., NAGAO, M., MATSUYAMA, T., McALLISTER, D., and ISHII, S. (1989). Cryopreserved articular chondrocytes grow in culture, maintain cartilage phenotype, and synthesize matrix components, *J. Orthop. Res.* **7**, 344–351.

SCHACHAR, N.S. and McGANN, L.E. (1986). Investigations of low temperature storage of articular cartilage for transplantation, *Clin. Orthop.* **208**, 146–150.

SUN, J., WANG, L., WARING, M.A., WANG, C., WOODMAN, K.K. and SHEIL, A.G. (1997). Simple and reliable methods to assess hepatocyte viability in bioartificial liver support system matrices, *Artif. Organs* **21**, 408–413.

TOMFORD, W.W., FREDERICKS, M.S. and MANKIN, H.J. (1982). Cryopreservation of intact articular cartilage, *Trans. Orthop. Res. Soc.* **7**, 176–180.

ULUDAG, H. and SEFTON, M.V. (1990). Colorimetric assay for cellular activity in microcapsules, *Biomaterials* **11**, 708–712.

VISTICA D.T., SKEHAN, P., SCUDIERO, D., MONKS, A., PITTMAN, A. and BOYD, M.R. (1991). Tetrazolium-based assays for cellular viability: A critical examination of selected parameters affecting formazan production, *Can. Res.* **51**, 2515–2520.

VIVIENTE, E., BUJIA, J., TORREGROSA, C., OSETE, J.M., MEDINA, A., SPREKELSEN, C. and WILMES, E. (1996). Cellular viability of cryopreserved cartilage grafts, *Acta. Otorrinolaringol Exp.* **47**, 263–267.

WAYNE, J.S., AMIEL, D., KWAN, M.K., WOO, S.L., FIERER, A. and MEYERS, M.H. (1990). Long-term storage effects on canine osteochondral allograft, *Acta. Orthop. Scand.* **61**(6), 539–545.

4.4 THE EFFECTS OF CRYOPRESERVATION AND IRRADIATION ON HUMAN PATELLAR TENDON ALLOGRAFTS

S. REZAIAMIRI, C. DAVIS,
A.F. TENCER & E.U. CONRAD

Biomechanics Laboratory of the Department of Orthopaedics
Harborview Medical Center and the University of Washington
325 Ninth Avenue, Mail Stop 359798
Seattle, WA 98104, USA

D.M. STRONG

Puget Sound Blood Center/Northwest Tissue Center
921 Terry Avenue
Seattle, WA 98108, USA

1. Introduction

Allograft patellar tendons present one option for reconstruction of the torn anterior cruciate ligament (ACL) of the knee (Bessette and Hunter, 1990; Fu *et al*, 1991; Noyes and Barber-Westin, 1996). Compared to an autograft, the principle advantage of an allograft is that it eliminates the necessity for harvesting the graft during surgery, and with it the resulting potential for morbidity at the donor site. Also, allografts allow a wider choice of graft type, shape and size. In animal studies, revascularisation, healing, and attainable tensile strength of allograft reconstructions have been found to be comparable to autografts in most (Arnoczky *et al*, 1982, 1986; Goertzen *et al*, 1992; Nikoloau *et al*, 1986; Shino *et al*, 1984) but not all cases (Jackson *et al*, 1991). Shino *et al* (1988) also reported success with cryopreserved allografts in the repair of the ACL in competitive athletes.

Irradiation is used to reduce the antigenicity of allografts as well as their potential for disease transmission (Spire *et al*, 1985). Also, freezing or freeze drying is commonly used to allow long-term storage of the tissue. Since a primary function of an allograft is to support load during joint function, questions have been raised about the effects of processing techniques on the tensile properties of allograft tendons.

Butler *et al* (1987) showed that after exposure to ethylene oxide and freeze drying, followed by rehydration, patellar-tendon-bone allografts had tensile modulus and strength values about 1/3 of those of fresh frozen and rehydrated tissue, while irradiation of frozen tissue alone produced no changes in properties. In contrast, the results of others indicate that irradiation of frozen grafts significantly decreases mechanical properties (Haut and Powlison, 1989; Paulos *et al*, 1987). Haut and Powlison stated that irradiation denatures collagen by scission of polypeptide chains, but the effect is dose dependent and is minimised in wet tissue. The effect of dose dependency of irradiation on allograft tissue properties was confirmed by Gibbons *et al* (1991) whose results showed significant changes with a dose of 30 kGy but not 20 kGy. Further, no significant differences were noted between 20 kGy irradiated and non-treated frozen allografts after six months of implantation (Butler *et al*, 1991).

The effects of various protocols for assuring sterility of allografts is controversial. Freeze drying, irradiation with 29 kGy and exposure to ethylene oxide have been found to delay but not eliminate expression of retroviral infection (Conway *et al*, 1990; Withrow *et al*, 1990). On the other hand, 25 kGy has been adopted by the International Atomic Energy Agency as the required dose for medical product sterilisation (Meryman, 1983).

Recently, Maeda *et al* (1991) presented results of mechanical testing of tendon allografts which were treated by a combination of solvent preservation, dehydration, and irradiation, which has been reported to be effective in preventing viral transmission (Spire *et al*, 1985). They found that tissues which were irradiated first followed by solvent treatment showed little change in both tensile stress and modulus, compared with frozen controls, but when treated in the reverse order, the decreases in tensile properties were significant.

Considering that irradiation, as demonstrated in most studies, degrades the tensile properties of allografts, we hypothesised that it may be possible to enhance tissue properties by improving the method of freezing. Cryopreservation is a methodology which reduces the water that leaves the cell for the extracellular space during freezing. The use of cryoprotectants, such as dimethylsulfoxide (Me_2SO), protects cells from both dehydration effects and intracellular ice formation under controlled-rate freezing. This might result in less damage to tissue than that resulting from conventional freezing. This study was performed to determine the following: (a) Does irradiation of conventionally frozen allografts affect tissue tensile properties? (b) Does cryopreservation alone affect allograft tensile properties compared with conventional freezing?

2. Materials and Methods

2.1. Specimen preparation

All tissues used were acquired from the Northwest Tissue Center (Seattle, Washington). Allografts were harvested from qualified donors (males or females ages 16–70 who did not have any known history of physical or physiological disorders that would alter the mechanical properties of the harvested tendons), maintaining a patellar bone-patellar tendon-tibial bone unit, and stored in tissue culture media (modified X-VIVO with Bacitracin and Polymycin, Whittaker Bio Products, Walkersville, Maryland) for up to 24 hours at 4°C before treatment.

Paired allografts were randomly tested in one of the following three ways:

(i)   Fresh frozen to −80°C at an uncontrolled rate. The cooling rate under these conditions approximates 2–3°C/min.

(ii) Cryopreserved by placing tissue in culture media containing Me_2SO to a final concentration of 7.5% and control rate frozen, as previously described (Gjerset et al, 1992).

(iii) Fresh frozen to −80°C at an uncontrolled rate, and then irradiated (while still frozen) at a dose level of 17.5 ± 0.35 kGy, as previously described (Conrad et al, 1995).

2.2. Experimental groups

Since it has been demonstrated that there is no significant difference in tensile properties between right and left tendons from the same donor (Gibbons et al, 1991), this was not repeated in order to conserve specimens. Sixteen specimens were used to determine if there is a difference in tensile properties between the lateral and medial halves of each whole tendon. Left medial halves were compared to left lateral halves, and right medial halves to right lateral halves (LM vs. LL and RM vs. RL) (Table 1). Each pair came from the same donor and was frozen.

Table 1. Experimental groups used in the experiment.

Group	Preservation Method	Matching Group	Number
Lateral vs. Medial	Fresh frozen	RL vs. RM	16
		LL vs. LM	16
Irradiated vs. Frozen	Right, frozen and irradiated	RM vs. LM	4
	Left, frozen	RL vs. LL	4
Cryopreserved vs. Frozen	Right, frozen	RL vs. LL	11
	Left, cryopreserved	RM vs. LM	11

RL = Right Lateral Halves; RM = Right Medial Halves; LL = Left Lateral Halves; LM = Left Medial Halves.

After establishing that there were differences in the properties between medial and lateral sizes of the same tendon, we assessed the effects of irradiation. This group consisted of four additional matched pairs (each pair from the same donor) where the right tendon of each pair was first frozen and then irradiated, and the left tendon was only frozen. The comparison was made in two subgroups, left and right medial halves and left and right lateral halves (LM vs. RM and LL vs. RL).

The effects of cryopreservation on the biomechanical properties of allograft patellar tendons were determined in the same manner as irradiation. Eleven additional tendon pairs were harvested and the right tendon of each pair was cryopreserved, while the left was frozen. Comparisons were made between contralateral halves (LM vs. RM and LL vs. RL).

2.3. Tendon failure testing

On the day of the experimental trials, all tissues to be tested were removed from the freezer and allowed to thaw in a water bath at room temperature to permit rehydration. The ligaments and their bony attachments were dissected longitudinally into medial and lateral halves. Next, each specimen was cut into an hourglass shape using a cutting dye, with the narrowest width equal to 0.5 cm. Three drill holes (0.076 inch) were made through each cortical bone end. Twenty gauge wire were passed through the holes. Bolts, 6.35 mm in diameter × 50.8 mm long, were wired to the bone ends and then the bone ends were placed in liquid polymethyl methacrylate (PMMA) in a mold. The mold was placed in an ice water bath to dissipate the heat generated from the PMMA as it solidified in order to reduce the potential for damage to the tissue by overheating.

Width and thickness measurements were made of the cross-section at the narrowest part of the tendon using a caliper (model no. 505-647-050, Enco Manufacturing, Chicago, IL) assuming it to be rectangular in shape. Measurements were taken three times each and averaged with the tendon under a load of 108 N in a materials testing machine (model 858, Bionix, MTS Systems, Minneapolis, MN).

As shown in Fig. 1, the bone-tendon-bone units secured in PMMA were fastened to grips of a material testing machine (Bionix 858, MTS Systems, Minneapolis, MN). Tendons were marked with at least three parallel lines perpendicular to the tendon fibers using Indian ink. The centre line was made at the narrowest point of the tendon with the other lines on either side at least 0.5 cm away. A video camera (Ikegama ITC-730A, 30 frames/sec, Ikegama Corporation, Maywood, NJ) was used to record the elongation of each specimen under load and a scale placed beside the tendon was used in the analysis to determine tensile elongation.

A tensile strain rate of 100% per second was selected. The test system was controlled by a personal computer (PC Tech 80286-10) and software (LabTech Notebook, release 4.1.2). Grip-to-grip displace-

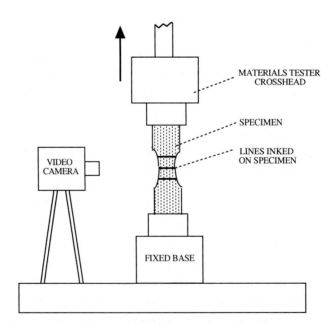

Fig. 1. Schematic diagram of the apparatus for loading allografts in tension.

ment data and load were sampled at 100 HZ, at the same time that the video camera recorded the elongation of the central part of the specimen to failure.

2.4. Calculation of failure stress, modulus and energy to failure

The system used to analyse specimen elongation included the video camera, a video cassette recorder (Panasonic AG-6200, Panasonics Broadcast and Television Systems, Secaucus, NJ) with single frame display capability, a video frame freezer (Hotronic AF-75, Hotronics Corporation, Campbell, CA), a colour decoder (DEC-110, For-A Corporation, Boston, MA) to convert NTC signals to RGB, a video image digitiser (NuVista Plus, True Vision Inc., Indianapolis, IN) to capture and digitise the images, and a Macintosh IIcx (Apple Computer Corp., Cupertino, CA) with software to display single frame images and determine changes in specimen length during loading (Image release 1.43, National Institutes of Health, Bethesda, MD).

The video analysis permitted the strain of the specimen to be determined. The video imaging was timed to the recorded force. Using the initial cross-sectional dimension measurements permitted the calculation of an "effective stress." Stress-strain curves were thus developed for each specimen from which tissue properties were determined. The modulus of elasticity was determined from the slope of the linear region of the stress-strain curve. Energy to failure was determined from the area under the stress-strain curve up to failure, and the maximum stress was also determined from the force and tendon cross-sectional area.

2.5. Data analysis

Statistical analysis and testing of hypotheses were performed using a non-parametric Wilcoxon signed rank test for small samples without the requirement for normal distribution of the data (Statview II, Abacus Concepts, Berkeley, CA).

3. Results

3.1. Lateral vs. medial halves of the same allograft tendon

As shown in Fig. 2, only the failure stress was found to be significantly different. Lateral tendons were 23% (right) to 34% (left) stronger than medial tendons. However, there were no differences in stiffness or strain energy.

3.2. Cryopreserved vs. frozen allografts

As Fig. 3 shows, medial cryopreserved tendons were 53.3% and lateral cryopreserved were 21.5% stronger than their frozen counterparts. The mean strain energy of cryopreserved tendons was 295% (medial) and 364% (lateral) greater than those which were frozen. Differences in the stiffness were not significant.

3.3. Irradiated frozen vs. frozen allografts

Irradiation resulted in numerically lower values for mechanical properties; however, large interspecimen variability and small sample size limited the detection of those which were statistically

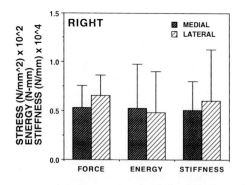
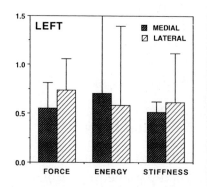

Fig. 2. Tensile properties of allograft tendons, comparing medial and lateral halves of the same specimen, (a) right side, (b) left side.

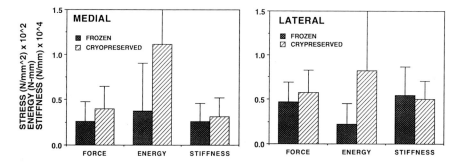

Fig. 3. Tensile properties of allograft tendons comparing cryopreservation to freezing, (a) medial halves, (b) lateral halves.

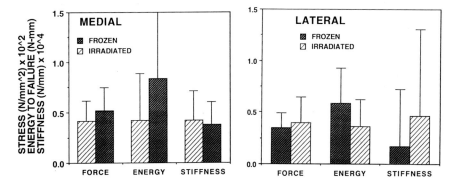

Fig. 4. Tensile properties of allograft tendons comparing freezing and irradiation to freezing without irradiation, (a) medial halves, (b) lateral halves.

significant. Irradiated tendons were 80.5% (medial) and 87.7% (lateral) as stiff as frozen tendons. The stifness and strain energy were not significantly changed (Fig. 4).

4. Discussion

Autografts and allografts are alternative tissues for anterior cruciate ligament (ACL) reconstruction, with allografts gaining in popularity as more research data is gathered to support their advantages over autografts. The advantages include decreased surgical time, because no additional time is required to harvest the graft, lack of morbidity at the graft site, and a wider choice of graft type, shape and size. Minimising the risk of transmission of disease with an allograft requires careful screening of donors and/or sterilisation. The effectiveness of sterilisation remains controversial concerning HIV (Maeda et al, 1991; Fideler et al, 1994; Spire et al, 1985; van Winkle et al, 1967), however, levels used in these experiments have been shown to inactivate HCV (Conrad et al, 1995).

In this study we have focussed on the effects of various treatment techniques to which allografts could be subjected, specifically cryopreservation for long-term storage and irradiation for sterilisation. This study was designed to determine the individual effects of each treatment method. It is common practice in tissue banks to split patellar tendons to increase the availability of grafts and reduce waste. We first compared medial and lateral sides of the same tendon to determine differences. Our results showed that lateral tendon halves had greater tensile force to failure than did medial halves. Gibbons et al (1991) also showed that lateral goat tendon halves have greater stress to failure and modulus than do medial halves. One explanation for this finding may be that the stresses on the lateral side of normal patellar tendon are greater because there is a force component acting to displace the patella laterally. This would place additional tension on the lateral side of the tendon. The clinical implication of this result is that using the lateral part of the patellar tendon results in a stronger graft without increasing its stiffness. The long-term clinical outcome comparing these components has not been studied.

We found that irradiation of frozen tendons at 17.5 kGy reduced their failure stress. This result agrees with the findings of Haut and Powlison (1989) who, after irradiating specimens to 20 kGy, found significant decreases in strength (27.5%) and modulus (56.2%). Alternatively, Gibbons et al (1991) reported no changes in properties due to 20 kGy of irradiation in goat patellar tendons. Our study and that of Haut and Powlison (1989) were performed using human allograft specimens. Rasmussen *et al* (1994) demonstrated significant changes during failure testing with doses of 40 kGy.

We found that cryopreservation results in an improvement in the allograft maximum stress to failure and energy to failure compared with conventional freezing. When tissues are cryo-preserved, they are first stored in a cryoprotectant (7.5% Me_2SO). Cryoprotectants function by reducing the water content of the cell but still maintaining near-normal cell ion/solute concentrations. Grout (1991) indicates that in a 0.154 M NaCl/glycerol (a cryoprotectant similar to Me_2SO) mixture, the NaCl concentration will increase 15 times if frozen to $-15°C$, but if glycerol is added at a 1:1 ratio by weight the concentration only increases to nine times at the same temperature. It is postulated that cell damage results from freezing due to osmotic dehydration caused by water freezing out of solution into the hyper-tonic extracellular space and causing cell shrinkage. It is possible that the stress placed on the cell during shrinkage is what causes irreversible membrane damage and cell death (Meryman, 1983). Thus, cryo-preservation attempts to reduce the amount of cell shrinkage and intracellular hyperosmolarity by applying a cryoprotectant and controlled freezing which provide time for water to exit the cell to avoid intracellular ice formation.

Evidence of tissue damage from extracellular ice has been shown in smooth muscle studies to be due to the formation of ice between muscle bundles trapping and cutting the fibers (Grout, 1991). As the ice crystals grow and compress the tissues/fibers between, large structures which cannot move to accommodate the ice are crushed. Ice crystals which form during slow-rate freezing become very large due to the formation of multiple nucleation sites. As the freezing rate is increased, fewer nucleation sites arise and therefore the ice crystals are smaller and not as able to trap and crush tissues and fibers. This theory would argue for faster rates of freezing to reduce the size of ice crystals. However, cryopreservation procedures used in this study employ a cryoprotectant compound and relatively slow rates of cooling ($1°C$/min). This procedure protects cells from hypertonicity, intracellular ice and changes ice crystal formation. Standard freezing protocols, used in most tissue banks, employ the simple step of placing the tissue into a −80°C freezer. Due to the bulk of the tissue and the packaging, this approach results in tissue freezing at a rate of less than 1°C/min but without the benefit of cryoprotectant, thus ice crystal formation may explain the differences between groups.

The studies cited (Butler et al, 1987; Gibbons et al, 1991; Haut and Powlison, 1989; Paulos et al, 1987) consider the frozen allograft to represent the control state, since other studies have shown that there is no difference in mechanical properties between fresh and frozen/ thawed but not dehydrated tissue (Paulos et al, 1987). The results presented here concerning the differences in properties due to cryopreservation dispute that assumption. Although these differences have been shown to be significant using laboratory biomechanical measurements, the significance in clinical outcome requires further study.

5. Summary

In summary, we formed the following conclusions from this study:
(a) The lateral half of the patellar tendon is stronger in tension than the medial half.
(b) Cryopreservation results in patellar tendons that are stronger and able to absorb more energy before failing than tendons preserved by slow, uncontrolled freezing.
(c) Irradiation at 17.5 kGy decreases patellar tendon strength.
(d) Clinical studies comparing these preservation techniques are needed.

6. Acknowledgements

The authors gratefully acknowledge the support of the Department of Orthopaedics of the University of Washington and the Northwest Tissue Center in Seattle. We also recognise the Media Center of the University of Washington for their assistance with the video image analysis.

7. References

ARNOCZKY, S.P., TARVIN, G.B. and MARSHALL, J.L. (1982). Anterior cruciate ligament replacement using patellar tendon. An evaluation of graft revascularisation in the dog, *J. Bone Joint Surg.* **64**, 217–224.

ARNOCZKY, S.P., WARREN, R.F. and ASHLOCK, M.A. (1986). Replacement of the anterior cruciate ligament using a patellar tendon allograft, *J. Bone Joint Surg.* **68**, 376–385.

BESSETTE, G.C. and HUNTER, R.E. (1990). The anterior cruciate ligament, *Orthopaedics* **13**, 551–562.

BUTLER, D.L., NOYES, F.R., WALZ, K.A., *et al* (1987). Biomechanics of human knee ligament allograft treatment, *Trans 33rd Meeting of the Orthopedic Research Society* **12**, 238.

BUTLER, D.L., OSTER, D.M., FEDER, S.M., GROOD, E.S. and NOYES, F.R. (1991). Effects of gamma irradiation on the biomechanics of patellar tendon allografts of the ACL in the goat, *Trans 37th Meeting of the Orthopedic Research Society* **16**, 205.

CONRAD, E.U., GRETCH, D.R., OBERMEYER, K.R., MOOGK, M.S., SAYERS, M., WILSON, J.L. and STRONG, D.M. (1995). Transmission of the hepatitis C virus by tissue transplantation, *J. Bone Joint Surg.* **77**, 214–224.

CONWAY, B., TOMFORD, W.W., HIRSCH, M.S., *et al* (1990). Effects of gamma radiation on HIV-1 in a bone allograft model, *Trans 36th Meeting of the Orthopedic Research Society* **15**, 225.

FIDELER, B.M., VANGSNESS Jr, C.T., MOORE, T., LI, Z. and RASHEED, S. (1994). Effects of gamma irradiation on the human immunodeficiency virus. A study in frozen human bone-patellar ligament-bone grafts obtained from infected cadaver, *J. Bone Joint Surg.* **76**, 1032–1035.

FU, F.H., GREENWALD, A.S., OLSON, E.J., *et al* (1992). The science of anterior cruciate ligament implants, *Scientific Exhibit, Trans 58th Meeting of the American Academy of Orthopedic Surgeons.*

GJERSET, G., NELSON, K.A. and STRONG, D.M. (1992). Methods of cryopreserving cells. In: *Manual of Clinical Laboratory Immunology.* N.R. Rose, E.C. deMacario, J.L. Fahey, H. Friedman and G.M. Penn, eds., American Society for Microbiology, Washington, D.C., pp 61–67.

GIBBONS, M.J., BUTLER, D.L., GROOD, E.S., BYLSKI-AUSTROW, D.I., LEVY, M.S. and NOYES, F.R. (1991). Effects of gamma irradiation on the initial mechanical and material properties of goat bone-patellar tendon-bone allografts, *J. Orthop. Res.* 9(2), 209–218.

GOERTZEN, M.J., DELLMAN, A., GRUBER, J., *et al* (1992). Neurovascular anatomy of anterior cruciate ligament allografts revealed by metallic impregnation and vascular injection techniques, *Trans 38th Meeting of the Orthopedic Research Society* 17, 666.

GROUT, B.W.W. (1991). The effects of ice formation during cryopreservation of clinical systems. In: *Clinical Applications of Cryobiology.* CRC Press, Boca Raton, pp 81–94.

HAUT, R.C. and POWLISON, A.C. (1989). Order of irradiation and lyophilization on the strength of patellar tendon allografts, *Trans 35th Meeting of the Orthopedic Research Society* 14, 514

JACKSON, D.W., GROOD, E.S., GOLDSTEIN, J., *et al* (1991). Autograft and allograft — an experimental study in goats, *Trans 37th Meeting of the Orthopedic Research Society* 16, 208.

MAEDA, A., INOUE, M., NAKATA, K., *et al* (1991). Changes of mechanical properties after solven preservation and/or gamma irradiation for tendon allografts, *Trans 37th Meeting of the Orthopedic Research Society* 16, 201.

MERYMAN, H.T. (1983). Principles of cryopreservation and the current role of frozen red blood cells in blood banking and clinical medicine. In: *Cryopreservation of Tissue and Solid Organs for Transplantation.* American Association of Tissue Banks.

NIKOLOAU, P.K., SEABER, A.V., GLISSON, R.R., RIBBECK, B.M. and BASSETT, F.H. (1986). Anterior cruciate ligament allograft transplantation. Long-term function, histology, revascularisation, and operative technique, *Am. J. Sports. Med.* **14**, 348–360.

NOYES, F.R. and BARBER-WESTIN, S.D. (1996). Reconstruction of the anterior cruciate ligament with human allograft. Comparison of early and late results, *J. Bone Joint Surg.* **78**, 524–537.

PAULOS, L.E., FRANCE, E.P., ROSENBERG, T.D. *et al* (1987). Comparative material properties of allograft tissues for ligament replacement: Effects of type, age, sterilisation and preservation, *Trans 33rd Meeting of the Orthopedic Research Society* **12**, 129.

RASMUSSEN, T.J., FEDER, S.M., BUTLER, D.L. and NOYES, F.R. (1994). The effects of 4 Mrad of gamma-irradiation on the initial mechanical properties of bone-pellar tendon-bone grafts, *J. Arthro. Rel. Surg.* **10**(2), 188–197.

SHINO, K., INOUE, M., HORIBE, S., NAGANO, J. and ONO, K. (1988). Maturation of allograft tendons transplanted into the knee. An arthroscopie and histological study, *J. Bone Joint Surg.* **70**, 556–560.

SHINO, K., KAWASAKI, T., HIROSE, H., GOTOH, I., INOUE, M. and ONO, K. (1984). Replacement of the anterior cruciate ligament by an allogeneic tendon graft. An experimental study in the dog, *J. Bone Joint Surg.* **66**, 672–681.

SPIRE, B., DORMONT, D., BARRE-SINOUSSI, F., MONTAGNIER, L. and CHERMANN, J.C. (1985). Inactivation of lymphadenopathy-associated virus by heat, gamma rays, and ultraviolet light, *Lancet* **1**, 188–189.

VAN WINKLE, W., BORICH, A.M. and FOGARTY, M. (1967). Destruction of radiation resistant microorganisms on surgical sutures by 60Co irradiation under manufacturing conditions. In: *Radiosterilisation of Medical Products*. International Atomic Energy Agency, Vienna, pp 169–180.

WITHROW, S.J., OULTON, S.A., SUTO, T.L., *et al* (1990). Evaluation of the antiretroviral effect of various methods of sterilizing/ preserving corticocancellous bone, *Trans 36th Meeting of the Orthopedic Research Society* **15**, 226.

Chapter 5

OSSEOUS AND OSTEOCHONDRAL TRANSPLANTATION

The Navy's successful experience with freeze drying bone allografts during the 1970s led investigators at the Navy to develop this application for a variety of other tissues as well. In addition, with the breakout of the Korean War in 1950, there was a growing demand for tissues. As reports of the success of these various applications appeared in the medical literature, civilian institutions began to request access to tissues. A logical extension to this programme was developed to enable both Navy and civilian physicians to reciprocally benefit through collaboration. A "graft registry" was established in 1952 to collect clinical data and access the benefits of tissue transplantation. This was also the beginning of many collaborations throughout the United States. In this chapter two of these major collaborators report on progress in their fields. Dr. Henry Mankin pioneered the use of large osseous and osteochondral allografts in the replacement of bone for management of bone tumours. More recently,

Dr. Alan Gross, also an early collaborator, has pioneered the use of "fresh" osteochondral allografts for osteochondral defects of the knee. Dr. Gross was a contributor in the 1975 proceedings of the Navy Tissue Bank, and both Drs. Mankin and Gross were contributors at the 1997 Symposium in honour of Dr. Sell.

D.M.S.

5.1 LONG-TERM RESULTS OF ALLOGRAFT REPLACEMENT IN THE MANAGEMENT OF BONE TUMOURS: A RETROSPECTION

H.J. MANKIN, M.C. GEBHARDT & W.W. TOMFORD

The Orthopaedic Oncology Unit and Bone Bank
Orthopaedic Service, Massachusetts General Hospital
Children's Hospital, Harvard Medical School
55 Fruit Street
Boston, MA 02114-2696, USA

1. Introduction

At an allograft conference held in Washington, D.C. on April 13–15, 1981, sponsored and chaired by the late Kenneth W. Sell, M.D., Ph.D., members of the Massachusetts General Hospital Orthopaedic Oncology Unit reported data from a series of allografts performed at that hospital over the past ten years (Mankin, 1983). The first procedure in that series was performed in November 1971 and by 1981, 121 allografts had been implanted: 42 for giant cell tumour, 28 for chondrosarcoma, five for parosteal osteosarcoma and three each for central osteosarcoma and fibrosarcoma. The early results as reported (Mankin, 1983) showed that of the 45 high-grade tumours, four patients had died (9%), seven had metastases (15%) and five had sustained a local recurrence (11%). The infection rate was 14.5%, the fracture rate 10.4% and the rate for non-union at the host-donor junction site was 10%. Fifty-six patients who showed no complications did well, but the overall score for the series was 79% excellent or good, 10.5% fair and 10.5% failures.

In a chapter entitled "Perspectives on Bone Allograft Biology" in the volume resulting from the meeting (Mankin and Friedlaender, 1983), Drs. Friedlaender and Mankin wrote these words: *"Despite the problematic and confusing findings in animal species, the clinical long term success with osteochondral allografts in humans provides a substantial incentive not only for further study but for continued application and expanded use of allografts in reconstructive orthopaedic procedures including traumatic, degenerative and neoplastic diseases..."*

In the 16 years that followed that presentation, the Orthopaedic Oncology Unit and the Bone Bank of the Massachusetts General Hospital have continued to explore the field of allograft transplantation, chiefly in relation to limb-sparing surgery for tumours of the bone. In the early days of treatment of bone tumours, the approach was extraordinarily simple — amputate the limb or radiate the lesion and pray that the patient survived. It should be clearly noted that for osteosarcoma and Ewing's tumour the patient's fate was almost inexorably sealed prior to the onset of therapy and limb-sparing surgery played no real role. Today, the treatment is far more complex by standards of that prior time based on two major factors: the successful use of adjuvant and neoadjuvant chemotherapy to prolong and in most cases sustain life; and the use of a large number of new techniques that make limb-sparing surgery not only feasible but most often successful. Amputations for patients with osteosarcoma or Ewing's sarcoma are very infrequent and most orthopaedic oncologic centres have within their armamentarium an array of limb-sparing surgical techniques suited for almost all tumour situations (Delloye *et al*, 1988; Dick *et al*, 1985; Eckardt *et al*, 1991; Jofe *et al*, 1988; Mnaymneh and Malinin, 1989; Sim *et al*, 1987). Based on improved adjuvant therapy, the patients now live longer and indeed, not only outliving their sarcomas (Eilber *et al*, 1987; Goorin *et al*, 1985; Link *et al*, 1986; Rosen *et al*, 1982; Winkler *et al*, 1988), but in some cases, also outliving the devices inserted as limb-sparing replacements. Since there is currently a finite duration for the survival of the skeletal replacement part, the problem has shifted from survival of the amputated dying patient to survival of the limb replacement part in an otherwise healthy patient.

Methods of limb-sparing surgery include the use of autograft segments (Enneking *et al*, 1980a; Enneking and Shirley, 1977) — a reliable but severely limited system. Custom metallic implants became the method of choice following the development of competent hip and knee replacements, and certainly provided and still provide the most satisfactory early functional restoration (Bos *et al*, 1987; Bradish *et al*, 1987; Chao and Sim, 1985; Eckardt *et al*, 1991; Kotz *et al*, 1986; Malawer and McHale, 1989). As noted above, however, they do not seem to hold up as well as initially promised, particularly in the young patient (Bos *et al*, 1987; Horowitz *et al*, 1991; Stauffer, 1991).

Bone allografts, on the other hand, are an ancient treatment and have had considerable appeal to physicians over the centuries. According to legend at least, the first of such procedure was performed by the Saints Cosmas and Damian who, in the sixth century, performed a "miraculous" limb transplant which has been the subject of numerous artistic renderings during the Renaissance (Rinaldi, 1987). Macewen is credited with the first report of an allograft transplant (Macewen, 1881), but it was not until the reports by Lexer shortly after the beginning of this century (Lexer, 1908, 1925) that orthopaedists began to consider the technique as a practical one.

A major discovery in the late 1950s by Herndon, Chase and Curtiss (Curtiss *et al*, 1959; Herndon and Chase, 1954) showed that freezing an allograft segment significantly reduced what was considered to be an immune response and hastened incorporation. Shortly thereafter, using the freezing and thawing technique several investigators reported large series of allografts in the surgical management of bone tumours. Ottolenghi in Argentina (Ottolenghi, 1966), Volkov in the USSR (Volkov, 1970), and Parrish in the US (Parrish, 1973, 1966) presented a series of well studied cases and the reports all showed considerable promise. The results remained unpredictable, however, presumably on the basis of the immune response. Infection fractures and non-union were all too frequently encountered and were difficult to treat.

Because of curiosity about the nature of these problems with alloimplants and because the early successes of the metallic implants had begun to fade (Bos et al, 1987; Eilber et al, 1987; Horowitz et al, 1991; Simon et al, 1986; Stauffer, 1991), several investigators began to perform experimental studies designed to improve methods of implantation (Delloye et al, 1988; Dick et al, 1985; Jofe et al, 1988; Makley, 1985; Mnaymneh et al, 1985; Mnaymneh and Malinin, 1989), better define and ameliorate the effect of the immune response (Burwell, 1969; Czitrom et al, 1986; Goldberg et al, 1985; Horowitz et al, 1991), and make banking safe and sensitive to the patient's requirements (Conway et al, 1990; Doppelt et al, 1981; Tomford et al, 1989, 1990).

Since 1971, the Orthopaedic Oncology Unit at the Massachusetts General Hospital (MGH) has been performing allograft implantation using fresh frozen cadaveric allogeneic segments in which the cartilage of the osteoarticular grafts has been cryopreserved with glycerol or dimethylsulfoxide (Me$_2$SO) prior to freezing. To date, we have performed over 970 of such procedures mostly for patients with aggressive or malignant bone tumours, and have from time to time reported on not only the current status of the patients (Cheng and Gebhardt, 1991; Jofe et al, 1988; Mankin, 1983; Mankin et al, 1982, 1987; Mankin and Friedlaender, 1983). but also on the technology, banking procedures (Conway et al, 1990; Doppelt et al, 1981; Tomford, 1983; Tomford et al, 1989, 1990) and major complications (Berrey, Jr. et al, 1990; Lord et al, 1988; Tomford et al, 1990).

This report is an update of the MGH data for the clinical series of 912 grafts (specifically excluding the 58 grafts involving the hemipelvis which by and large present different problems both in performance of the surgery and in complications). This provides an opportunity to compare the data with those reported for the first 181 patients at the allograft conference in Washington 16 years earlier.

2. Background

The immune response to even frozen allograft bone is well recognised but not very well defined in humans. The response is known to be species dependent (Goldberg *et al*, 1985; Stevenson, 1991), quite variable in extent (Burwell, 1969; Czitrom *et al*, 1986; Friedlaender *et al*, 1983; Horowitz and Friedlaender, 1991), and sometimes exerts a deleterious effect on the operative procedure (Friedlaender *et al*, 1997). Antibodies can be detected to bone grafts and although less for frozen bone than fresh the response is still sufficient to alter the end results in animal systems (Goldberg *et al*, 1985; Stevenson, 1991). Experimental studies have demonstrated a variable response to the immune reaction ranging from rapid dissolution of the graft (very rare in humans (Berrey, Jr. *et al*, 1990)) to "walling off" of the segment with almost no vascular invasion (Burchardt, 1987; Friedlaender *et al*, 1997; Goldberg *et al*, 1985; Mankin *et al*, 1982; Mnaymneh and Malinin, 1989; Stevenson, 1991). Some tentative evidence has been advanced which seems to demonstrate that the high infection rate is a manifestation of the immune response as well (Hernigou *et al*, 1991; Lord *et al*, 1988; Tomford *et al*, 1990).

Non-union at the host-donor junction sites and allograft fractures, both of which represent major complications of the procedure, are also believed to reflect the immune status of the graft (Berrey, Jr. *et al*, 1990). As has been clearly noted by all clinical studies the triad of infection, non-union and allograft fracture represent the major complications of the procedure and account for most of the graft failures of the surgical procedure (Berrey, Jr. *et al*, 1990; Lord *et al*, 1988; Loty *et al*, 1990; Mankin, 1983; Mnaymneh *et al*, 1985; Tomford *et al*, 1990).

In a similar fashion cartilage is known to be antigenic and in fact has been shown to evoke a profound cellular and humoral antibody response (Czitrom *et al*, 1986). It is thought, however, that the cartilage matrix pore size is so small that antigen cannot pass out nor can cells or antibody enter, provided the matrix is intact (Czitrom *et al*, 1986). If the cartilage is altered by surface injury or subchondral bone fracture, it is presumed that the immune response to the matrix and cells is a major event in the development of joint disease. Cryopreservation with DMSO seems to help reduce the likelihood of such cartilage destruction although even the most rigorous and complex of techniques have thus far been unsuccessful in maintaining cell viability in the *in vivo* human system (Schachar and McGann, 1991; Tomford, 1983). Of greater concern is the evident fact that a poor fit of the graft, which leads to surface cartilage loss or microfractures of the underlying subchondral bone, is likely to lead to an early form of osteoarthritis. In our series, about 20% of the distal femoral or proximal tibial grafts have required resurfacing procedures at a mean of over five years (see below).

3. Bone Banking

Most of the grafts implanted in our patients came from the MGH Bone Bank, which was established in 1974. The bank uses a set of guidelines which help to guarantee that the parts are disease free, appropriate in shape and of proper size (Doppelt *et al*, 1981; Friedlaender and Tomford, 1991; Tomford *et al*, 1989). Prior to procurement, donors are screened by discussion with the donor's treating physician and/or family and a careful chart review for evidence of occult malignancy, infection of any sort, toxic substance ingestion, drug abuse or risk factors for AIDS (Friedlaender and Tomford, 1991). All procurements are performed under sterile conditions in an operating room and almost always will follow procurement of living organs by other harvest teams. The MGH Bone Bank teams consist for the most part of physicians skilled in the technique who move rapidly to obtain the long bone and pelvic parts. Swabs from each of the individual parts are cultured separately for bacteria and heart blood samples cultured and screened for Hepatitis B and C and tested for HIV by determination of antibodies and antigen and performing PCR studies (Buck *et al*, 1989; Strong *et al*, 1991; Tomford *et al*, 1989). The bones are stripped of soft tissue, except for ligaments and tendinous attachment sites and especially the posterior capsule and collateral ligaments of the knee joint; capsular, iliopsoas and gluteus medius attachment sites on the proximal femur; and the rotator cuff and deltoid and pectoral insertions of the proximal humerus. The cartilage is immersed in 8% DMSO in an effort to maintain cellular viability during the freezing and thawing process (Schachar and McGann, 1991; Tomford, 1983). Following the reconstruction of the cadaver with wooden dowels and plaster of Paris, the allograft parts are wrapped in gas-sterilised polyethylene bags and appropriate cloth outerwraps and labelled. Prior to freezing slowly to −80°C, all parts are X-rayed in two planes with a metal marker taped to the outer wrap. Wherever possible blood and a lymph node are obtained and stored, and under ideal circumstances a full autopsy is performed on the remaining parts.

Allograft parts remain in the freezer until needed and a computerised inventory is maintained. No part is used until all the tests have been returned supporting the sterile and virus-free status of the part. At the time of contemplated surgery, the part with best fit is selected on the basis of comparison of the X-ray of the allograft and that of the patient (the latter obtained with the same sizing device used for the donor parts in place). Following resection of the tumour the part is brought into the operating room and thawed rapidly by immersion in warm Ringer's lactate (60°C) (Schachar and McGann, 1991; Tomford, 1983). Additional cultures are obtained at the time of thaw and are useful in retrospective analysis of infections as well as prophylactic treatment of the patient post operatively.

4. The Patient Series

From November 24, 1971 until August 20, 1997, the Orthopaedic Oncology Service at the Massachusetts General Hospital has performed 970 allograft transplants including 58 in the pelvis. Because the problems of local recurrence, severity of disease and risk of infection are different for the pelvic grafts, they are excluded from this study. This brings the number to 912, of which 470 are males and 442 females and the mean age is 31.5 ± 17.3 years with a range from three to 79 years.

The operative procedures conformed to principles of performance of limb-sparing surgery for benign and malignant bone tumours and almost always included the soft tissue surrounding the bony lesion, and the scar of the prior biopsy or surgery, and a large segment of normal bone on either side of the lesion. In 167 cases, the margin was described as intralesional or was not recorded. The margin was marginal in 273 and wide for 472, but none in this series were defined as radical (Enneking et al, 1980b). Twenty-nine percent of the patients received either pre- and post-operative or post-operative chemotherapy and 9% received radiation post operatively.

The diagnoses for which the 912 procedures were performed are shown in Table 1 and it should be evident that a considerable number of the patients had either benign or low-grade disease. In fact, 312 of the patients (34%) were classified as Stage 0, including the 129 giant cell tumours and 158 patients with non-tumourous conditions (see Table 1). Forty of the patients (4%) were classified as Stage IA; 172 (17%) as Stage IB; 14 as Stage IIA (2%); 320 (35%) as Stage IIB; and 69 (8%) patients as having a Stage III lesion (Enneking et al, 1980b). Central osteosarcoma was the most prevalent tumour diagnosis (215 cases) followed by 135 cases of giant cell tumour, 129 chondrosarcomas, 55 parosteal osteosarcomas, and 41 Ewing's sarcoma. Eighty-four grafts were introduced as salvage procedures for failed total joint replacement or allografts.

The anatomical sites for the transplants are shown in Table 2 and, as can be noted, 487 (53%) of the grafts are osteoarticular (mostly distal femur, proximal tibia, proximal humerus, proximal femur and distal radius), and 226 are intercalary (25%) (mostly femur, tibia and humerus). Allograft and prosthesis including the hip and knee account for an additional 123 patients (14%) and most of the remaining 76 patients (8%) had allograft-arthrodeses of the shoulder or knee.

It should be clearly evident that not all of these 912 patients could be followed closely over the 26 years of this study. Ninety-five of the patients are dead of disease (10.4%) and 159 (17.4%) of them had a graft failure or local recurrence which required removal and replacement of the part or amputation (in only 55 patients (6%) the limb was amputated and of these 17 (2%) were for tumour recurrence). A total of 96 patients (10.5%) who did not represent failures of the process were lost to follow-up at an average time of 7.2 ± 5.0 years. Since the duration of follow-up for most of these 96 patients exceeds the time when complications occur (see below) none of them are excluded from the study.

Table 1. Allograft transplantation: diagnoses for 912 patients treated from 11/71 to 8/97.

Tumours:	
Central osteosarcoma	215
Giant cell tumour	135
Chondrosarcoma	129
Parosteal osteosarcoma	55
Ewing's sarcoma	41
Fibrosarcoma or MFH	38
Metastatic carcinoma	34
Adamantinoma	23
Soft tissue sarcoma	18
Osteoblastoma	12
Desmoplastic fibroma	10
Chondroblastoma	7
Aneursymal bone cyst	7
Angiosarcoma	7
Lymphoma	5
Chondromyxoid fibroma	3
Ossifying fibroma	3
Myeloma	3
Additional diagnoses	8
Non-tumourous conditions:	
Failed allo or TJR	84
Massive osteonecrosis	32
Traumatic loss	19
Fibrous dysplasia	13
Others	10

Table 2. Allograft transplantation: anatomical sites and types for 912 procedures performed between 11/71 to 8/97.

Osteoarticular (487):	
Distal femur	225
Proximal tibia	101
Proximal humerus	65
Proximal femur	37
Distal radius	24
Distal humerus	16
Distal tibia	8
Proximal ulna	5
Scapula	2
Intercalary (226):	
Femur	98
Tibia	73
Humerus	43
Radius	5
Fibula	3
Ulna	3
Allograft-Prosthesis (123):	
Proximal femur	69
Distal femur	33
Proximal tibia	11
Entire femur	4
Entire humerus	1
Allograft Arthrodesis (76):	
Distal femur	35
Proximal humerus	27
Proximal femur	8
Proximal tibia	3
Distal tibia	2
Distal radius	1

5. Results

The 912 patients which comprise this series were seen as regularly as was deemed necessary over the 26 years of the study and evaluated for evidence of local recurrence or complications of the procedure. Some of them were followed by corresponding with the primary physician from another setting while, as noted above, 96 patients were lost to follow-up at a mean time of 7.2 ± 5.0 years. The scoring system utilised to evaluate their results was one originally proposed by us some years ago and remains our standard method of study (Mankin *et al*, 1982). The system is based on analysis of functional capacity. Patients were scored as **excellent** (no evident disease (NED), return to virtually full function of the part without pain or significant disability, could do non-contact sports); **good** (NED, modest to moderate limitation of function, no pain or major disability, limited sports activities); **fair** (NED, major limitations with a brace or support such as crutches, walker or cane required, some tolerable pain, no sports, about half did not return to prior work activity); and **failure** (dead as a direct consequence of a local recurrence or amputation of the part or removal of the graft for recurrence or complication). The scoring system has been compared several times with that derived by analysis using the Enneking MSTS system (Enneking, 1987) and the one utilised in this study is a bit harsher but certainly easier for house officers and fellows to apply. The advantage to this system is that it is dependent on function; and one is able to not only compare the various anatomical regions, but the results of implantation of intercalary with osteoarticular segments or with grafts used in an arthrodesis or as part of an allograft plus prosthesis system.

The results for the 840 subjects who were followed for two or more years are shown in Table 3. As can be noted 72% of the 450 patients with osteoarticular grafts were characterised as excellent or good while 28% were graded as fair or failure. The 200 patients with intercalary grafts fared considerably better with 84% currently graded acceptable. The 115 patients with allo-prosthesis showed a 74% acceptable score, while those 75 with an allo-arthrodesis did relatively

Table 3. Allograft transplantation: results for 840 patients followed for two or more years (11/71 to 8/95).

Type of graft	Excellent	Good	Fair	Failure
Ostearticular (450)	88	234	23	105
	20%	52%	5%	23%
Intercalary (200)	83	84	4	29
	42%	42%	2%	15%
Allo-prosthesis (115)	23	62	3	27
	20%	54%	3%	23%
Allo-arthrodesis (75)	2	38	5	30
	3%	51%	7%	40%
Total series (840)	196	418	35	191
	23%	50%	4%	23%
If 40 tumour failures are deleted				
Total series (800)	196	418	35	151
	25%	52%	4%	19%

poorly, with only 54% presenting a good or excellent score. The overall score for the series of 840 patients showed a figure for "acceptable" (excellent or good) at 73%, but if the 40 tumour failures are deleted from the series of 800 patients climbs to 77% (31% excellent and 49% good).

As described earlier, the complications of the operative procedure are the principal cause of failure (Table 4). The success or failure of an operation on a patient with a malignant bone tumour must first be considered on the basis of control of the neoplastic process. As noted in Table 4, for the 357 patients with high-grade tumours, 24% died of disease, 35% had metastases and 9% sustained a local recurrence. These values are not inconsistent with any system for dealing with high-grade tumours such as osteosarcoma and Ewing's sarcoma and

Table 4. Allograft transplantation: tumor complications in 840 cases 11/71 to 8/95.

Tumour Complications in 357 Patients with High-Grade Tumours	
Death	86 (24%)
Metastasis	124 (35%)
Recurrence	32 (9%)
Allograft Complications for All 840 Procedures	
Infection	100 (12%)
Fracture	161 (19%)
Non-union	147 (18%)
Unstable joint	30 (5%)

are to a large extent independent of the allograft surgery (with perhaps the exception of a local recurrence) (Dick *et al*, 1985; Eckardt *et al*, 1991; Eilber *et al*, 1987; Friedlaender, 1983; Horowitz *et al*, 1991; Kotz *et al*, 1986; Malawer and McHale, 1989; Simon *et al*, 1986). More characteristic of the allogeneic transplant procedure itself, however, are four major complications: infection, fracture, non-union and instability of the joint which can be noted to be a major issue for the patients. Infection occurred in 100 of the 840 patients (12%), fracture in 161 (19%), non-union in 147 (18%) and unstable joint in 30 (5%). Since some of the patients presented with more than one complication, the numbers listed above are not additive and in fact, 485 of the 840 (58%) patients had none of the allograft complications; and looking at the entire series, 388 (46%) had no complications at all. It should be noted that of this latter group, 96.4 remain good or excellent at a mean time of 8.6 ± 5 years following their surgery.

Re-operations were plentiful in this group but reflected not only the allograft complications but also the problems related to tumours. Of the 840 patients, 448 (53%) did not require additional surgery, but 261 had one, 88 had two and 43 had three or more additional operative procedures. Of the 392 reoperations, 160 were for open reduction and internal fixation and 55 were amputations, of which 17 were for recurrent disease. This provides an amputation rate for the procedure of 6.5% and for allograft complications of 4.5%. Amongst the 213 patients with distal femoral and 92 patients with proximal tibial osteoarticular grafts, 56 (18.4%) had subsequent total knee replacements; and of 36 patients with proximal femoral osteoarticular grafts, eight (22%) subsequently required total hip replacements. The results of these operations led to a satisfactory score ("good" for all but one "excellent") for over 75% percent of the patients. The mean time to performance of such surgery was 5.4 ± 2.2 years.

The ultimate analytic tools for a series of cases such as this are the Kaplan-Meier Life Table Analysis and Cox regression systems, both of which demonstrate that infection, fracture, non-union, local recurrence, type of graft and tumour stage had a significant impact on the results. Figure 1 is a plot depicting the outcome for the entire series. It demonstrates that most of the failures (both allograft and tumours) occur by five years and that the curve declines little after that point, which strongly suggests that once the problems of infection (almost all appear by one year) (Hernigou et al, 1991; Lord et al, 1988; Tomford et al, 1990) and fracture (most of which occur by three years) (Berrey, Jr. et al, 1990) are no longer issues, the graft becomes "stable" and lasts at least throughout the 20-over years of additional observation afforded by this analysis. Specifically, age of the patient (Fig. 2) and site of the graft (Fig. 3) did not provide a significant difference to the outcome of the procedure. In Fig. 4, it is clearly evident that the four types of graft, osteoarticular, intercalary, allograft with prosthesis and allograft-arthrodesis have a difference in outcome, strongly suggesting that allograft-arthrodesis is not as successful a procedure as the other three. It also points out that the largest percentage of failures for all four types of grafts occur in the first three years, and following five or so years, the grafts become relatively stable.

Both the stage of the tumour (Fig. 5) and diagnosis (Fig. 6) have an effect on outcome. Patients with Stages II or III disease or more malignant diagnoses have a statistically significantly poorer result for

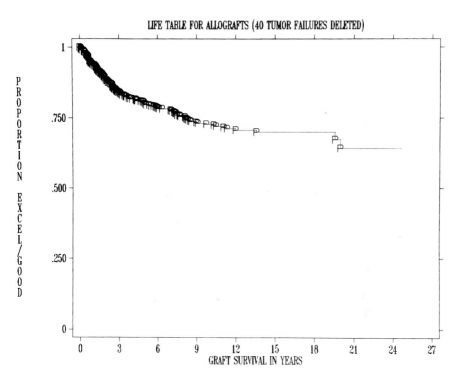

Fig. 1. The overall series as demonstrated by a life table plot (Kaplan-Meier). Note that the tumour failures are deleted in order to assess the outcome of the alloimplants themselves. As can be noted, most of the failures occur in the first five years and that following this period the grafts become "stable" at an approximately 75% good or excellent status.

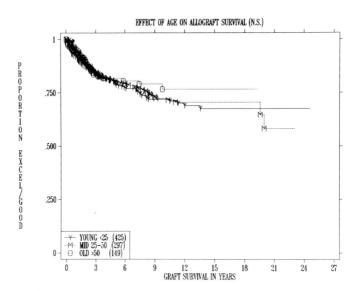

Fig. 2. Life table (Kaplan-Meier Plot) comparing the effect of age on survival. As can be noted, young, mid and older age groups did not display a significant difference in outcome.

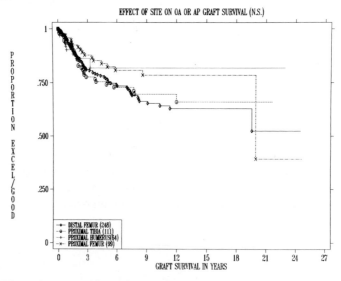

Fig. 3. Effect of site of operative procedure on survival. This plot compares the graft survival for distal femoral, proximal tibial, proximal humeral and proximal femoral osteoarticular, and allo-prosthetic grafts. As can be noted the differences are not significant.

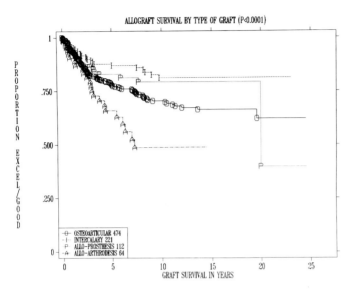

Fig. 4. The effect of type of graft on allograft survival. It is evident that the intercalary grafts have the best outcome and that the allo-arthrodeses have the poorest. This difference is highly significant.

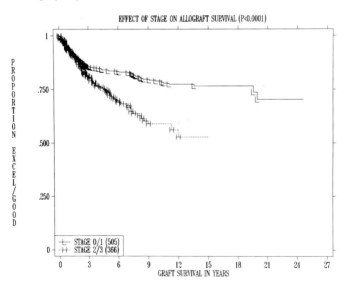

Fig. 5. This graphic demonstrates the effect of stage of the tumour on outcome. It is evident that it is highly statistically significant ($p = 0.00001$). Stage 0–1 cases have a mean survival of over 80%, while the average for those of higher grade is approximately 72%.

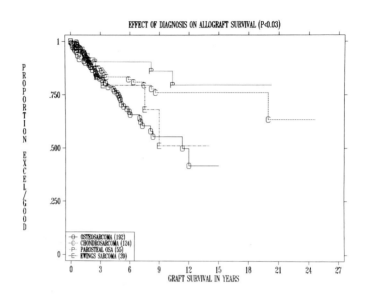

Fig. 6. The effect of the four most prevalent malignant diagnoses in the series is shown in this plot. It should be evident that osteosarcoma has the poorest prognosis, while parosteal osteosarcoma the best. The data are significant at $p < 0.03$.

the allograft, presumably related to the increased frequency of recurrence, the extent of the surgery, and/or the effect of adjuvant chemotherapy and radiation on allograft incorporation. The effect of the allograft complications can be appreciated by analysis of Fig. 7 which clearly demonstrates the high failure rate associated with infection and the still damaging but considerably less pernicious effect of fractures and non-unions.

The "bottom line" is best defined in terms of the results for the entire series at five years, ten years and 15 years following the surgery. When these data are reviewed it is noted that of 694 grafts in place longer than five years, 502 (72%) are still rated as good or excellent; and of 379 in place for more than ten years, the percentage remains more or less the same. For the 141 patients who have had their graft in place for 15 or more years, 99 (69%) are still successful and for 44 which were implanted 20 or more years ago, 29 (66%) are still rated excellent or good.

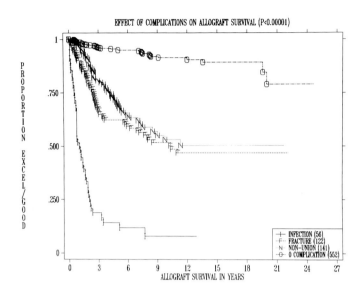

Fig. 7. Effect of allograft complications on the success of the procedure. If no complications supervene, the mean score for good or excellent results is over 95%. Infection reduces the mean success rate to 16%, fracture to 65% and non-union to approximately the same. Note that most of the infections occur in the first year and most of the fractures by five years. These data are highly significant.

6. Discussion

From the data presented above it is apparent that in our series as well as in those from other clinical units, massive allografts are an effective method of dealing with connective tissue tumours and some benign but destructive conditions affecting the skeleton (Cheng and Gebhardt, 1991; Dick *et al*, 1985; Jofe *et al*, 1988; Loty *et al*, 1990; Makley, 1985; Mankin, 1983; Mankin *et al*, 1982; Mankin and Friedlaender, 1983; Mnaymneh *et al*, 1985; Mnaymneh and Malinin, 1989). Regardless of how the series are reported it seems that somewhere between 70–80% of the patients do reasonably well, and that after the first three to five years the grafts become stable and have only exceptional events that lead to failure. It is also evident that these results vary somewhat with the type of graft and the stage of the lesion (and hence complexity of the surgery and relative necessity for adjuvant chemotherapy). The three principal factors which appear to most significantly affect the end results are recurrence, infection and fracture. Together these account for the majority of the failures.

Of considerable importance in analysing these data is that the failure rate is clearly highest in the first year and then diminishes rather sharply until at the fourth or fifth year. At that time, the system becomes stable and then remains so throughout the 20 over years of this study. Most of the non-unions and infections occur in the first year and the bulk of the fractures are noted before the third to the fifth year depending on the type of graft and presumably, to some extent, its length and the type of fixation used. Few failures occur after the fifth year suggesting that the grafts establish an equilibrium state with the host; possibly not getting any better in terms of function over the years, but more importantly not getting any worse. The exception to this rule appears to be the need for a joint resurfacing in about 18% of the patients with proximal femoral, distal femoral or proximal tibial osteoarticular grafts at an average of five years following the initial surgery. Even with this procedure, the success rate still remains above the 65% level.

7. Conclusions

The data presented offer for consideration two burning questions. The first of these is what have we learnt about the allograft procedure over the last 16 years since our presentation at the conference in Washington in April, 1981? The second burning question is obviously what can we do over the next 16 years to make things better?

In response to the first question, some axioms about the procedure can be stated as follows:

• Allografts are like the little girl with the curls...when they are good they are very good...but when they are bad they are horrid!

- No matter what you do or how you do it, 80% excellent and good is the best you get right now...and that is probably because infection, fracture and non-union are immunologically directed.
- Grafts are replaced with host bone... but very s–l–o–w–l–y, and it is our impression that the job is never really done. Further, the slow and unpredictable rate of replacement is at least in part the cause of fracture.
- One of the most essential items is to have access to a good bank. You must get clean parts of the right size in a timely fashion.
- Patients must be carefully chosen for the procedure. We cannot really do the procedure for patients that are too young because allografts do not grow, or for those that are too old because the patient may not tolerate the length of time until function is restored; or for patients who are going to get a very long and difficult course of radiation and chemotherapy...the grafts just do not do as well.
- The surgeon must work rapidly, maintain as high a degree of sterility as possible, and follow the patients for a long time — it is the only way we will learn about the procedure.
- It is essential to have viable muscle over the allograft ... gastrocnemius, rectus and latissimus flaps are very helpful and will reduce the infection rate.
- One should be careful about creating defects in the bone. They will probably never heal and serve as stress risers forever. If holes are necessary, they should be filled with screws or polymethyl-methacrylate.
- As tempting as it is, one should never transplant both sides of a joint. Without a competent synovial nervous system to give sensation to the joint, it is highly likely to develop into a Charcot's arthropathy.
- Adding autograft to the host-donor junction site does not seem to decrease non-union rate of the host-donor junction sites.
- If the allograft has been in place for three or more years, a small number of fractured grafts may heal so it is worth a brief trial of plaster before performing open reduction or other treatment.

- Infected grafts are doomed. They should be removed and an antibiotic-impregnated polymethylmethacrylate spacer inserted and antibiotics administered. After a few months, another allograft or a metallic implant should be introduced. The salvage rate for such a procedure is quite high.
- Although DMSO is still used to preserve the viability of the chondrocytes, it is highly unlikely that they survive after transplant. Despite that, the cartilage holds up rather well and thus far only a small number of our osteoarticular grafts have required metallic resurfacing.
- Chemotherapy and radiation reduce the graft competence but the end result is still better than 50%.

The second burning question in all this is "can these results be improved?" If one accepts the thesis that most of the complications are immunologically directed (and hence represent a form of "rejection") the logical approach to the problem is to attempt to improve the results either by immunosuppression or by better matching of the donor and host. The former is difficult to justify for two reasons. The first and most obvious is that the currently utilised immunosuppressive agents have a mortality rate of their own. Thus, one finds oneself in the awkward role of advocating "life-threatening" drugs for a "limb-threatening" disease. Furthermore, treating a patient with a high-grade sarcoma with an immunosuppressive drug interferes with the immune system and is thus likely to increase the rate of growth or dissemination of micro-metastases and therefore further increase the risk to the patient's life.

A better match is clearly advantageous for certain animal systems (Czitrom et al, 1986; Friedlaender et al, 1983; Goldberg et al, 1985; Horowitz and Friedlaender, 1991; Stevenson, 1991) and in theory would be of great advantage for humans, particularly in terms of the potential for successful implantation of vascularised grafts. The issue which faces us, at least in theory, is that a perfect match may not really be desirable since such a graft is likely to undergo the devastating changes seen in the osteoarticular form of osteonecrosis of bone (only rarely seen in frozen cadaveric allogeneic implants). The second problem with matching is a practical one. It would seem to be very difficult to match not only for size and shape (believed to be essential to achieve good results!) and also major histocompatibility complex. A recent preliminary study showed that either pre- or post-transplant sensitisation to histocompatibility class II antigens appeared to augur poorly for the grafting procedure (Friedlaender *et al*, 1997). If these data are confirmed by longer observation of the series, it should be possible with networking of a number of large banks to obtain such a limited match and thus improve results.

Additional ways to improve the current results would include further attention to DMSO cryopreservation of the cartilage. Currently, the best obtainable is far less than the 50% viability for *ex vivo* intact cartilage segments (Schachar and McGann, 1991; Tomford, 1983) (in sharp contrast with the almost 100% viability achievable by freezing and thawing matrix-free cells in culture with the same concentration of DMSO (Tomford, 1983)). These data support the contention that the passage of DMSO through the matrix to reach the cell is not free and will require some special techniques (Schachar and McGann, 1991).

It is evident, however, that the system remains imperfect and that complicating events such as infection, fracture and non-union make the outcome not only unpredictable but at times may lead to failure ultimately. However, it should be apparent that "failure" is a relative term particularly since of the 170 patients whose grafts failed for reasons of allograft complications (rather than as a result of tumour recurrence), 79% were salvaged by subsequent surgery. The number of amputations for non-tumour related complications for the entire series of 912 patients is only 38 (4%) and even adding in the 17 amputations related to tumour failures brings that value to 6%.

Research continues in a number of areas as described above. With more interest and more scientists studying the problem, it is likely that some major breakthrough will occur. Reduction or at least "control" over the immune response will provide a better graft which will be less prone to complications and late failure. With improved networking in banking, a greater number of allogeneic segments will be available for each patient and perhaps allow a simple major histocompatibility complex (MHC) match. Improvement in surgical technique continues to make the operative procedure more predictable and safer for the patient; and standardised, meticulous control of banking procedures should reduce bacterial and virus transmission to an acceptable level. Ultimately, it is hoped that a sufficiently predictable and high rate of success can be achieved to allow those words, written by us in 1981, "...*the clinical long term success with osteochondral allografts in humans provides a substantial incentive not only for further study but for continued application and expanded use of allografts in reconstructive orthopaedic procedures including traumatic, degenerative and neoplastic diseases...*" to be truer with each passing year.

8. References

BERREY, B.H., JR., LORD, C.F., GEBHARDT, M.C. and MANKIN, H.J. (1990). Fractures of allografts. Frequency, treatment, and end-results, *J. Bone Joint Surg. (Am)* **72**, 825–833.

BOS, G., SIM, F., PRITCHARD, D., SHIVES, T., ROCK, M., ASKEW, L. and CHAO, E. (1987). Prosthetic replacement of the proximal humerus, *Clin. Orthop.* 178–191.

BRADISH, C.F., KEMP, H.B., SCALES, J.T. and WILSON, J.N. (1987). Distal femoral replacement by custom-made prostheses. Clinical follow-up and survivorship analysis, *J. Bone Joint Surg. (Br)* **69**, 276–284.

BUCK, B.E., MALININ, T.I. and BROWN, M.D. (1989). Bone transplantation and human immunodeficiency virus. An estimate of risk of acquired immunodeficiency syndrome (AIDS), *Clin. Orthop.* 129–136.

BURCHARDT, H. (1987). Biology of bone transplantation, *Orthop. Clin. North Am.* **18**, 187–196.

BURWELL, R.G. (1969). The fate of bone grafts. In: *Recent Advances in Orthopaedics.* G.A. Apley, ed., Churchill, London, pp 115–207.

CHAO, E.Y. and SIM, F.H. (1985). Modular prosthetic system for segmental bone and joint replacement after tumor resection, *Orthopedics* **8**, 641–651.

CHENG, E.Y. and GEBHARDT, M.C. (1991). Allograft reconstructions of the shoulder after bone tumor resections, *Orthop. Clin. North Am.* **22**, 37–48.

CONWAY, B., TOMFORD, W.W., HIRSCH, M.S., SCHOOLEY, R.T. and MANKIN, H.J. (1990). Effects of gamma irradiation on HIV-1 in a bone allograft model, *Trans. Orthop. Res. Soc.* **15**, 225.

CURTISS, P.H., POWELL, A.E. and HERNDON, C.H. (1959). Immunological factors in homogeneous bone transplantation. III. The inability of homogeneous rabbit bone to induce circulating antibodies in rabbits, *J. Bone Joint Surg.* **41A**, 1482–1488.

CZITROM, A.A., LANGER, F., McKEE, N. and GROSS, A.E. (1986). Bone and cartilage allotransplantation. A review of 14 years of research and clinical studies, *Clin. Orthop.* 141–145.

DELLOYE, C., DE NAYER, P., ALLINGTON, N., MUNTING, E., COUTELIER, L. and VINCENT, A. (1988). Massive bone allografts in large skeletal defects after tumor surgery: A clinical and microradiographic evaluation, *Arch. Orthop. Trauma Surg.* **107**, 31–41.

DICK, H.M., MALININ, T.I. and MNAYMNEH, W.A. (1985). Massive allograft implantation following radical resection of high-grade tumors requiring adjuvant chemotherapy treatment, *Clin. Orthop.* **197**, 88–95.

DOPPELT, S.H., TOMFORD, W.W., LUCAS, A.D. and MANKIN, H.J. (1981). Operational and financial aspects of a hospital bone bank, *J. Bone Joint Surg. (Am.)* **63**, 1472–1481.

ECKARDT, J.J., EILBER, F.R., ROSEN, G., MIRRA, J.M., DOREY, F.J., WARD, W.G. and KABO, J.M. (1991). Endoprosthetic replacement for stage IIB osteosarcoma, *Clin. Orthop.* **270**, 202–213.

EILBER, F., GIULIANO, A., ECKARDT, J., PATTERSON, K., MOSELEY, S. and GOODNIGHT, J. (1987). Adjuvant chemotherapy for osteosarcoma: A randomized prospective trial, *J. Clin. Oncol.* **5**, 21–26.

ENNEKING, W.F. (1987). A system for evaluation of the surgical management of musculoskeletal tumors. In: *Limb Salvage in Musculoskeletal Oncology*. W.F. Enneking, ed., Churchill Livingstone, New York, pp 145–150.

ENNEKING, W.F., EADY, J.L. and BURCHARDT, H. (1980a). Autogenous cortical bone grafts in the reconstruction of segmental skeletal defects, *J. Bone Joint Surg.(Am.)* **62**, 1039–1058.

ENNEKING, W.F. and SHIRLEY, P.D. (1977). Resection-arthrodesis for malignant and potentially malignant lesions about the knee using an intramedullary rod and local bone grafts, *J. Bone Joint Surg. (Am.)* **59**, 223–236.

ENNEKING, W.F., SPANIER, S.S. and GOODMAN, M.A. (1980b). Current concepts review. The surgical staging of musculoskeletal sarcoma, *J. Bone Joint Surg. (Am.)* **62**, 1027–1030.

FRIEDLAENDER, G.E. (1983). Immune responses to osteochondral allografts. Current knowledge and future directions, *Clin. Orthop.* **174**, 58–68.

FRIEDLAENDER, G.E., MANKIN, H.J. and SELL, K.W. (1983). *Osteochondral Allografts*. Little Brown and Co., Boston.

FRIEDLAENDER, G.E., STRONG, D.M., SPRINGFIELD, D.S. and MANKIN, H.J. *(unpublished data)*.

FRIEDLAENDER, G.E. and TOMFORD, W.W. (1991). Approaches to the retrieval and banking of osteochondral allografts. In: *Bone and*

Cartilage Allografts. G.E. Friedlaender and V.M. Goldberg, eds., American Academy of Orthopaedic Surgeons, Park Ridge, IL, pp 185–192.

GOLDBERG, V.M., POWELL, A., SHAFFER, J.W., ZIKA, J., BOS, G.D. and HEIPLE, K.G. (1985). Bone grafting: Role of histocompatibility in transplantation, *J. Orthop. Res.* **3**, 389–404.

GOORIN, A.M., ABELSON, H.T. and FREI, E., 3D (1985). Osteosarcoma: Fifteen years later, *N. Engl. J. Med.* **313**, 1637–1643.

HERNDON, C.H. and CHASE, S.W. (1954). The fate of massive autogenous and homogenous bone grafts incuding articular surfaces, *Surg. Gynec. Obstet.* **98**, 273–290.

HERNIGOU, P., DELEPINE, G. and GOUTALLIER, D. (1991). Infections after massive bone allografts in surgery of bone tumors of the limbs. Incidence, contributing factors, therapeutic problems, *Rev. Chir. Orthop. Reparatrice. Appar. Mot.* **77**, 6–13.

HOROWITZ, M.C. and FRIEDLAENDER, G.E. (1991). The immune response to bone grafts. In: *Bone and Cartilage Allografts.* G.E. Friedlaender and V.M. Goldberg, eds., American Academy of Orthopaedic Surgeons, Park Ridge, IL, pp 85–102.

HOROWITZ, S.M., GLASSER, D., HEALEY, J.H. and LANE, J.M. (1991). Prosthetic and extremity survivorship in limb salvage. How long do the reconstructions last? Presentation at 58th Annual Meeting of AAOS, Anaheim, CA, March 12, 1991.

JOFE, M.H., GEBHARDT, M.C., TOMFORD, W.W. and MANKIN, H.J. (1988). Reconstruction for defects of the proximal part of the femur using allograft arthroplasty, *J. Bone Joint Surg. (Am.)* **70**, 507–516.

KOTZ, R., RITSCHL, P. and TRACHTENBRODT, J. (1986). A modular femur-tibia reconstruction system, *Orthopedics.* **9**, 1639–1652.

LEXER, E. (1908). Die Verwendung der freien Knochenplastik nebst Versuchen uber Gelenkversteifung und Gelenktransplantation, *Arch. f. Klin. Chir.* **86**, 939–954.

LEXER, E. (1925). Joint transplantation and arthroplasty, *Surg. Gynec. Obstet.* **40**, 782–809.

LINK, M.P., GOORIN, A.M., MISER, A.W., GREEN, A.A., PRATT, C.B., BELASCO, J.B., PRITCHARD, J., MALPAS, J.S., BAKER, A.R. and KIRKPATRICK, J.A. (1986). The effect of adjuvant chemotherapy on relapse-free survival in patients with osteosarcoma of the extremity, *N. Engl. J. Med.* **314**, 1600–1606.

LORD, C.F., GEBHARDT, M.C., TOMFORD, W.W. and MANKIN, H.J. (1988). Infection in bone allografts. Incidence, nature, and treatment, *J. Bone Joint Surg. (Am.)* **70**, 369–376.

LOTY, B., COURPIED, J.P., TOMENO, B., POSTEL, M., FOREST, M. and ABELANET, R. (1990). Bone allografts sterilised by irradiation. Biological properties, procurement and results of 150 massive allografts, *Int. Orthop.* **14**, 237–242.

MACEWEN, W. (1881). Observations concerning transplantation of bones, illustrated by a case of inter-human osseous transplantation whereby over two-thirds of the shaft of the humerus was restored, *Proc. Roy. Soc. London* **32**, pp 232–234.

MAKLEY, J.T. (1985). The use of allografts to reconstruct intercalary defects of long bones, *Clin. Orthop.* 58–75.

MALAWER, M.M. and McHALE, K.A. (1989). Limb-sparing surgery for high-grade malignant tumours of the proximal tibia. Surgical technique and a method of extensor mechanism reconstruction, *Clin. Orthop.* **239**, 231–248.

MANKIN, H.J., DOPPELT, S.H., SULLIVAN, T.R. and TOMFORD, W.W. (1982). Osteoarticular and intercalary allograft transplantation in the management of malignant tumours of bone, *Cancer* **50**, 613–630.

MANKIN, H.J. (1983). Complications of allograft surgery. In: *Osteochondral Allografts.* G.E. Friedlaender, H.J. Mankin and K.W. Sell, eds., Little Brown and Co., Boston, pp 259–274.

MANKIN, H.J. and FRIEDLAENDER, G.E. (1983). Perspectives on bone allograft biology. In: *Osteochondral Allografts.* G.E. Friedlaender, H.J. Mankin and K.W. Sell, eds., Little Brown and Co., Boston, pp 3–8.

MANKIN, H.J., GEBHARDT, M.C. and TOMFORD, W.W. (1987). The use of frozen cadaveric allografts in the management of patients with bone tumors of the extremities, *Orthop. Clin. North Am.* **18**, 275–289.

MNAYMNEH, W., MALININ, T.I., MAKLEY, J.T. and DICK, H.M. (1985). Massive osteoarticular allografts in the reconstruction of extremities following resection of tumours not requiring chemotherapy and radiation, *Clin. Orthop.* **197**, 76–87.

MNAYMNEH, W. and MALININ, T. (1989). Massive allografts in surgery of bone tumours, *Orthop. Clin. North Am.* **20**, 455–467.

OTTOLENGHI, C.E. (1966). Massive osteoarticular bone grafts. Transplant of the whole femur, *J. Bone Joint Surg. (Br.)* **48**, 646–659.

PARRISH, F.F. (1966). Treatment of bone tumors by total excision and replacement with massive autologous and homologous grafts, *J. Bone Joint Surg. (Am.)* **48**, 968–990.

PARRISH, F.F. (1973). Allograft replacement of all or part of the end of a long bone following excision of a tumor, *J. Bone Joint Surg. (Am.)* **55**, 1–22.

RINALDI, E. (1987). The first homoplastic limb transplant according to the legend of Saint Cosmas and Saint Damian, *Ital. J. Orthop. Traumatol.* **13**, 393–406.

ROSEN, G., CAPARROS, B., HUVOS, A.G., KOSLOFF, C., NIRENBERG, A., CACAVIO, A., MARCOVE, R.C., LANE, J.M., MEHTA, B. and URBAN, C. (1982). Preoperative chemotherapy for osteogenic sarcoma: Selection of postoperative adjuvant chemotherapy based on the response of the primary tumor to preoperative chemotherapy, *Cancer* **49**, 1221–1230.

SCHACHAR, N.S. and McGANN, L.E. (1991). Cryopreservation of articular cartilage. In: *Bone and Cartilage Allografts.* G.E. Friedlaender and V.M. Goldberg, eds., American Academy of Orthopaedic Surgeons, Park Ridge, IL, pp 211–230.

SIM, F.H., BEAUCHAMP, C.P. and CHAO, E.Y. (1987). Reconstruction of musculoskeletal defects about the knee for tumor, *Clin. Orthop.* **221**, 188–201.

SIMON, M.A., ASCHLIMAN, M.A., THOMAS, N. and MANKIN, H.J. (1986). Limb-salvage treatment versus amputation for osteosarcoma of the distal end of the femur, *J. Bone Joint Surg. (Am.)* **68**, 1331–1337.

STAUFFER, R.N. (1991). Problems with using metallic implants for replacement of bony defects. In: *Bone and Cartilage Allografts.* G.E. Friedlaender and V.M. Goldberg, eds., American Academy of Orthopaedic Surgeons, Park Ridge, IL, pp 295–299.

STEVENSON, S. (1991). Experimental issues in histocompatability of bone grafts. In: *Bone and Cartilage Allografts.* G.E. Friedlaender and V.M. Goldberg, eds., American Academy of Orthopaedic Surgeons, Park Ridge, IL, pp 45–54.

STRONG, D.M., SAYERS, M.H. and CONRAD, E.U., III (1991). Screening tissue donors for infectious markers. In: *Bone and Cartilage Allografts.* G.E. Friedlaender and V.M. Goldberg, eds., American Academy of Orthopaedic Surgeons, Park Ridge, IL, pp 193–209.

TOMFORD, W.W. (1983). Cryopreservation of articular cartilage. In: *Osteochondral Allografts.* G.E. Friedlaender, H.J. Mankin and K.W. Sell, eds., Little Brown and Co., Boston, pp 215–218.

TOMFORD, W.W., DOPPELT, S.H. and MANKIN, H.J. (1989). Organization, legal aspects and problems of bone banking in a large orthopaedic center. In: *Bone Transplantation.* M. Aebi and P. Regazzoni, eds., Springer Verlag, Berlin, pp 145–150.

TOMFORD, W.W., THONGPHASUK, J., MANKIN, H.J. and FERRARO, M.J. (1990). Frozen musculoskeletal allografts. A study of the clinical incidence and causes of infection associated with their use, *J. Bone Joint Surg. (Am.)* **72,** 1137–1143.

VOLKOV, M. (1970). Allotransplantation of joints, *J. Bone Joint Surg. (Br.)* **52,** 49–53.

WINKLER, K., BERON, G., DELLING, G., HEISE, U., KABISCH, H., PURFURST, C., BERGER, J., RITTER, J., JURGENS, H. and GEREIN, V. (1988). Neoadjuvant chemotherapy of osteosarcoma: Results of a randomized cooperative trial (COSS-82) with salvage chemotherapy based on histological tumour response, *J. Clin. Oncol.* **6,** 329–337.

5.2 LONG-TERM RESULTS OF FRESH OSTEOCHONDRAL ALLOGRAFTS FOR OSTEOCHONDRAL DEFECTS OF THE KNEE SECONDARY TO TRAUMA OR OSTEOCHONDRITIS DISSECANS

A.E. GROSS, M.T. GHAZAVI & A. DAVIS

Mount Sinai Hospital
600 University Avenue, Suite 476A
Toronto, Ontario M5G 1X5 Canada

1. Introduction

Reconstruction of osteochondral defects of the knee in young active patients has always been a major challenge in orthopaedic surgery. The purpose of this paper is to present the surgical technique and long-term results including survivorship analysis of fresh small fragment osteochondral allografts of the knee in young active patients with osteochondral defects secondary to trauma or osteochondritis dissecans.

McDermott et al (1985) reviewed 100 patients who received fresh, small-fragment osteochondral allografts for articular defects about the knee. The diagnoses included osteoarthritis, spontaneous osteonecrosis of the knee, steroid-induced avascular necrosis of the femoral condyles, osteochondritis dissecans, and trauma. Grafts done for post-traumatic changes in the joint did best. Those done for primary osteoarthritis did poorly. Meyers and co-workers also had poor results with fresh grafts placed into osteoarthritic knees (Meyers *et al*, 1989; Convery *et al*, 1991). Garret (1987) produced excellent results for patients treated for traumatic defects and osteochondritis dissecans. It is the opinion of the senior author (AEG) that post-traumatic defects and osteochondritis dissecans of the knee are the best indications for grafting (McDermott *et al*, 1985; Gross, 1992; Zukor *et al*, 1989; Oakeshott *et al*, 1988).

Beaver *et al* (1992), using Meier-Kaplan survivorship analysis, demonstrated that younger patients (< 60 years) in the post-traumatic group have longer surviving grafts that older patients (> 60 years) in the same group. Fortunately, the great majority of post-traumatic patients are in their second and third decades.

Unipolar/unicompartmental grafts are the most successful when considering the tibiofemoral articulation (McDermott *et al*, 1985; Gross, 1992; Zukor *et al*, 1980, 1989; Oakeshott *et al*, 1988; Beaver *et al*, 1992). Patients should, therefore, be referred for surgery before secondary changes occur on the non-traumatised side.

If there is an associated deformity secondary to the joint defect, then an osteotomy is performed to decompress the compartment into which the graft is inserted. If the defect involves the medial femoral condyle and there is a secondary varus deformity, then a proximal tibial valgus osteotomy is performed. If the defect is in the lateral tibial plateau and there is a secondary valgus deformity, then a distal femoral varus osteotomy is performed. The osteotomy is usually done at the same time as the allograft.

2. Procurement

Donors are located by the Multiple Organ Retrieval and Exchange Programme of Toronto and must meet the criteria outlined by the American Association of Tissue Banks and be under 30 years of age. Procurement is carried out within 24 hours of the death of the donor (usually immediately after life support is terminated after the other organs have been harvested). The knee is excised with the capsule intact in the operating room and then kept in Ringer's lactate with added cefazoline and bacitracin at 4°C. The recipient is admitted to hospital and the graft is inserted within 24 hours of the recovery.

3. Surgical Technique

The surgical approach is direct mid-line allowing access for the insertion of the allograft and if necessary the osteotomy. The damaged articular surface is resected to a horizontal bed of bleeding cancellous bone and the graft is shaped and inserted using cancellous screws for rigid fixation. If the meniscus has been excised or is significantly damaged, an allograft meniscus is inserted and fixed to the capsule by interrupted sutures.

The graft is not used to correct alignment and should not be placed in a compartment which is bearing more than physiological load. If a deformity exists, as is often the case, an osteotomy can be performed six months prior to the allograft or simultaneous with the allograft if the osteotomy involves the opposite side of the joint. For example, if a patient has a lateral tibial plateau fracture and an associated valgus deformity, a distal femoral varus osteotomy and lateral tibial plateau allograft can be carried out at the same time. If the patient suffers from loss of the medial femoral condyle and an associated varus deformity, a valgus osteotomy of the tibia and an allograft of the medial femoral condyle can be performed at the same time. If however, a fracture of the medial plateau is associated with varus, a valgus osteotomy of the proximal tibia should be performed at least six months prior to the allograft. See figures of cases 1(a) and (b), and cases 2(a)–(d).

Postoperatively continuous passive motion (CPM) is used to maximise cartilage nutrition. The patients wear a long leg brace with an ischial ring and a knee lock for one year.

4. Materials

Between 1972 and 1992, 126 knees of 123 patients with osteochondral defects secondary to trauma (111 cases), or osteochondritis dissecans

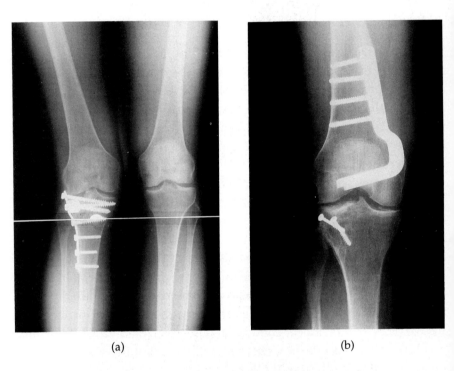

(a)   (b)

Fig. 1. (a) Standing X-ray of both knees in a 35-year old female with fracture of the right lateral tibial plateau treated by open reduction and internal fixation two years previously. Note the loss of bone and cartilage of the lateral plateau with the secondary valgus deformity, (b) Standing X-ray of the right knee ten years after fresh osteochondral allograft to replace lateral tibial plateau, and a distal femoral varus osteotomy to correct valgus.

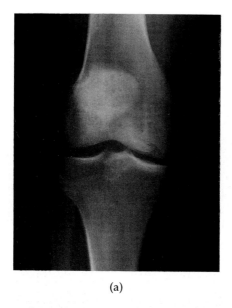

(a)

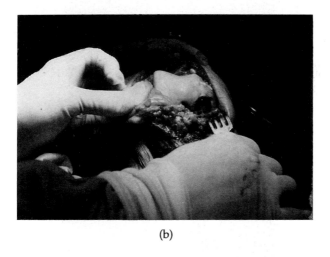

(b)

Fig. 2. (a) Pre-op X-ray of the right knee of a 22-year old male with post-traumatic osteochondritis dissecans of medial femoral condyle, (b) Intra-operative photograph showing area of osteochondritis of medial femoral condyle, (c) Intra-operative photograph with fresh osteochondral allograft in place, (d) Post-op X-ray eight years after fresh osteochondral allograft to replace medial femoral condyle.

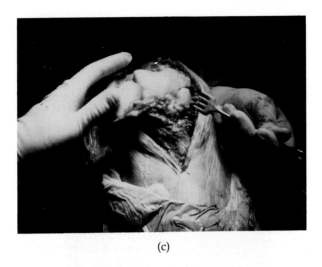

(c)

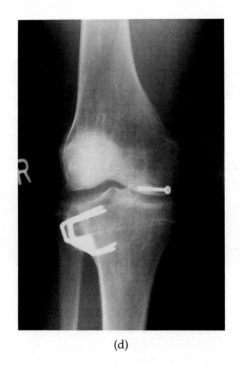

(d)

Fig. 2. *(Continued)*.

(15 cases) were reconstructed using fresh small-fragment osteochondral allografts. The average age was 35 years (range = 15–64), and the gender distribution was 81 males and 42 females.

The location of defects was as follows: tibial plateau (55 lateral, six medial and two combined medial and lateral), femoral condyle (27 medial and 23 lateral), bipolar tibial and femoral (seven lateral and one medial compartment), and patellofemoral (one in the patellar groove of the femur and one in the patella).

The grafts which were 8–40 mm thick were fixed to good bleeding cancellous bone after resecting the defect. In 47 cases the meniscus was included in the transplant. 68 knees underwent osteotomy to correct alignment (37 distal femoral, 31 upper tibial). Patients were assessed clinically pre- and post-operation using a rating score based on subjective and objective criteria. Radiographic assessment included alignment, graft union, fracture and resorption, joint space narrowing, and osteoarthritis.

5. Results

The average follow up was 7.5 years (range = 1–22 years). A failure was defined as a decrease in knee score or the need for further surgery.

Survivorship analysis (Kaplan-Meir) demonstrated 95% successful results at five years (95% confidence limits = 87–98), 71% success rate at 10 years (95% confidence limits = 56–83), and 66% successful results at 20 years (95% confidence limit = 50–81). Among 18 failures one had an arthrodesis, eight cases had total knee replacement (TKR.), the graft was removed in one case and eight cases failed because of a decrease in score but still retain their grafts. The success rate was 85%.

Complications included three stiff knees, one wound haematoma and one patellar tendon rupture. Log-rank analysis revealed a statistically significant relationship of failure of bipolar grafts ($P < 0.05$) and workers compensation patients ($P = 0.0396$), but no significant relationship to other factors like osteotomy, meniscus transplant, sex, and medial or lateral side of the knee.

Also, analysis of variance in successful cases did not show any statistically significant effect of patient's age, sex, post-operative complications, or magnitude of pre-operative scores. Radiographic assessment of 18 failed cases showed four collapsed grafts, seven cases with loss of joint space, and ten cases with significant osteoarthritis.

Except for two cases of questionable union, all grafts solidly united to the host bone six to twelve months after surgery. Among clinically successful cases, we noted five cases of mild graft collapse (less than 3 mm), 11 cases of decreased joint space, and 18 cases of osteoarthritic changes. Among the cases who demonstrated negative radiographic changes, 11 cases were malaligned with overstressing of the graft.

6. Discussion

The rationale for fresh osteochondral allografts is clinical and experimental evidence of maintenance of viability and function of chondrocytes following fresh transplantation. There is also histological evidence that the bony part of these grafts can be replaced by host bone in a uniform fashion in two to three years (Oakeshott et al, 1988).

The survivorship in this study with long-term follow up (95% at five years, 77% at ten years, and 66% at 20 years) is very encouraging. The statistically significant relationship of failures to workers compensation patients and bipolar grafts have been the guidelines for better selection of patients and for doing the procedure in unipolar cases.

Although most failed cases showed radiographic changes of collapse (four cases), joint space narrowing (seven cases) and osteoarthritis (ten cases), similar changes were found in some successful cases.

The development of radiographic changes in 11 cases who were not properly aligned to shift the weight from the transplant indicates the importance of realignment osteotomy. Overall, the high success rate in long-term follow up of this uncomplicated procedure which not only does not compromise salvage surgery but facilitates it by restoring bone stock, makes it an appropriate procedure for unipolar osteochondral defects of the knee secondary to trauma or osteochondritis dissecans in properly selected patients.

Fresh osteochondral allografts have also been used for pure chondral defects by using precision instruments to create a bony defect under the chondral defect. This allows the use of the bony part of the graft for fixation and anchorage of the cartilage (Garret, 1986). There has been recent interest in the use of autologous tissue for resurfacing joints. Both periosteum (O'Driscoll and Salter, 1986) and chondrocytes (Brittberg *et al*, 1994) are used. These techniques have the advantage of not exposing the patients to the theoretical risk of an immune response, but even more importantly exposure to bacteria or viruses carried by the donor. These autologous techniques are more appropriate for surface chondral defects whereas the technique used in this paper addresses the problem of major traumatic defects involving both cartilage and bone. Using proper screening protocols the risk of transmitting HIV is one in one million six hundred and sixty-seven thousand six hundred (Buck *et al*, 1989). The risk for Hepatitis C has not been reported yet for bone and cartilage but there has been case reports of transmission (Conrad *et al*, 1995; Tomford, 1995). The risk of transmitting Hepatitis C in properly screened blood is one in one hundred and three thousand, Hepatitis B one in sixty three thousand, and HTLV one in six hundred and forty-one thousand (Schreiber *et al*, 1996). This same article states that the risk of transmitting HIV in properly screened blood is one in 493 000. These figures represent the worst possible risks of disease transmission by allograft transplantation and should be used for unprocessed tissue (fresh or deep frozen without irradiation or freeze drying). In our opinion these risks are justified in patients with major bone and or cartilage defects causing significant disability. In patients with pure chondral defects the disability is not as great and the loss of tissue is not of the same magnitude. Autologous techniques may be more appropriate under these circumstances (Brittberg *et al*, 1994).

7. References

BEAVER, R.J., MAHOMED, M., BACKSTEIN, D., DAVIS, A., ZUKOR, D.J. and GROSS, A.E. (1992). Fresh osteochondral allografts for post-traumatic defects in the knee, a survivorship analysis, *J. Bone Joint Surg.* **74B**, 105–110.

BRITTBERG, M., LINDAHL, A., NILSSON, A., OHLSSON, C., ISAKSSON, O. and PETERSON, L. (1994). Treatment of deep cartilage defects in the knee with autologous chondrocyte transplantation, *N. Engl. J. Med.* **331**, 889–895.

BUCK, B.E., MALININ, T.I. and BROWN, M.D. (1989). Bone transplantation and human immunodeficiency virus. An estimated risk of acquired immunodeficiency syndrome, *Clin. Orthop.* **240**, 129–136.

CONRAD, E.U., GRETCH, D.R., OBERMEYER, K.R., MOOGK, M.S., SAYERS, M., WILSON, J.J. and STRONG, D.M. (1995). Transmission of the hepatitis-C virus by tissue transplantation, *J. Bone Joint Surg.* **77A**, 214–224.

CONVERY, F.R., MEYERS, M.H. and AKESON, W.H. (1991). Fresh osteochondral allografting of the femoral condyle, *Clin. Orthop.* **273**, 139–145.

GARRET, J. (1987). Osteochondral allografts for treatment of chondral defects of the femoral condyles: Early results, Proceedings of the Knee Society, *Am. J. Sports Med.* **15**, 387.

GARRET, J.C. (1986). Treatment of osteochondral defects of the distal femur with fresh osteochondral allografts; a preliminary report, *Arthroplasty* **2**, 222–226.

GROSS, A.E. (1992). Use of fresh osteochondral allografts to replace traumatic join defects. In: *Allografts in Orthopaedic Practice*. A.A. Czitrom, A.E. Gross, eds., William & Wilkins, Baltimore, pp 78–82.

McDERMOTT, A.G.P., LANGER, F., PRITZKER, K.P.H. and GROSS, A.E. (1985). Fresh small osteochondral allografts, *Clin. Orthop.* **197,** 96.

MEYERS, M.H., AKESON, W. and CONVERY, F.R. (1989). Resurfacing of the knee with fresh osteochondral allograft, *J. Bone Joint Surg.* **71A,** 704–713.

O'DRISCOLL, S.W. and SALTER, R.B. (1986). The repair of major osteochondral defects in joint surfaces by neochondrogenesis with autogenous osteoperisoteal grafts stimulated by continuous passive motion: An experimental investigation in the rabbit, *Clin. Orthop.* **208,** 131–140.

OAKESHOTT, R.D., FARINE, I., PRITZKER, K.P.H., LANGER, F. and GROSS, A.E. (1988). A clinical and histological analysis of failed fresh osteochondral allografts, *Clin. Orthop.* **233,** 283–294.

SCHREIBER, G.B., BUSCH, M.P., KLEINMAN, S.H. and KORELITZ, J.J. (1996). The risk of transfusion-transmitted viral infections. *N. Engl. J. Med.* **334,** 1685–1689.

TOMFORD, W.W. (1995). Transmission of disease through transplantation of musculoskeletal allografts, *J. Bone Joint Surg.* **77A,** 1742–1754.

ZUKOR, D.J., OAKESHOTT, R.D. and GROSS, A.E. (1980). Osteochondral allograft reconstruction of the knee — part 2: Experience with successful and failed fresh osteochondral allografts, *Am. J. Knee Surg.* **2**(4), 182–191.

ZUKOR, D.J., PAITICH, B., OAKESHOTT, R.D., LANGER, F and GROSS, A.E. (1989). Reconstruction of post traumatic articular surface defects using fresh small-fragment osteochondral allografts. In: *Bone Transplantation.* M. Aebi, P. Regazzoni, eds., Springer-Verlag, Berlin, pp 293–305.

Chapter 6

THE CONTRIBUTION OF TISSUE BANKING IN CARDIOVASCULAR SURGERY AND NEUROSURGERY

6.1 Neurosurgical Applications of Allogeneic Tissue
   D.J. Prolo and S.A. Oklund (*San Jose, California, USA*)

6.2 Cardiovascular Tissue Transplantation
   M.H. Goldman *et al* (*University of Tennessee Graduate School of Medicine, Knoxville, USA*)

As described in the introduction to the previous chapter, many investigators benefited from collaborations with the United States Navy and from the ensuing development of applications in their own particular specialties. Dr. Donald Prolo, who reports in this chapter on neurosurgical applications of allogeneic tissue, is an example of such a collaborator. Dr. Prolo also received funding by the Navy during his early experimentation with allogeneic tissue and was a major contributor to the understanding of sterilisation effects on tissues.

As previously described, many clinical applications were reported during the 1950s. The year 1952 marks the first clinical evaluations of arterial allografts at the Naval Hospital in Bethesda. Their success resulted in such a demand for arterial grafts that the Navy sent out a request to all Navy hospitals for assistance in procurement. By the end of 1952, the Navy Tissue Bank was regularly storing skin (both freeze-dried and stored in nutrient media), bone, blood vessels, cartilage and nerves. Dr. Mitchell Goldman reports on the history and recent advances in the application of tissue in cardiovascular surgery. Dr. Goldman and Dr. Prolo were both presenters at the 1997 Symposium honouring Dr. Sell.

D.M.S.

6.1 NEUROSURGICAL APPLICATIONS OF ALLOGENEIC TISSUE

D.J. PROLO & S.A. OKLUND

203 DiSalvo Avenue
San Jose, CA 95128

1. Introduction

It is a transcendent honour for Dr. Sally Oklund and me to participate in a symposium dedicated to the memory of Dr. Kenneth W. Sell, our supreme intellectual and material benefactor and the father of tissue transplantation. Moreover, it is a privilege to remember and recount the pervasive influence of Dr. Sell in fostering neurosurgical applications of allogeneic tissues. Dr. Sell's contributions have been anchored in science. As this tale unfolds, they will be recognised as flowing from his intuitive genius to nurture and guide an inchoate discipline.

Stanford of the late 1960s was vibrant with excitement over the culmination of discoveries of Dr. Norman Shumway first in canine then human cardiac allogeneic transplantation. From this environment of seemingly unlimited possibilities for transplantation, my interest was aroused in the transfer of tissue between humans, notably skull, dura mater and peripheral nerves. The death of a beautiful young girl in 1970 following cranioplasty with a prefabricated acrylic plate ultimately catalysed my decision to investigate the use of potentially viable human skull to repair skull defects. In 1970 we began actively studying the biological properties of autogeneic cranium removed to relieve cerebral swelling, preserved frozen, then replaced orthotopically to repair skull defects. Concurrently, Drs. Mansfield Smith and William Angell were researching transplantation of human auditory ossicles and human heart valves, respectively. Under the visionary leadership of Dr. Smith a symposium on tissue transplantation was convened at the Institute for Medical Research, January 1973, at Santa Clara Valley Medical Center in San Jose. Drs. Ken Sell and Marshall Urist were among the 30 attending physicians and scientists. Dr. Sell demonstrated commanding knowledge of the entire universe and potential of tissue transplantation. He recognised the need for physicians throughout the United States to develop this field with research and clinical applications. The Navy Tissue Bank had been the only source of allogeneic tissue; he anticipated the need for 30 such banks to serve the American population. As Commanding Officer of the Naval Medical Research Institute and former Director of the Navy Tissue Bank, he coaxed others to develop the field of tissue transplantation. His work and words were seminal on that occasion, at the Tissue Bank Symposium, August 13–15, 1975 in Washington, DC and at the American Association of Tissue Banks first annual meeting in 1977. He inspired a renewed surge of purpose and motivated all his audiences to develop the science and clinical practice of tissue transplantation. Among his many contributions this Galilean foresight endures to bring him honour.

At that meeting in 1973 he encouraged me to submit to the Naval Research Institute a proposal for funding studies on the transplantation of canine and human cranium. From his stimulus my interest intensified in this work already ongoing. The Neuroskeletal Transplantation Laboratory subsequently formed which received grants of US$228 072 from the Naval Medical Research Institute, administered through the Office of Naval Research, between 1976 and 1983. The hidden hand of Dr. Kenneth W. Sell has blessed this laboratory with the material resources and intellectual guidance over the last quarter century of its existence. Through Dr. Sell's prescience the American Association of Tissue Banks formed in 1976 as a professional organisation dedicated to promoting the scientific development of tissue transplantation, clinical investigation of tissue use and standards across America for this emerging field.

In 1980 there were three national repositories for bone and dura: the Navy Tissue Bank, University of Miami Tissue Bank (formed in 1972) and our laboratory (also formed for investigation in 1972). Tissue banks proliferated during the 1980s. Entrepreneurial efforts dominated the landscape as various laboratories sought hegemony of access to the treasured human gifts of tissue and thereby market control. Not surprisingly turf battles erupted. Our laboratory (renamed Western Transplantation Services in 1988) did not escape. We were under constant assault from external forces threatening our survival. Although time and professional service were contributed without compensation since 1972 at the nonprofit Institute where our laboratory was housed, in April 1990 that Institute engineered displacement of the authors and sale of Western Transplantation Services (WTS) to another Bay Area institution. After restraining orders, a preliminary injunction, and finally a court trial, on December 20, 1990 a jury returned a verdict for WTS with compensatory and punitive damages against that Institute. Dr. Kenneth Sell's intervention with deposition testimony, October 18, 1990, given at Emory University in Atlanta, provided the crucial link in the chain of historical information in preserving and perpetuating our laboratory at that critical juncture.

Permissibly one may now pass retrospective judgment on the wisdom of Dr. Sell's spiritual and tangible support of our laboratory for the purpose of extending to the neurosurgical community the benefits of allogeneic tissue. Since 1979 we have published 27 papers on tissue transplantation in peer-reviewed journals and textbooks. More are in progress. Since 1976 our laboratory has distributed nearly 100 000 grafts of bone, dura mater, fascia lata and corneas without one report of transmissible disease. What were our discoveries?

2. Delayed Cranioplasty/Remodelling of Skull

Our first publication (Prolo *et al*, 1979) examined the biological response of explanted skull frozen for preservation, then replaced as a cranial autograft. The repair of membranous bone of skull was found similar to remodelling of endochondral bone of the appendicular skeleton. In 53 patients undergoing delayed cranioplasty with auto-geneic skull frozen from three weeks up to 19 months, 48 patients had very successful results. Academic neurosurgeons use this paper in instructing residents in training of the healing sequences of replaced human cranium after craniotomy.

3. Ethylene Oxide Sterilisation

In 1980 (Prolo et al, 1980) we published experiments showing the effectiveness of gaseous ethylene oxide (EO) in sterilising bone, dura mater and fascia lata. After three years of investigation, we demonstrated this alkylating agent eradicated surface microorganisms and diffused interstitially through hard and soft tissues to eliminate bacteria in wet bone, dura and fascia. Desorption of ethylene oxide and its by-products, ethylene chlorohydrin and ethylene glycol, occurred during lyophilisation over 72 hours. With a contamination rate of 10–22% in aseptically procured bone and a clinical infection rate of 6.9% in unsterilised allografts, the case for terminal sterilisation of bone was made at a conference organised by Dr. Sell at the National Institutes of Health, April 13–15, 1981 (Prolo and Oklund, 1983).

4. Neurosurgeon's Role in Transplantation; Morality of Brain Death Determinations

The pivotal role of neurosurgeons in provision of viable organs and tissues for transplantation was expressed in a series of papers (Prolo, 1979, 1980, 1981a, 1985a, 1996a). Examination of the writings of Aristotle and Aquinas supported the moral probity of equating brain death with death to the organism as a whole after escape of the integrating rational principle or intellectual soul (Prolo, 1981b).

5. Allografts in Anterior Cervical Fusion

Effectiveness of EO-sterilised allogeneic corticocancellous cylindrical grafts of ilium and femoral head were reported in the 115 patients of 14 surgeons (Prolo, 1981a). Out of 166 cervical interspaces receiving allografts, 160 fused. This 96% fusion rate was identical with that reported for fresh autografts. This data was reported as part of a presentation to the plenary session of the Congress of Neurological Surgeons in 1980 entitled "Use of Transplantable Tissues in Neurosurgery."

6. Yellow Bone/Tetracycline

In "The Significance of Yellow Bone" (Oklund *et al*, 1981), we reported in the *Journal of the American Medical Association (JAMA)* the high frequency of tetracycline staining of cadaver bone procured for transplantation. Though no deleterious effects of tetracycline being released from bone was then known, a subsequent letter to the editor of *JAMA* revealed that mobilisation of tetracycline from the skeleton in the hyperdynamic state of pregnancy resulted in hepatotoxicity and death of one patient (Bhagavan *et al*, 1982).

7. Experimental Canine Cranioplasty

The mongrel canine skull was adopted as an ideal model for approximating constraints for successful cranioplasty in the human. Whereas, underlying central nervous system tissue is aregenerative, cranial bone can regenerate to some extent. However, the adult skull provides the "worst case" condition for repair of bone. This biologically inactive character of the adult skull led an earlier investigator, Barth (Barth, 1893), to conclude mistakenly from studies on dogs that all elements of fresh transplanted bone die and must be replaced by surrounding tissue. Three-quarters of a century later, we selected 18-mm adult canine skull defects as an ideal experimental model to assay various auto- and allografts quantitatively for effectiveness after various treatments. Random-point analysis of microradiographs prepared from thin sections and analysis of identical bone sections labelled for newly formed bone with tetracycline for six months before sacrifice allowed assessment of the biological effectiveness of implants treated with various sterilisation techniques.

8. Sterilisation/Osteoinduction in Skull

Our first study (Prolo et al, 1982) compared lyophilised allogeneic 18-mm canine discs sterilised with ethylene oxide ($n = 9$), gamma irradiation ($n = 7$), methanol/chloroform/iodoacetic acid ($n = 7$) with those aseptically harvested and lyophilised only ($n = 33$) — the latter a common method of procurement and preservation.

Urist had reported that bone treated with methanol/chloroform/ iodoacetic acid retained the osteoinductive bone morphogenetic protein (BMP) (Urist, 1980). He called this AAA bone autolysed, antigen-extracted, allogeneic bone. Our criteria for evaluating implants at six months included volume of defect filled, radiodensity, extent of fusion around the circumference, revascularisation and remodelling. Bone discs sterilised with methanol/chloroform/ iodoacetic acid remodelled at a superior rate ($p < 0.01$). Radiation sterilisation resulted in decreased density and inferentially diminished protection to the brain ($p < 0.025$). Ethylene oxide/lyophilised and lyophilised only implants provided comparable repair. This observation validated our clinical method of preparing allografts for human use. An acceptable canine cranioplasty was achieved in 86% of the methanol/chloroform/iodoacetic acid/lyophilised implants. All other alloimplants served as osteoconductive templates with successful canine cranioplasty occurring in 56% to 58%.

9. Canine Cranioplasty with AAA Grafts

Defects in adult canine skull larger than 17 mm do not heal spontaneously. In a second series of experiments (Oklund et al, 1986) fresh canine autografts were compared to frozen autografts, antigen-extracted, autolysed, partially demineralised auto- and allografts (AAA grafts). Quantitative reproducible observations demonstrated fresh calvarial autografts were superior to all processed implants in volume/percent fill of defect, mm^2 new cortical bone, mm^2 new and old cortical bone, and cortical bone porosity. Frozen autografts were about 75% as effective as fresh autografts, and partially demineralised AAA grafts only 50% as effective. Fresh cancellous bone added to allografts to provide responding bone marrow cells to the putatively preserved BMP in the AAA graft did not improve long-term repair. Remodelling of grafts appeared consistent with osteoconductive invasion by peripheral host endosteal and diploic elements. Host external periosteum and dura contributed less. Central osteoinductive recruitment of mesenchymal cells from muscle or dura did not occur appreciably in adult dogs. Partially demineralised dog calvarial grafts were resorbed without acting as a template for new bone formation. This study proved convincingly that surface demineralisation, antigen extraction and autolytic digestion of autografts and allografts with or without fresh iliac bone did not improve calvarial regeneration in adult dogs compared to fresh autografts.

10. Composite Autogeneic Human Cranioplasty

In parallel with the above experimental series in canine cranioplasty, a human clinical investigation attempted arrest of the pervasive resorption observed in many frozen autografts following delayed cranioplasty. Burwell (Burwell, 1966) reported enhanced osteogenesis in allografts supplemented with fresh cancellous autografts. Frozen autogeneic bone frequently undergoes aseptic necrosis when reimplanted in cranial defects. In six patients the addition of fresh iliac corticocancellous bone impacted into full or partial thickness holes and craters at 2 cm intervals through the centre and periphery of the frozen autograft did not enhance remodelling. Length of time frozen and sterilisation with ethylene oxide or irradiation did not influence healing of the graft. Resorption occurred in both fresh and frozen autogeneic bone. Autogeneic skull repaired through osteoconductive remodelling. Phase 1 resorption of autograft was non-osteoclastic; Phase 2 resorption coupled to new bone formation did not occur in those grafts which diminished in size (Prolo and Oklund, 1984).

11. Human Skull Allografts

Undemineralised, ethylene oxide sterilised 15 mm allografts successfully fill bur hole sites at craniotomy and cranioplasty in humans (Prolo *et al*, 1984). Among 45 patients between 10–88 years of age with post-operative observation from six months to five years, 115 allogeneic discs successfully filled bur hole defects without instances of resorption or rejection. Discs were incorporated through osteoconductive remodelling from adjacent diploe.

12. Nonosteoclastic Resorption of Skull

Trephination dates from Neolithic times (10 000–7000 BC) (Stula, 1984) and is the oldest known operation. Skull allografts called "rondells" (round discs) were discovered among Neolithic Celtic remains. It is interesting that our focussed research on round discs of allogeneic skull to replace skull defects was apparently a preoccupation of the prehistoric Celts.

Disillusionment with human bone cranioplasty over this century has followed the recurrent experience that orthotopic transplantation of bone to skull is almost invariably accompanied by a striking propensity for resorption. Processing of autogeneic and allogeneic skull including freezing, chemical exposures such as demineralisation, ethylene oxide sterilisation, and irradiation can weaken matrix proteins and mineral bonds that can lead to ingravescent non-osteoclastic resorption of the graft. Successful autografts and allografts remodel through non-osteoclastic resorption coupled with new bone formation.

In 1991 (Prolo and Oklund, 1991) we reported our careful microscopic observations on the biological fate of explanted frozen autogeneic skull plates in two females ages two and 64. After 10 months and six years *in situ*, respectively, these plates resorbed, requiring the patients to undergo acrylic cranioplasty. Microscopic analysis of the residual shrunken plate removed from the two-year old revealed new bone formation, including marrow. Study of the devitalised plate in the 64-year old showed ghosts of residual lamellar matrix that suggested decomposing collagen. Extremely rare islands of new bone were lying within less necrotic matrix. No osteoclasts were seen in either specimen. A unique acellular non-osteoclastic resorption antedated invasion of these two autografts by osteoprogenitor cells. This aseptic necrosis was unrelated to remodelling and characterised the initial response of these autografts placed in an orthotopic cranial bed.

Calciolysis or passive diffusion of bone mineral occurs in unremodelled skull implants leading to necrosis of exposed matrix proteins and variable resorption of the template. Skull grafts that heal do so by osteoconductive invasion of the template from the margins of the defect, rather than through osteoinductive trans-duction of mesenchymal cells from overlying muscle or underlying dura mater.

13. Human Skeletal Growth and Development

In 1990 a summary of skeletal growth and development was published in the *CRC Handbook of Human Growth and Developmental Biology* (Oklund and Prolo, 1990).

14. Contributions on Bone Healing in Spinal Fusion and Human Cranioplasty

Multiple chapters in textbooks and journals were prepared for discussion of bone healing and grafting in spinal surgery. (Prolo, 1981a, 1989, 1990, 1996b, 1996c; Prolo and Rodrigo, 1985; Rodrigo and Prolo, 1988; Prolo and Oklund, 1993,1995). The history and methodology of human cranioplasty has been published twice. (Prolo, 1985b, 1996d).

Table 1. Economic and functional rating scale.

ECONOMIC RATING

   E1 Complete invalid
   E2 No gainful occupation (including ability to do housework or
       continue retirement activities)
   E3 Able to work but not at previous occupation
   E4 Working at previous occupation on part-time or limited
       status
   E5 Able to work at previous occupation with no restrictions of
       any kind

FUNCTIONAL RATING

   F1 Total incapacity (or worse than before operation)
   F2 Mild to moderate level of low-back pain and/or sciatica
       (or pain same as before operation but able to perform all
       daily tasks of living)
   F3 Low level of pain and able to perform all activities except
       sports
   F4 No pain but patient has had one or more recurrences of low-
       back pain or sciatica
   F5 Complete recovery, no recurrent episodes of low-back pain
       able to perform all previous sports activities

15. Evaluating Results of Lumbar Spine Operations

In 1986 criteria were proposed for evaluating semi-quantitatively
pre- and post-operatively the economic and functional status of
patients undergoing treatment of lumbar spine disorders. (Table 1)
(Prolo *et al*, 1986). This outcome rating scale has since been used
extensively in the literature by authors assessing results of their
therapies in both the lumbar and cervical spine. A device manufacturer
has used it to document efficacy of the lumbar interbody fusion cage
for the Food and Drug Administration (Ray, 1997). The scale represents

a modification of the one used by Urist and Dawson (Urist and Dawson, 1981). It was initially applied to 34 patients undergoing posterior lumbar interbody fusion. Application of this rating scale demonstrated an 85% favourable response with a fusion incidence of 94%.

16. Evolutionary Healing of Cranial Grafts: Fresh Autograft, Demineralised Autolysed Antigen-extracted Allografts (AAA) and AAA Bone Powder

In 20 mm ungrafted defects of adult mongrel dogs, less than 20% of the defect volume is filled with new bone by six months (manuscript in preparation). The greatest rate of spontaneous filling of the defect occurs during the first six weeks (Table 2). Greater ingrowth occurs from the thicker medial than from the thinner lateral skull (Table 3) next to the defect, suggesting that endosteal cells of the diploic marrow contribute most to this repair rather than the dura mater or periosteum.

Both fresh autografts and demineralised AA allografts incorporate totally by six months, but autografts achieve this more rapidly. At six months autografts filled the entire defect; AA allografts filled less than 80%.

Table 2. Ungrafted defect at six weeks, 12 weeks and six months.

	Volume (%) of Defect Filled	New Bone (mm²)
6 Weeks	13.3 ± 3.41 (8)[a]	5.8 ± 1.59 (8)
12 Weeks	10.8 ± 3.31 (8)	5.9 ± 2.20 (8)
6 Months	19.7 ± 3.92 (8)	9.4 ± 1.77 (8)

[a]Mean ± standard error of the mean with number of defects observed in parentheses. The volume defect filled by new bone and the amount of new bone was greater at six months than at 12 or six weeks, $p < 0.025$.

Table 3. Distance new bone grew in from the medial and the lateral skull (mm).

	Ingrowth from Lateral Skull	Ingrowth from Medial Skull
6 Weeks	1.5 ± 0.5 (7)[a]	2.7 ± 0.5 (7)
12 Weeks	1.5 ± 0.5 (7)	2.3 ± 0.6 (7)
6 Months	2.0 ± 0.4 (14)	2.7 ± 0.2 (14)

[a]Mean ± standard error of the mean with the number of defects observed in parentheses. Spontaneous Repair of four defects, two at six months, one at 12 and six weeks each were two standard deviations above their group means, and, therefore, were not included in statistical evaluation. The difference between lateral and medial skull by the t-test for correlated data was significant ($t = 4.479$, $p < 0.01$).

In both the fresh autografts and AA allografts new bone formation sequentially progressed from the periphery to central areas of the graft by osteoconductive "creeping substitution." Pre-existing vascular channels in the cortical bone of the autograft were conduits for remodelling. In partially demineralised cortical bone of allografts and trabecular bone of autografts and allografts, extensive fields of new bone centripetally remodelled the graft from periphery to centre.

Allogeneic bone powder consisting of particles of various sizes was prepared under the same conditions as allogeneic skull disks. Smaller pieces were totally demineralised while large spicules retained mineral. Such grafts at 12 weeks fill less than 70% of the defect. Remodelling occurs over the external surface of the graft, and new bone appears to surround mineralised bone powder. Demineralised bone resorbs without promoting osteogenesis. New bone formation occurred around mineralised bone in the canine calvaria. Our observations coincide with those of Niederwanger and Urist that demineralised freeze-dried bone powder from four commercial banks implanted into Swiss-Webster and athymic mice induced none to minimal new bone or cartilage (Niederwanger and Urist, 1997).

17. Observations with Bone Morphogenetic Protein (BMP) in Cranial Defects at Six Months

Implants of human BMP within polylactic acid (PLA) wafers were provided by Dr. Marshall Urist (manuscript in preparation). In four of the five dogs the BMP implant was associated with considerably more new bone than the PLA-only control or the ungrafted defect. Skull trabeculae in the diploic space surrounding the BMP implant accumulated considerable tetracycline label. New bone also grew over and under the BMP implant. However, little new bone was able to penetrate the PLA carrier so that a defect, partially filled with the PLA wafer, remained.

18. Preliminary Long-term Results of over 300 Patients Undergoing Posterior Lumbar Interbody Fusion (PLIF)

Since 1981 over 300 patients have undergone PLIF with ethylene oxide (EO) sterilised/corticocancellous allografts prepared in our laboratory (manuscript in preparation). Extensive study will generate multiple perspectives and publications regarding indications, co-morbities, time course of fusion and outcome results using the economic/functional scale described above (Table 1).

With the application of the ordinal economic/functional rating scale in 215 patients analysed, 85% of patients achieved excellent or good results; 95% achieved solid fusion with EO-sterilised bone. In 310 patients none has become infected.

19. Conclusion

With faith in our potential for extending tissue transplantation to the neurosurgical community, Dr. Kenneth Sell called upon us to serve as one instrument of his grand design. We have proven the effectiveness and safety of ethylene oxide-sterilised allografts thousands of times in achieving interbody spinal fusions. We have confirmed the inimical environment of the skull in achieving experimental and human cranioplasty. In both the human and canine skull demineralisation of a bone implant consistently promotes non-osteoclastic resorption; mineralised calvaria slowly remodels, primarily through osteo-conductive "creeping substitution." Our experience with Dr. Urist's bone morphogenetic protein strongly suggests the ideal implant for cerebral protective and cosmetic cranioplasty will be autolysed, antigen extracted allogeneic largely mineralised bone impregnated with BMP. We hope our modest contributions have fulfilled Kenneth Sell's expectations.

Philosophers have long argued over the fundamental principles of morality and why one should obey them. Thomas Hobbes believed self-interest is the ultimate motive of all actions and is ultimately the sole good. Others argue that benevolence or the disinterested desire for the welfare of others as a basic a part of human nature as self-interest, and that by intuition benevolence should prevail over self-interest.

In 1759 a professor of Moral Philosophy in Glasgow published *The Theory of Moral Sentiments* (Smith, 1759). Adam Smith wrote that men when acting on enlightened self-interest and with sympathy for their fellow man serve not only their own best interests, but also the good of the community as a whole. They are guided in this as if by an "invisible hand" to promote an end which was not part of their intention.

The last quarter century reflects the invisible hand extending the boundaries of tissue transplantation. The era was introduced and blessed by the visible hand of Dr. Kenneth Sell presiding over its scientific birth. With passage of time the field has evolved with less science and more entrepreneurism. While the standards and rigours of tissue banking have risen, the science is in large part disengaged from tissue banks and rests in the universities which no longer operate tissue banks. For example, the epochal discovery of the bone morphogenetic protein at the University of California Los Angeles (UCLA) by Marshall Urist is the single largest accomplishment in tissue transplantation this century. With success in this industry now firmly ensconced in large multi-institutional commercial banks, it is fitting to celebrate the vision and pragmatic success of the one who simply began it all — Dr. Kenneth W. Sell.

20. References

BARTH, A. (1893). Ueber histologische befunde nach knochen-implantationen, *Arch. Klin. Chir.* **46**, 409–417.

BHAGAVAN, B.S., WENK, R.E., McCARTHY, E.F., GEBHARDT, F.C. and LUSTGARTEN, J.A. (1982). Long-term use of tetracycline, *JAMA* **247**, 2780.

BURWELL, R.G. (1966). Studies in the transplantation of bone: VIII. Treated composite homografts, autografts of cancellous bone: An analysis of inductive mechanisms in bone transplantation, *J. Bone Joint Surg. (Br.)* **48B**, 532–566.

NIEDERWANGER, M. and URIST, M.R. (1997). Demineralised bone matrix supplied by bone banks for a carrier of recombinant human bone morphogenetic protein (rh BMP-2): A substitute for autogeneic bone grafts, *J. Oral Implantology.* **XXII**, 210–215.

OKLUND, S.A., PROLO, D.J. and GUTIERREZ, R.V. (1981). The significance of yellow bone: Evidence for tetracycline in adult human bone, *JAMA* **246**, 761–763.

OKLUND, S.A., PROLO, D.J., GUTIERREZ, R.V. and KING, S.E. (1986). Quantitative comparisons of healing in cranial fresh autografts, frozen autografts, and processed autografts and allografts in canine skull defects, *Clin. Orthop.* **205**, 269–291.

OKLUND, S.A. and PROLO, D.J. (1990). Human skeletal growth and development. In: *CRC Handbook of Human Growth and Developmental*

Biology. Meisami, E. and Timiras P.S., eds., CRC Press, Inc., Boca Raton, Vol. 2, Part B, pp 53–67.

PROLO, D.J. (1979). Current thoughts on standards by a neurosurgeon. In: *American Association of Tissue Banks, Proceedings of the 1977 Annual Meeting.* K.W. Sell, V.P. Perry and M.M. Vincent, eds., American Association of Tissue Banks, Rockville Maryland, pp 115–116.

PROLO, D.J., BURRES, K.P., McCLAUGHLIN, W.T. and CHRISTENSEN, A.H. (1979). Autogenous skull cranioplasty: Fresh and preserved (frozen) with consideration of the cellular response, *Neurosurgery* **4**, 18–29.

PROLO, D.J. (1980). The neurosurgeon in transplantation: Provision and use of cadaver tissues and organs, *Neurosurgery* **6**, 342–343.

PROLO, D.J., PEDROTTI, P.W. and WHITE, D.H. (1980). Ethylene oxide sterilisation of bone, dura mater and fascia lata for human transplantation, *Neurosurgery* **6**, 529–539.

PROLO, D.J. (1981a). Use of transplantable tissue in neurosurgery. In: *Clinical Neurosurgery.* P.W. Carmel, ed., Williams and Wilkins, Baltimore, Vol. 28, pp 407–417.

PROLO, D.J. (1981b). The moral legitimacy of organ transplantation, *Neurosurgery* **8**, 510–512.

PROLO, D.J., PEDROTTI, P.W., BURRES, K.P. and OKLUND, S. (1982). Superior osteogenesis in transplanted allogeneic canine skull following chemical sterilisation, *Clin. Orthop.* **168**, 230–242.

PROLO, D.J. and OKLUND, S.A. (1983). Sterilisation of bone by chemicals. In: *Osteochondral Allografts Biology, Banking and Clinical Applications.* G.E. Friedlaender, H.J. Mankin, K.W. Sell, eds., Little Brown and Co., Boston, Chapter 22, pp 233–238.

PROLO, D.J., GUTIERREZ, R.V., DeVINE, J.S. and OKLUND, S. (1984). Clinical utility of allogeneic skull discs in human crainotomy, *Neurosurgery* **14**, 183–186.

PROLO, D.J. and OKLUND, S.A. (1984). Composite autogeneic human cranioplasty: Frozen skull supplemented with fresh iliac corticocancellous bone, *Neurosurgery* **15**, 846–851.

PROLO, D.J. (1985a). Transplantation of cadaver tissues and organs. In: *Neurosurgery*. R.H. Wilkins and S.S. Rengachary, eds., McGraw-Hill, New York, Part XV, Chapter 351, pp 2598–2601.

PROLO, D.J. (1985b). Cranial defects and cranioplasty. In: *Neurosurgery*. R.H. Wilkins and S.S. Rengachary, eds., McGraw-Hill, New York, Part VIII, Chapter 204, pp 1647–1656.

PROLO, D.J. and RODRIGO, J.J. (1985). Contemporary bone graft physiology and surgery, *Clin. Orthop.* **200**, 322–342.

PROLO, D.J., OKLUND, S.A and BUTCHER, M. (1986). Toward uniformity in evaluating results of lumbar spine operations. A paradigm applied to posterior lumbar interbody fusions, *Spine* **11**, 601–606.

PROLO, D.J. (1989). Osteosynthesis in lumbar interbody fusion. In: *Lumbar Interbody Fusion*. P.M. Lin and K. Gill., eds., Aspen Publishers, Inc., Rockville, MD, pp 71–78.

PROLO, D.J. (1990). Biology of Bone Fusion. In: *Clinical Neurosurgery*. P.M. Black., ed., Williams and Wilkins, Baltimore, Vol. 36, Chapter 10, pp 135–146.

PROLO, D.J. and OKLUND, S.A. (1991). The use of bone grafts and alloplastic materials in cranioplasty, *Clin. Orthop.* **268**, 270–278.

PROLO, D.J. and OKLUND, S.A. (1993). Report on the use of bank bone. In: *Spinal Trauma: Current Evaluation and Management. Neurosurgical Topics*. G.L. Rea and C.A. Miller, eds., *American Association of Neurological Surgeons*, Park Ridge, Illinois, Chapter 14, pp 213–218.

PROLO, D.J. and OKLUND, S.A. (1995). Bone healing and grafting in spinal surgery. In: *Techniques of Spinal Fusion and Stabilisation*. P.W.

Hitchon, V.C. Traynelis and S.S. Rengachary, eds., Thieme, New York, Chapter 6, pp 72–78.

PROLO, D.J. (1996a). Transplantation of cadaver tissues and organs. In: *Neurosurgery, 2nd ed.* R.H. Wilkins and S.S. Rengachary, eds., McGraw-Hill, New York, Chapter 442, pp 4253–4256.

PROLO, D.J. (1996b). Morphology and metabolism of fusion of the lumbar spine. In: *Neurological Surgery, 4th ed.* J.R. Youmans, ed., W.B. Saunders, Philadelphia, Chapter 109, pp 2449–2460.

PROLO, D.J. (1996c). Biology of bone. In: *Principles of Spinal Surgery.* A.H. Menezes and V.H.K Sonntag, eds., McGraw-Hill, New York, Chapter 9, pp 141–149.

PROLO, D.J. (1996d). Cranial defects and cranioplasty. In: *Neurosurgery, 2nd ed.* R.H. Wilkins and S.S. Rengachary, eds., McGraw-Hill, New York, Chapter 275, pp 2783–2795.

RAY, C.D. (1997). Threaded titanium cages for lumbar interbody fusions, *SPINE* **22**, 667–680.

RODRIGO, J.J. and PROLO, D.J. (1988). Allografts. In: *Operative Orthopedics.* M.W. Chapman, ed., Lippincott Co, Philadelphia, Chapter 71, pp 911–928.

SMITH, A. (1759). The Theory of Moral Sentiments. Macfie and D.D. Raphael, eds., Clarendon Press, 1974, Oxford.

STULA, D. (1984). *Cranioplasty Indications, Techniques and Results.* Springer-Verlag, New York, pp 1–112.

URIST, M.R. (1980). Bone transplants and implants. In: *Fundamental and Clinical Physiology of Bone.* M.R. Urist, ed., J.B. Lippincott Co, Philadelphia, pp 331–368.

URIST, M.R. and DAWSON, E. (1981). Intertransverse process fusion with the aid of chemosterilised autolysed antigen-extracted allogeneic (AAA) bone, *Clin. Orthop.* **154**, 97–113.

6.2 CARDIOVASCULAR TISSUE TRANSPLANTATION

M.H. GOLDMAN, S.L. STEVENS, M.B. FREEMAN,
M.P. OMBRELLARO, D.A. WEATHERFORD, T.R. REEVES,
V.L. ROWE, L. STEWART & T.T. REDDICK

The Division of Vascular and Transplantation Surgery
Department of Surgery
The University of Tennessee Graduate School of Medicine
1924 Alcoa Highway
Knoxville, Tennessee 37920, USA

1. Introduction

On August 13, 1975, Dr. Kenneth W. Sell opened the symposium commemorating the 25th anniversary of the United States Navy Tissue Bank entitled "Tissue Banking For Transplantation" with the call for an organisation to meld the concepts of tissue preservation, organ transplantation, and tissue bank organisation (Sell, 1976). He emphasised on uniform standards for procurement, graft selection, labelling, preservation, storage, use and performance in order to insure sterility, efficacy, availability; exclude disease transmission; and make a "maximum effort to insure that tissues or organs to be used are the best available." With this charge, he founded the American Association of Tissue Banks (AATB). He emphasised on the exchange of scientific information and rapid implementation of new developments. It is of note that he did not mention market share, competitive edge, proprietary information, patents, or profit in his launching of the AATB. That bit of wisdom would be left to those who benefited from his prescience yet found refuge behind the rhetoric of commercial competition. Dr. Sell followed a concept that was the result of 70 years of investigation predicated on the seminal work in preservation, transplantation and vascular surgery of the Nobel Laureate, Alexis Carrel. In addition to pioneering techniques of suturing, organ transplantation, cardiac repair, tissue preservation and tissue culture, and cryopreservation, Carrel initiated studies on vascular grafting, especially promoting the use of venous allografts (Carrel, 1905). He introduced and experimented with many forms of preservation including freezing, cooling and drying (Carrel, 1910). Dr. Sell's interest in the whole gamut of tissue transplantation led the transplantation laboratory at the Naval Medical Research Institute (NMRI) toward a series of experiments seeking to elucidate whether preserved cadaver vascular structures could be used as vascular substitutes.

2. Factors Important in the Function of Cardiovascular Grafts

The vascular graft, it was felt, had to be biocompatible, flexible, non-thrombogenic, conduct blood flow, be porous enough to permit ingrowth of tissue, allow for anastomotic integrity, and have durability (Table 1). Arteries, both fresh and cryopreserved, albeit in a rudimentary fashion, had shown early promise, but suffered from deterioration, aneurysm formation and lack of availability (Gross et al, 1948, 1949; Fisher et al, 1948; Kremer, 1953; Hufnagal et al, 1953). The concept of cadaver organ and tissue donation would wait for a few more generations before promulgation. It is of consequence that, in decrying the long-term durability or patency of allograft arteries, failure as a result of progression of disease was not differentiated from graft failure. It may be that much of the "graft loss" seen early on was from disease progression. In addition, synthetic grafts had come to the fore as suitable

Table 1. Features of a vascular graft.

Biocompatible
Flexible
Non-thrombogenic
Porous but not leaky
Anastomotic integrity
Durable
Available and not costly

for large vessel replacement, while the saphenous and cephalic vein autograft became the tissue of choice for medium and small vessel substitution. There seemed to be little impetus to look toward cadaver sources for alternatives. In fact, fresh cadaver grafts from limbs of war casualties had been found to have poor results when used as small vessel grafts to salvage limbs of contemporary injured soldiers (Jeger, 1915). After the advent of anticoagulation, the heart-lung machine, antibiotics and transfusion, cardiovascular surgery became dependent on the autogenous vein for small vessel bypass or replacement. However, the need for another stand-in for the venous autograft has recently become apparent as veins in some patients were found to be inadequate or depleted and synthetic grafts proved to be inferior in situations requiring small arterial conduits. No substitute was available for the venous circulation.

In reconsidering cadaver allografts as potential sources for small conduits the issues of thrombogenicity, durability, antigenicity, cost and availability had to be weighed in the context of whether cryopreserved tissue, which retained functional cellular elements, was desirable. Endothelium was felt to be necessary for anti-thrombogenicity, to provide local paracrine effects and to prevent intimal hyperplasia. Smooth muscle cells were viewed as important in promoting elasticity and maintaining the structural and functional integrity of the graft (Wolinsky and Glagov, 1964). Cryopreserved veins seemed to be an ideal candidate. Morphologic work showed that endothelium was not adversely affected by cryopreservation and in spite of the fact that some cells were lost during processing, fibrinolytic, endothelin and prostacyclin production was maintained (Sachs et al, 1982; Brockbank et al, 1990; Malone et al, 1980; Showalter et al, 1989). However, it was demonstrated that when cryopreserved veins were implanted into the arterial circulation, endothelium was denuded. (Calhoun et al, 1977; Faggioli et al, 1994). Moreover, all endothelial function was not normal after cryopreservation (Ligush et al, 1991). Cryopreserved arterial segments had been shown to have reduced contractile force and compliance, both endothelial and smooth muscle cell functions (Muller-Schweinitzer, 1994; Muller-Schweinitzer et al, 1997). They also had a propensity to fracture on thawing (Pegg et al, 1996). It seemed that the method of cryopreservation, the duration of storage and the method of thawing were important in providing functional and stable grafts (Table 2) (Brockbank, 1994; Elmore et al, 1991, 1992; Stevens et al, 1990). Preservation with a chondroitin sulphate-based methodology including dimethylsulfoxide (Me$_2$SO) was superior to Me$_2$SO alone in retaining normal morphology and some endothelial function. In contrast was the fact that the cryopreserved endothelium may have rendered the veins more contractile and hypothetically more susceptible to vasospasm (Elmore et al, 1991).

Table 2. Factors important in the function of cryopreserved cardiovascular tissue.

Procurement and handling
Equilibration medium and time
Cryopreservation technique
Duration of storage
Thawing technique
Immunogenicity

3. Immunogenicity of Cardiovascular Grafts

It was not completely compelling that transplanted cryopreserved endothelium would not induce an allogeneic immune response in the engrafted host. Early hypotheses that endothelium was weakly immunogenic or that cryopreservation might mitigate immunogenicity were based on patency as endpoints and did not rigorously confirm that viable endothelium was being transplanted (Schwartz *et al*, 1967; Harjola *et al*, 1969; Thiede *et al*, 1979; Ladin *et al*, 1982). Much contrary information was available. It was well known in the transplantation literature that endothelial cells expressed Class I major histocompatibility locus antigens, could be induced to express Class II antigens and could act as antigen presenting cells (Goldman *et al*, 1984, 1979; Pober *et al*, 1986; Ferry *et al*, 1987; Vetto and Burger, 1971; Burger and Vetto, 1982; Marin *et al*, 1990; Savage *et al*, 1993; Hirschberg *et al*, 1975). Also, histocompatibility matching and endothelial activation made a difference in animal models with respect to graft survival, evidence of acute rejection and chronic rejection (Calhoun *et al*, 1977; Stevens *et al*, 1990; Orosz, 1994). The lack of endothelium seemed to increase allograft patency while immunosuppression seemed to increase cryopreserved and fresh vessel transplant patency (Galumbeck *et al*, 1987; Miller *et al*, 1993; Augelli *et al*, 1991; Bandlien *et al*, 1983; Wagner *et al*, 1995). Not all studies confirmed that immunosuppression could abrogate the immune response to vascular grafts (Land and Messmer, 1996). The balance between transplanting a functional thrombosis protective endothelium and an immunologically active and response-promoting endothelium hung on how viable and functional the endothelial cells were in the early hours and days after transplantation; how fast repopulation by native cells occurred; how much immune response was generated; how much intimal hyperplasia and medial thickening was due to immune injury, preservation injury or lack of endothelial cells; and whether endothelium had a role in the long-termed integrity of the graft (Land and Messmer, 1996). Endothelial repopulation of the grafts occurred within two to three months. The hypothesised mechanisms included ingrowth from the anastomotic ends, fall out from circulating stem cells or ingrowth of capillaries through the walls of the graft. Capillary ingrowth seemed to affect midgraft hyperplasia while end ingrowth affected anastomotic hyperplasia. Capillary ingrowth was related to the porosity of the graft. Grafts, which were non-porous by virtue of having a wrap, tended to have less capillary ingrowth and retarded endothelialisation (Table 3).

Table 3. Effect of porosity, wrapping (w) and no wrap (nw) on capillary ingrowth and endothelialisation of the midgraft in two kinds of PTFE when placed endovascularly in canine aorta. The wrap is a non-porous PTFE coating.

Porosity (microns)	Endothelialisation (%)	Capillary ingrowth/40 ×
30 w	24	19
30 nw	70	50
60/20 w	24	38
60/20 nw	80	45

Smooth muscle cells may play a role in initiating or at least providing antigen for the recipient host to recognise and are known to be viable and functional after cryopreservation (Ricotta et al, 1979). Their role in contributing to immunogenicity, intimal thickening, and long-term integrity and function has not been thoroughly explored in the context of cryopreserved vascular allografts (Theobald et al, 1993). Intimal thickening is affected by many factors relating to the interplay of endothelial cells and smooth muscle cells. Shear stress changes, modulated by endothelial cell receptors, leads to activation and migration of smooth muscle cells (Dobrin et al, 1989; Morinaga et al, 1987). Anastomotic, immune, hypoxic, and denuding injury all activate processes ultimately resulting in vascular thickening which appears to be similar morphologically to chronic rejection (Land

and Messmer, 1996; Hayry, 1995). It seems that the development of anastomotic thickening may occur independently of the thickening in midgraft. It may be independent of the neointima formation seen in midgraft and may represent an injury response to the anastomotic procedure, effects of shear stress, or effects of compliance mismatch (DeWeese, 1978; Ombrellaro *et al*, 1995). Midgraft hyperplasia may be more closely dependent on re-endothelialisation and cytokine- and adhesion molecule-mediated interchanges between endothelial cells, smooth muscle cells and leukocytes (Ombrellaro *et al*, 1996; Weatherford *et al*, 1997). Curtailing the immune response with adequate immunosuppression until repopulation of both endothelial and smooth muscle cells by host origin cells may confer better patency and function but a satisfactory regimen in humans has not been found (Vischjager *et al*, 1996; Carpenter and Tomaszewski, 1997).

4. Preservation of Cardiovascular Grafts

Intimal hyperplasia and progression of native disease leading to graft thrombosis have been the most likely causes of the rather poor extended results achieved by cryopreserved cadaver allograft vessels both in the aortocoronary and in the peripheral positions (Vischjager *et al*, 1996; Carpenter and Tomaszewski, 1997; Shah *et al*, 1993; Laub *et al*, 1992; Sellke *et al*, 1989; Ochsner *et al*, 1984; Gelbfish *et al*, 1986). Patency rates have varied from 40–60% at one year with poorer results for infrapopliteal anastomoses. Cryopreserved veins, in the peripheral position, may not fare much better than synthetics and may be more costly (Table 4). Aneurysm formation has been a factor, although enough time may not have passed to assess the full impact of arterial pressure on the degenerative and reparative events *in vivo* (Schmitz-Rixen *et al*, 1988; Martin *et al*, 1994). Since aneurysmal dilatation occurs in autografted saphenous veins, it may be difficult to pick out a difference unless a comparative clinical study was performed (Szilagyi *et al*, 1973; Stanley *et al*, 1973). Early thrombosis may represent poor preservation of endothelium or technical misadventure. Of notable exception is the utility of cadaver veins in infected areas where

Table 4. Primary graft patency of cryopreserved allograft and other graft types in the infrageniculate position.

Graft Type	12 Months (%)
* Reverse saphenous vein	84
* *In situ* vein	80
* Arm vein	83
* Human umbilical vein	77
* PTFE	68
+ Cryopreserved allograft	41

References:
+ (Carpenter and Tomaszewski, 1997; Posner *et al*, 1996).
* (Dalman and Taylor, 1994).

prosthetic material is contraindicated (Fujitani *et al*, 1992; Snyder *et al*, 1987). However, unless the immunogenicity of the vascular material can be modified, the use of cryopreserved allograft vessels for bypass, valves for venous disease, and heart valves for cardiac surgery may be limited.

It was in the search for an allograft conduit that was not immunogenic that Dr. Sell supported the lyophilised vein project at the tissue bank of the Naval Medical Research Institute in Bethesda, MD, in 1978 (Goldman *et al*, 1981). Previous experience with lyophilised bone had shown that lyophilisation rendered the tissue less immunogenic. Lyophilised arterial segments had been used successfully in the past, but had been abandoned because of lack of tissue or because of degenerative changes (Creech *et al*, 1956; Brown *et al*, 1953). It was hoped that the lyophilised veins, essentially collagen and other structural protein tubes, would be non-immunogenic while remaining non-thrombogenic, patent and durable. Initial studies in ACI to Fischer rats demonstrated that lyophilised veins did not induce an antibody response when transplanted across a major histocompatibility barrier (Goldman *et al*, 1979). The veins, when allografted in dogs, were seen to reendothelialise and repopulate with smooth muscle-like cells, also to develop collagen profiles that indicated some scarring rather than native type collagen. Patency in the dog inferior vena cava (IVC), aorta, carotid artery, and as mesocaval shunts was excellent. Aneurysmal dilatation was not seen after 12–18 months (Goldman *et al*, 1978; Gottlob *et al*, 1982). It was felt that the increased porosity of the lyophilised veins allowed for more rapid neointima formation and greater durability, giving some credence to the capillary ingrowth theory (Muto *et al*, 1986). However, save one study using lyophilised veins as dialysis access grafts, the veins were rarely used clinically (Merrill *et al*, 1979). More recent work in our laboratory has led to the finding that lyophilisation does not disturb the function of venous valves. Lyophilised vein valves retain their competency and do not leak even under supraphysiologic back pressure (Reeves *et al*, 1997). It seems that lyophilised vein valves could be best suited for venous reconstruction for venous incompetence (Nash, 1988). They would be readily available and would not have the immune potential that cryopreserved venous valves might have.

The issue of immunogenicity surrounds the use of cryopreserved allograft heart valves as well (Cochran and Kunzelman, 1989; Baskett *et al*, 1996). Retrospective clinical studies with human cryopreserved valve grafts have reported reasonable intermediate length function with graft survivals of 89–100% at 7.5 years in the aortic position and 94% at 3.5 years in the pulmonic position (Shapira and Shemin, 1994; Doty *et al*, 1993; McGiffin *et al*, 1988; Kirklin *et al*, 1987; O'Brien *et al*, 1987). Allografts have also been used successfully for complete or partial mitral valve replacement (Acar *et al*, 1996). Freedom from thromboembolism seems to be a major advantage. The loss of valve function has been ascribed to immunologic events including ABO and HLA mismatching leading to degeneration or calcification (Yankah *et al*, 1995). Cryopreserved allografts have been shown to elicit in the recipient both broad- and donor-specific IgM and IgG to class I and class II HLA antigens, and to have induced increased alloreactivity in host T cells to donor lymphocytes (Shaddy *et al*, 1996; Hogan *et al*, 1996; Fischlein *et al*, 1995; Hoekstra *et al*, 1994). Some studies of post-cryopreservation and of explanted valves show absence of viable endothelial or smooth muscle cells leading to questions similar to those asked about cryopreserved vein grafts (Lupinetti *et al*, 1993; Schoen *et al*, 1995). Others have shown persistence of donor cells in explanted aortic valve replacements removed for technical malalignment (O'Brien *et al*, 1987). Is it better to have a viable endothelial layer and smooth muscle substrata remaining immunogenic or to have a non-viable stroma? The method of cryopreservation may play a significant role in determining how viable and therefore how immunogenic the valves are (Cochran and Kunzelman, 1989; McNally *et al*, 1989). It remains that cryopreserved valves do have a role in young people, in women who wish to have children and can not be on anticoagulation, pulmonic valve replacement, and in patients with endocarditis.

Therefore, what is the current status of cryopreserved cardio-vascular tissue and how has it changed since Dr. Sell's original research application (US Navy allocation for research moneys) providing resources to study vein transplantation for the repair of battle casualties at NMRI? Cryopreserved cardiovascular allograft tissues are still in a research era and should be handled as such. Xenografts have not been concertedly addressed and may pose further immunologic problems. Scientifically-valid clinical protocols using cryopreserved allografts should be undertaken. They should involve open comparison of cryopreservation techniques and contemporary comparison of alternative therapies so that outcomes may be genuinely analysed (Grunkemeier and Bodnar, 1995). Both clinical and fundamental work needs to be performed to answer the questions of the roles of viability, immunogenicity, immunosuppression, host environment and cryopreservation techniques in order that a graft which is acceptable, non-thrombogenic, and durable may be available. As initially envisioned by Dr. Sell in 1975, the goals of the American Association of Tissue Banks — setting standards in a free and scientific environment for provision of safe and efficacious tissue for the betterment of mankind — are still the guidelines which should shepherd advancements in cardiovascular tissue banking.

Acknowledgments

Supported in part by a grant from the Physicians Medical Education and Research Foundation, Knoxville, Tennessee.

References

ACAR, C., TOLAN, M., BERREBI, A., GAER, J., GOUEZO, R., MARCHIX, T., GEROTA, J., CHAUVAUD, S., FABIANI, J.N., DELOCHE, A. and CARPENTIER, A. (1996). Homograft replacement of the mitral valve. Graft selection, technique of implantation, and results in forty-three patients, *J. Thorac. Cardiovasc. Surg.* **111**, 367–378.

AUGELLI, N.V., LUPINETTI, F.M., EL KHATIB, H., SANOFSKY, S.J. and ROSSI, N.P. (1991). Allograft vein patency in a canine model. Additive effects of cryopreservation and cyclosporine, *Transplantation* **52**, 466–470.

BANDLIEN, K.O., TOLEDO-PEREYRA, L.H., BARNHART, M.I., CHOUDHURY, S.P., DIAZ-VELEZ, A., MCKENZIE, G.H. and CORTEZ, J.A. (1983). Improved survival of venous allografts following graft pretreatment with cyclosporine, *Transplant Proc.* **15**, 3084–3091.

BASKETT, R.J., ROSS, D.B., NANTON, M.A. and MURPHY, D.A. (1996). Factors in the early failure of cryopreserved homograft pulmonary valves in children: Preserved immunogenicity? *J. Thorac. Cardiovasc. Surg.* **112**, 1170–1178.

BROCKBANK, K.G., DONOVAN, T.J., RUBY, S.T., CARPENTER, J.F., HAGEN, P.O. and WOODLEY, M.A. (1990). Functional analysis of cryopreserved veins. Preliminary report, *J. Vasc. Surg.* **11**, 94–100.

BROCKBANK, K.G. (1994). Effects of cryopreservation upon vein function *in vivo*, *Cryobiology* **31**, 71–81.

BROWN, R.B., HUFNAGAL, C.A., PATE, J.W. and STRONG, W.R. (1953). Freeze-dried arterial homografts: Clinical application, *Surg. Gyn. Obst.* **97**, 657–661.

BURGER, D.R. and VETTO, R.M. (1982). Vascular endothelium as a major participant in T-lymphocyte immunity, *Cell Immunol.* **70**, 357–361.

CALHOUN, A.D., BAUR, G.M., PORTER, J.M., HOUGHTON, D.H. and TEMPLETON, J.W. (1977). Fresh and cryopreserved venous allografts in genetically characterised dogs, *J. Surg. Res.* **22**, 687–696.

CARPENTER, J.P. and TOMASZEWSKI, J.E. (1997). Immuno-suppression for human saphenous vein allograft bypass surgery: A prospective randomised trial, *J. Vasc. Surg.* **26**, 32–42.

CARREL, A. (1905). Anastomosis and Transplantation of Blood Vessels, *Am. Med.* **10**, 284–285.

CARREL, A. (1910). Latent life of arteries, *J. Exp. Med.* **12**, 146–176.

COCHRAN, R.P. and KUNZELMAN, K.S. (1989). Cryopreservation does not alter antigenic expression of aortic allografts, *J. Surg. Res.* **46**, 597–599.

CREECH, O.M., DEBAKEY, M.E. and COOLEY, D.A. (1956). Structural alterations in human aortic homografts in one to two and one-half years after transplantation, *Surg. Gyn. Obst.* **103**, 47–53.

DALMAN, R.L. and TAYLOR, L.M. (1994). Infrainguinal revascularisation procedures. In: *Basic Data Underlining Clinical Decision Making In Vascular Surgery.* J.M. Porter and L.M. Taylor, eds., Quality Medical Publishing Inc. St. Louis, pp 141–143.

DEWEESE, J.A. (1978). Anastomotic intimal hyperplasia. In: *Vascular Grafts.* P.N. Sawyer and M.J. Kaplitt, eds., Appleton-Century-Crofts, New York, pp 147–152.

DOBRIN, P.B., LITTOOY, F.N. and ENDEAN, E.D. (1989). Mechanical factors predisposing to intimal hyperplasia and medial thickening in autogenous vein grafts, *Surgery* **105**, 393–400.

DOTY, D.B., MICHIELON, G., WANG, N.D., CAIN, A.S. and MILLAR, R.C. (1993). Replacement of the aortic valve with cryopreserved aortic allograft, *Ann. Thorac. Surg.* **56**, 228–235.

ELMORE, J.R., GLOVICZKI, P., BROCKBANK, K.G. and MILLER, V.M. (1991). Cryopreservation affects endothelial and smooth muscle function of canine autogenous saphenous vein grafts, *J. Vasc. Surg.* **13**, 584–592.

ELMORE, J.R., GLOVICZKI, P., BROCKBANK, K.G. and MILLER, V.M. (1992). Functional changes in canine saphenous veins after cryopreservation, *Int. Angiol.* **11**, 26–35.

FAGGIOLI, G.L., GARGIULO, M., GIARDINO, R., PASQUINELLI, G., PREDA, P., FINI, M., CORBASCIO, M., STELLA, A., D'ADDATO, M. and RICOTTA, J.J. (1994). Long-term cryopreservation of autologous veins in rabbits, *Cardiovasc. Surg.* **2**, 259–265.

FERRY, B., HALTTUNEN, J., LESZCZYNSKI, D., SCHELLEKENS, H., MEIDE, P.H. and HAYRY, P. (1987). Impact of class II major histocompatibility complex antigen expression on the immunogenic potential of isolated rat vascular endothelial cells, *Transplantation* **44**, 499–503.

FISCHLEIN, T., SCHUTZ, A., HAUSHOFER, M., FREY, R., UHLIG, A., DETTER, C. and REICHART, B. (1995). Immunologic reaction and viability of cryopreserved homografts, *Ann. Thorac. Surg.* **60**, S122–S125.

FISHER, B., WILDE, R., ENGSTROM, P. and FISHER, E.R. (1948). Experimental reconstruction of the aortic bifurcation, *Surgery* **39**, 940–949.

FUJITANI, R.M., BASSIOUNY, H.S., GEWERTZ, B.L., GLAGOV, S. and ZARINS, C.K. (1992). Cryopreserved saphenous vein allogenic homografts: An alternative conduit in lower extremity arterial reconstruction in infected fields, *J. Vasc. Surg.* **15**, 519–526.

GALUMBECK, M.A., SANFILIPPO, F.P., HAGEN, P.O., SEABER, A.V. and URBANIAK, J.R. (1987). Inhibition of vessel allograft rejection by endothelial removal. Morphologic and ultrastructural changes, *Ann. Surg.* **206**, 757–764.

GELBFISH, J., JACOBOWITZ, I.J., ROSE, D.M., CONNOLLY, M.W., ACINAPURA, A.J., ZISBROD, Z., LIM, K.H., CAPPABIANCA, P. and CUNNINGHAM, J.N., JR. (1986). Cryopreserved homologous saphenous vein: Early and late patency in coronary artery bypass surgical procedures, *Ann. Thorac. Surg.* **42**, 70–73.

GOLDMAN, M.H., BRICKLEY-PARSONS, D., FOUTY, W.J., FLOERING, D.A., COLVIN, D.B., FORNEY, M.N. and FRENCH, D.C. (1978). Freeze-dried canine vena cava allografts as mesocaval shunts, *Trans. Am. Soc. Arti. Int. Organs*, **24**, 193–200.

GOLDMAN, M.H., STRONG, D.M., BRICKLEY-PARSONS, D., FLOERING, D.A., GAWITH, K. and FRENCH, D. (1979). Lyophilised veins as vascular substitutes, *Transplant. Proc.* **11**, 1510–1511.

GOLDMAN, M.H., FLOERING, D.A., FRENCH, D.R., GAWITH, K.E., FORGEY, J.D. and STRONG, D.M. (1981). Lyophilised veins as arterial interposition allografts, *Cryobiology* **18**, 306–312.

GOLDMAN, M.H., TUTTLE-FULLER, N., SALIM, J., BENDHEIM, S. and MOHANAKUMAR, T. (1984). Class I antibody induction by rat endothelium, *J. Surg. Res.* **36**, 327–331.

GOTTLOB, R., STOCKINGER, L. and GESTRING, G.F. (1982). Conservation of veins with preservation of viable endothelium, *J. Cardiovasc. Surg. (Torino)* **23**, 109–116.

GROSS, R.E., HURWITT, E.S., BILL, A.H. and PIERCE, E.C. (1948). Preliminary observations on the use of human arterial grafts in the treatment of certain cardiovascular defects, *N. Engl. J. Med.* **239**, 578–701.

GROSS, R.E., BILL, A.H. and PIERCE, E.C. (1949). Methods for preservation and transplantation of arterial grafts: Observations on arterial grafts in dogs: Report of transplantation of preserved arterial grafts in nine human cases, *Gurg. Gynecol. Obstet.* **88**, 689–701.

GRUNKEMEIER, G.L. and BODNAR, E. (1995). Comparative assessment of bioprosthesis durability in the aortic position, *J. Heart Valve Dis.* **4**, 49–55.

HARJOLA, P.T., SCHEININ, T.M. and TIILIKAINEN, A. (1969). Factors affecting early patency of human venous allografts in arterial reconstruction, *Ann. Clin. Res.* **1**, 169–176.

HAYRY, P. (1995). Aspects of allograft rejection. I: Molecular pathology of acute and chronic rejection, *Transplantation Rev.* **9**, 113–120.

HIRSCHBERG, H., EVENSEN, S.A., HENRIKSEN, T. and THORSBY, E. (1975). The human mixed lymphocyte-endothelium culture interaction, *Transplantation* **19**, 495–504.

HOEKSTRA, F., KNOOP, C., JUTTE, N., WASSENAAR, C., MOCHTAR, B., BOS, E. and WEIMAR, W. (1994). Effect of cryopreservation and HLA-DR matching on the cellular immunogenicity of human cardiac valve allografts, *J. Heart Lung Transplant.* **13**, 1095–1098.

HOGAN, P., DUPLOCK, L., GREEN, M., SMITH, S., GALL, K.L., FRAZER, I.H. and O'BRIEN, M.F. (1996). Human aortic valve allografts elicit a donor-specific immune response, *J. Thorac. Cardiovasc. Surg.* **112**, 1260–1266.

HUFNAGAL, C.A., RABIL, P.J. and REED, L. (1953). A method for the perservation of arterial homo and heterografts, *Surg. Forum* **4**, 162.

JEGER, E. (1915). Zur technik det blutgefassnaht, *Beitr. Klin. Chir.* **97**, 553–558.

KIRKLIN, J.W., BLACKSTONE, E.H., MAEHARA, T., PACIFICO, A.D., KIRKLIN, J.K., POLLOCK, S. and STEWART, R.W. (1987). Intermediate-term fate of cryopreserved allograft and xenograft valved conduits, *Ann. Thorac. Surg.* **44**, 598–606.

KREMER, K. (1953). Probleme der freien gefasstransplantation: Konservierungsmethoden zur aufbewahrung von gefasstransplanten, *Zentralbl. Chir.* **78**, 1857–1867.

LADIN, D.A., LINDENAUER, S.M., BURKEL, W.E. *et al* (1982). Viability, immunological reaction and patency of cryopreserved venous allografts, *Surg. Forum* **33**, 460–463.

LAND, W. and MESSMER, K. (1996). The impact of ischemia/reperfusion on specific and non-specific, early and late chronic events after organ transplantation, *Transplantation Rev.* **10**, 108–127.

LAUB, G.W., MURALIDHARAN, S., CLANCY, R., ELDREDGE, W.J., CHEN, C., ADKINS, M.S., FERNANDEZ, J., ANDERSON, W.A. and McGRATH, L.B. (1992). Cryopreserved allograft veins as alternative coronary artery bypass conduits: Early phase results, *Ann. Thorac. Surg.* **54**, 826–831.

LIGUSH, J., BERCELI, S.A., MOOSA, H.H., SHEPPECK, R.A., WARTY, V.S., ARMANY, M.A. and BOROVETZ, H.S. (1991). First results on the functional characteristics of cryopreserved human saphenous vein, *Cells and Materials* **1**, 359–368.

LUPINETTI, F.M., TSAI, T.T., KNEEBONE, J.M. and BOVE, E.L. (1993). Effect of cryopreservation on the presence of endothelial cells on human valve allografts, *J. Thorac. Cardiovasc. Surg.* **106**, 912–917.

MALONE, J.M., MOORE, W.S., KISCHER, C.W., KEOWN, K. and CONINE, R. (1980). Venous cryopreservation: Endothelial fibrinolytic activity and histology, *J. Surg. Res.* **29**, 209–222.

MARIN, M.L., HARDY, M.A., GORDON, R.E., REEMTSMA, K. and BENVENISTY, A.I. (1990). Immunomodulation of vascular endothelium: Effects of ultraviolet B irradiation on vein allograft rejection, *J. Vasc. Surg.* **11**, 103–111.

MARTIN, R.S., 3RD, EDWARDS, W.H., MULHERIN, J.L., JR., EDWARDS, W.H., JR., JENKINS, J.M. and HOFF, S.J. (1994). Cryopreserved saphenous vein allografts for below-knee lower extremity revascularisation, *Ann. Surg.* **219**, 664–670.

McGIFFIN, D.C., O'BRIEN, M.F., STAFFORD, E.G., GARDNER, M.A. and POHLNER, P.G. (1988). Long-term results of the viable cryopreserved allograft aortic valve: Continuing evidence for superior valve durability, *J. Card. Surg.* **3**, 289–296.

McNALLY, R., BARWICK, R., MORSE, B.S. and RHODES, P. (1989). Actuarial analysis of a uniform and reliable preservation method for viable heart valve allografts, *Ann. Thorac. Surg.* **48**, S82–S84.

MERRILL, R.H., MCLEOD, C.G., JR. and JARSTFER, B.S. (1979). The use of lyophilised vein grafts in vascular access for chronic hemodialysis, *Arti. Organs* **3**, 245–248.

MILLER, V.M., BERGMAN, R.T., GLOVICZKI, P. and BROCKBANK, K.G. (1993). Cryopreserved venous allografts: Effects of immuno-suppression and antiplatelet therapy on patency and function, *J. Vasc. Surg.* **18**, 216–226.

MORINAGA, K., EGUCHI, H., MIYAZAKI, T., OKADOME, K. and SUGIMACHI, K. (1987). Development and regression of intimal thickening of arterially transplanted autologous vein grafts in dogs, *J. Vasc. Surg.* **5**, 719–730.

MULLER-SCHWEINITZER, E. (1994). Applications for cryopreserved blood vessels in pharmacological research, *Cryobiology* **31**, 57–62.

MULLER-SCHWEINITZER, E., MIHATSCH, M.J., SCHILLING, M. and HAEFELI, W.E. (1997). Functional recovery of human mesenteric and coronary arteries after cryopreservation at −196 degrees C in a serum-free medium, *J. Vasc. Surg.* **25**, 743–750.

MUTO, Y., EGUCHI, H., MIYAZAKI, T., YUKIZANE, T., OKADOME, K. and SUGIMACHI, K. (1986). Modified vein allograft for small arterial reconstruction in dogs, *Jpn. J. Surg.* **16**, 225–230.

NASH, T. (1988). Long term results of vein valve transplants placed in the popliteal vein for intractable post-phlebitic venous ulcers and pre-ulcer skin changes, *J. Cardiovasc. Surg. (Torino)* **29**, 712–716.

O'BRIEN, M.F., STAFFORD, E.G., GARDNER, M.A., POHLNER, P.G. and McGIFFIN, D.C. (1987). A comparison of aortic valve replacement with viable cryopreserved and fresh allograft valves, with a note on chromosomal studies, *J. Thorac. Cardiovasc. Surg.* **94**, 812–823.

OCHSNER, J.L., LAWSON, J.D., ESKIND, S.J., MILLS, N.L. and DECAMP, P.T. (1984). Homologous veins as an arterial substitute: Long-term results, *J. Vasc. Surg.* **1**, 306–313.

OMBRELLARO, M.P., STEVENS, S.L., FREEMAN, M.B. and GOLDMAN, M.H. (1995). Intra-arterial stented grafts: The effect of intraluminal placement on prosthetic healing, *Surg. Forum* **46**, 373–377.

OMBRELLARO, M.P., STEVENS, S.L., KERSTETTER, K., FREEMAN, M.B. and GOLDMAN, M.H. (1996). Healing characteristics of intraarterial stented grafts: Effect of intraluminal position on prosthetic graft healing, *Surgery* **120**, 60–70.

OROSZ, C.G. (1994). Endothelial activation and chronic allograft rejection, *Clin.Transplant.* **8**, 299–303.

PEGG, D.E., WUSTEMAN, M.C. and BOYLAN, S. (1996). Fractures in cryopreserved elastic arteries, *Cryobiology* **33**, 658–659.

POBER, J.S., COLLINS, T., GIMBRONE, M.A., JR., LIBBY, P. and REISS, C.S. (1986). Inducible expression of class II major histocompatibility complex antigens and the immunogenicity of vascular endothelium, *Transplantation* **41**, 141–146.

POSNER, M.P., MAKHOUL, R.G., ALTMAN, M., KIMBALL, P., COHEN, N., SOBEL, M., DATTILO, J. and LEE, H.M. (1996). Early results of infrageniculate arterial reconstruction using cryopreserved homograft saphenous conduit (CADVEIN) and combination low-dose systemic immunosuppression, *J. Am. Coll. Surg.* **183**, 208–216.

REEVES, T.R., CEZEAUX, J.L., SACKMAN, J.E., CASSADA, D.C., FREEMAN, M.B., STEVENS, S.L. and GOLDMAN, M.H. (1997). The mechanical characteristics of lyophilised human saphenous vein valves, *J. Vasc. Surg.*, (in press).

RICOTTA, J.J., COLLINS, G.J. and RICH, N.M. (1979). Effects of aspirin and dextran on patency of bovine heterografts in the venous system, *Ann. Surg.* **189**, 116–119.

SACHS, S.M., RICOTTA, J.J., SCOTT, D.E. and DEWEESE, J.A. (1982). Endothelial integrity after venous cryopreservation, *J. Surg. Res.* **32**, 218–227.

SAVAGE, C.O., HUGHES, C.C., McINTYRE, B.W., PICARD, J.K. and POBER, J.S. (1993). Human CD4+ T cells proliferate to HLA-DR+ allogeneic vascular endothelium. Identification of accessory interactions, *Transplantation* **56**, 128–134.

SCHMITZ-RIXEN, T., MEGERMAN, J., COLVIN, R.B., WILLIAMS, A.M. and ABBOTT, W.M. (1988). Immunosuppressive treatment of aortic allografts, *J. Vasc. Surg.* **7**, 82–92.

SCHOEN, F.J., MITCHELL, R.N. and JONAS, R.A. (1995). Pathological considerations in cryopreserved allograft heart valves, *J. Heart Valve Dis.* **4**(Suppl 1), S72–S75.

SCHWARTZ, S.I., KUTNER, F.R., NEISTADT, A., BARNER, H., RESNICOFF, S. and VAUGHAN, J. (1967). Antigenicity of homografted veins, *Surgery* **61**, 471–477.

SELL, K.W. (1976). Tissue banking and transplantation in perspective. In: *Tissue Banking for Transplantation*. K.W. Sell and G.E. Friedlaender, eds., Grune and Stratton Inc. New York, pp 3–5.

SELLKE, F.W., MENG, R.L. and ROSSI, N.P. (1989). Cryopreserved saphenous vein homografts for femoral-distal vascular reconstruction, *J. Cardiovasc. Surg. (Torino)*. **30**, 838–842.

SHADDY, R.E., HUNTER, D.D., OSBORN, K.A., LAMBERT, L.M., MINICH, L.L., HAWKINS, J.A., McGOUGH, E.C. and FULLER, T.C. (1996). Prospective analysis of HLA immunogenicity of cryopreserved valved allografts used in pediatric heart surgery, *Circulation* **94**, 1063–1067.

SHAH, R.M., FAGGIOLI, G.L., MANGIONE, S., HARRIS, L.M., KANE, J., TAHERI, S.A. and RICOTTA, J.J. (1993). Early results with cryopreserved saphenous vein allografts for infrainguinal bypass, *J. Vasc. Surg.* **18**, 965–969.

SHAPIRA, O.M. and SHEMIN, R.J. (1994). Aortic valve replacement with cryopreserved allografts: Mid-term results, *J. Card. Surg.* **9**, 292–297.

SHOWALTER, D., DURHAM, S., SHEPPECK, R., BERCELI, S., GREISLER, H., BROCKBANK, K., MAKAROUN, M., WEBSTER, M., STEED, D. and SIEWERS, R. (1989). Cryopreserved venous homografts as vascular conduits in canine carotid arteries, *Surgery* **106**, 652–658.

SNYDER, S.O., WHEELER, J.R., GREGORY, R.T., GAYLE, R.G. and ZIRKLE, P.K. (1987). Freshly harvested cadaveric venous homografts as arterial conduits in infected fields, *Surgery* **101**, 283–291.

STANLEY, J.C., ERNST, C.B. and FRY, W.J. (1973). Fate of 100 aortorenal vein grafts: Characteristics of late graft expansion, aneurysmal dilatation, and stenosis, *Surgery* **74**, 931–944.

STEVENS, S.L., TYLER, J.D., FREEMAN, M.B., HOPKINS, F., LEWIS, T., BRAY, J., EDWARDS, A.L., BROCKBANK, K. and GOLDMAN, M.H. (1990). Factors affecting patency of venous allografts in miniature swine, *J. Vasc. Surg.* **12**, 361–366.

SZILAGYI, D.E., ELLIOTT, J.P., HAGEMAN, J.H., SMITH, R.F. and DALL'OLMO, C.A. (1973). Biologic fate of autogenous vein implants as arterial substitutes: Clinical, angiographic and histopathologic observations in femoro-popliteal operations for atherosclerosis, *Ann. Surg.* **178**, 232–246.

THEOBALD, V.A., LAUER, J.D., KAPLAN, F.A., BAKER, K.B. and ROSENBERG, M. (1993). "Neutral allografts" — lack of allogeneic stimulation by cultured human cells expressing MHC class I and class II antigens, *Transplantation* **55**, 128–133.

THIEDE, A., ENGEMANN, R., KORNER, H. and MULLER-RUCHHOLTZ, W. (1979). Comparison of the immunologic reactions of arterial transplants in the arterial system and of venous transplants in the venous system using inbred strains of rats, *Transplant. Proc.* **11**, 603–606.

VETTO, R.M. and BURGER, D.R. (1971). The identification and comparison of transplantation on canine vascular endothelium and lymphocytes, *Transplantation* **11**, 374–377.

VISCHJAGER, M., VAN GULIK, T.M., VAN MARLE, J., PFAFFENDORF, M. and JACOBS, M.J. (1996). Function of cryopreserved arterial allografts under immunosuppressive protection with cyclosporine A, *J. Vasc. Surg.* **24**, 876–882.

WAGNER, E., ROY, R., MAROIS, Y., DOUVILLE, Y. and GUIDOIN, R. (1995). Fresh venous allografts in peripheral arterial reconstruction in dogs. Effects of histocompatibility and of short-term immunosuppression with cyclosporine A and mycophenolate mofetil, *J. Thorac. Cardiovasc. Surg.* **110**, 1732–1744.

WEATHERFORD, D.A., OMBRELLARO, M.P., SCHAEFFER, D.O., STEVENS, S.L., SACKMAN, J.E., FREEMAN, M.B. and GOLDMAN, M.H. (1997). Healing characteristics of intraarterial stent grafts in an injured artery model, *Ann. Vasc. Surg.* **11**, 54–61.

WOLINSKY, H. and GLAGOV, S. (1964). Structural basis for the static mechanical properties of the aortic media, *Clin. Res. May.* **14**, 400–413.

YANKAH, A.C., ALEXI-MESKHISHVILI, V., WENG, Y., SCHORN, K., LANGE, P.E. and HETZER, R. (1995). Accelerated degeneration of allografts in the first two years of life, *Ann. Thorac. Surg.* **60**, S71–S76.

Chapter 7

BANKING AND CLINICAL USE OF HUMAN SKIN, BIOLOGICAL MEMBRANES AND ACELLULAR DERMIS

Many aspects of tissue banking had been included in Volume I of ADVANCES, with the exception of SKIN BANKING. This omission is rectified in this volume. Inclusion of papers dealing with this subject has a particular relevance to the tribute we seek to present for the life and work of Kenneth Sell. It was not until 1949, with the United States Tissue Bank, that modern day skin banking was heralded. This success, of course, drew upon the pioneering work of Thomas Gibson, Rupert Billingham and Peter Medawar in Glasgow and Oxford, UK, who demonstrated, for the first time, that allograft rejection was an immunological phenomenon, which Medawar terms as "actively acquired immunity." A simple experiment has shown that a "second set" of skin grafts from a parent to a burned child were rejected more quickly than the first set. Dr. Billingham was a good friend to Dr. Sell and was also a presenter at the 1975 Symposium. Dr. Kagan, who reviews human skin banking in this chapter, was a presenter at the 1997 Symposium.

The field has moved on to biological membranes, cultured keratinocytes, combinations of these, and now acellular human dermis. All are described in this chapter.

G.O.P.

7.1 HUMAN SKIN BANKING: PAST, PRESENT AND FUTURE

R.J. Kagan

University of Cincinnati College of Medicine
University Hospital Burn Special Care Unit
Ohio Valley Tissue & Skin Center
231 Bethesda Avenue
Cincinnati, Ohio 45267-0558, USA

1. Skin Banking: Past

Skin autografting was first described by Reverdin (Reverdin, 1871) and the clinical utility of allograft skin as a method of wound coverage followed shortly thereafter (Reverdin, 1872). Girdner (Girdner, 1881) was the first to report the use of allogeneic skin to cover a burn wound. However, it was not until five years later that Thiersch described the histological anatomy of skin engraftment and later popularised the clinical use of split thickness skin grafts (Thiersch, 1886).

Banking of human skin did not begin until the early 1900s. Wentscher reported the transplantation of human skin that had been refrigerated for 3–14 days (Wentscher, 1903); however it was not until the 1930s that blood and tissue banking took their place in the clinical practice of medicine. The clinical utility of allograft skin in burn wound coverage did not occur until 1938 when Bettman reported its success in the treatment of children with extensive full thickness injuries (Bettman, 1938). Webster and Mathews described the successful take of skin autografts stored for three weeks at 4–7°C (Webster, 1944; Mathews, 1945) yet it was not until 1949 that the United States Navy Tissue Bank was established, signalling the beginning of modern day skin banking.

Baxter explored the histological effects of freezing on human skin and identified the occurrence of ice crystal formation and tissue destruction (Baxter and Entin, 1948). This was followed in 1952 by the pioneering research of Billingham and Medawar demonstrating that skin could be effectively cryopreserved using glycerol (Billingham and Medawar, 1952). Taylor subsequently demonstrated that the utilisation of glycerol was associated with decreased ice crystal formation with freezing (Taylor, 1949). Shortly thereafter Brown and Jackson popularised the use of allogeneic human skin grafts as biological dressings for extensive burns and denuded tissue (Brown *et al*, 1953; Jackson 1954). By 1966, Zaroff reported the ten-year experience of the Brooke Army Medical Center with allograft skin in the treatment of thermally-injured patients (Zaroff *et al*, 1966). In their report, the authors described the mechanical and physiological benefits of allograft skin as a biological dressing. Later that year, Morris reported the beneficial effects of allogeneic skin in the treatment of infected ulcers and other contaminated wounds (Morris *et al*, 1966). In 1968, Cochrane reported the first successful clinical use of frozen autologous skin grafts having previously demonstrated the successful take of rat skin following controlled freezing in 15% glycerol and rapid rewarming prior to implantation (Cochrane, 1966). Shuck further extended the potential use of allogeneic skin to include traumatic wounds based upon the Vietnam war experience (Shuck *et al*, 1969). These increasing clinical uses of allograft skin led to further research into the mechanisms of its beneficial effects in wound healing, including the reduction of bacterial infection (Eade, 1958; Woods, 1960) and the stimulation of neovascularisation (O'Donaghue and Zarem, 1958).

Bondoc and Burke are credited with establishing the first functional skin bank in 1971 (Bondoc and Burke, 1971). Their experience with allograft skin led to a report of successful burn wound excision and allografting with temporary immunosuppression in children with massive injuries (Burke *et al*, 1975). Today, allograft skin remains an ideal temporary cover for extensive or excised cutaneous or soft tissue wounds, particularly when the use of autologous tissue is not clinically indicated or when sufficient autograft skin is not available.

2. Skin Banking: Present

2.1. Clinical uses of allograft skin

2.1.1. *Coverage of extensive full thickness wounds*

The clinical use of allograft skin in specialised burn care centres has been one of the driving forces behind the growth and development of skin banks in the United States. The general indications for its use in wound management are listed in Table 1. Allograft skin possesses

Table 1. Indications for allograft skin use in wound management.

Coverage of extensive wounds where autologous tissue is not available
Coverage of widely meshed skin autografts
Extensive partial thickness burns
Extensive epidermal slough
Testing for the ability to accept autograft
Template for the delayed application of keratinocytes

Table 2. Advantages of human allograft skin use.

Reduce water, electrolyte and protein loss
Prevent desiccation of tissue
Suppress bacterial proliferation
Reduce wound pain
Reduce energy requirements
Promote epithelialisation
Prepare wounds for definitive closure
Provide dermal template for epidermal grafts

many of the ideal properties of biological dressings and plays a major role in the surgical management of extensive wounds when autologous tissue may not be immediately available (Table 2). It reduces evaporative water loss and the drainage of protein-rich fluids, prevents wound desiccation, and suppresses microbial proliferation. Wound pain is lessened and is associated with better patient compliance with occupational and physical therapy. By restoring a physiological barrier at the wound surface, it reduces heat loss through the wound and mitigates the hypermetabolic stress response to burn injury. Fresh (viable) allograft skin represents the gold standard for biological dressings employed for temporary wound closure (Table 3). Its use has become critically important for the surgeon faced with the immediate coverage of excised massive burn wounds. Allogeneic grafts are best applied unmeshed in order to maximise their effects as a temporary wound cover. Meshing of fresh allograft skin is rarely performed because re-epithelialisation of the interstices by allogeneic epidermis is uncommon. The allografts become well-vascularised, stimulate neovascularisation in the underlying wound bed, and provide temporary wound closure while preparing the recipient site for permanent coverage with autologous skin. In addition, fresh (refrigerated) allografts tolerate modest wound contamination and adhere better to the freshly-excised subcutaneous fat than do cryopreserved grafts. The allogeneic skin is usually removed once the patient's donor sites are healed sufficiently for reharvesting or once autologous cultured skin is available for permanent wound closure.

Table 3. Advantages of fresh allograft skin.

Rapidity and strength of adherence to the wound
Control of microbial growth
Rapidity of revascularisation
Reproducible clinical results

When refrigerated (fresh) allograft is not available, cryopreserved skin is an excellent alternative for temporary wound coverage. Although frozen cryopreserved skin generally has less measurable viability than fresh skin, it is generally difficult to maintain continuous and ample stores of fresh skin beyond 14 days. It has therefore been a standard practice in skin banking to cryopreserve allograft skin that is not needed within 7–14 days rather than discard it. In fact, it is the potential and unpredictable demand for allograft skin in specialised burn care centres that has prompted the growth and development of local and regional skin banks throughout the world. Further research in allograft skin cryopreservation will be essential in order to maintain an ample supply of viable tissue for clinical use.

2.1.2. *Coverage of widely meshed skin autografts*

Another use of allograft skin has been its placement on top of widely expanded, meshed autologous skin grafts (Fig. 1). Originally, this technique was described utilising meshed allograft (Alexander *et al*, 1981). This method does not provide coverage for the entire wound; therefore most burn surgeons currently performing overlay allografting use non-meshed (sheet) allograft. This affords better protection of the open interstices of the autograft from desiccation and microbial contamination until epithelialisation is complete. While this technique may play a role in the management of massive excised full thickness injuries, it should be used with discretion since many surgeons have expressed concern that the overlying allograft may induce an inflammatory rejection response that can retard the rate of re-epithelialisation of the underlying autografts. Some have therefore advocated the use of lyophilised allograft for this purpose as it is less viable and less antigenic.

2.1.3. *Healing of partial thickness wounds*

Frozen allograft skin is an excellent wound cover when vascularisation and adherence is not desired. Because it is usually less viable than fresh skin, it functions more as a biological dressing than as a temporary

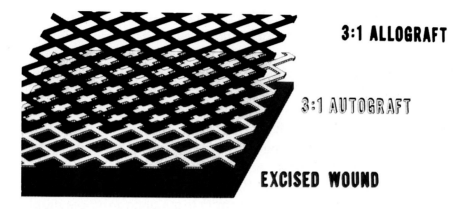

3:1 ALLOGRAFT

3:1 AUTOGRAFT

EXCISED WOUND

Fig. 1. Diagrammatic illustration of meshed allograft overlay technique as described by Alexander (1981). The allograft is generally meshed 1.5:1 or 3:1 while the underlying autograft may be meshed 3:1 or greater.

skin replacement. Its adherence to the underlying wound bed results in the relief of pain and the limitation of exudative and water losses, and reduces the need for frequent painful dressing changes. As the partial thickness wound re-epithelialises, the allograft slowly separates without disturbing the delicate autologous epithelium. Although this application is probably not cost effective in the management of small second-degree burns or skin graft donor sites, it is often beneficial in cases of extensive partial thickness wounds where its ability to prevent desiccation and promote epithelialisation may reduce hospital stay and/or the need for autografting. In addition, cryopreserved allograft is an excellent biological dressing for the management of patients with extensive cutaneous wounds resulting from drug reactions or superficial skin disorders (i.e. toxic epidermal necrolysis, Stevens-Johnson syndrome, Staphylococcal scalded skin syndrome). When used for superficial wounds of this nature, allograft skin should be applied prior to exposing the wound to topical antibiotics since these agents tend to have an adverse affect on allograft adherence to the wound surface.

2.1.4. Testing for later acceptance of autograft

Both cryopreserved and fresh allograft have been used by physicians for the care of a variety of cutaneous and soft tissue wounds. In these instances, allograft is used to provide a temporary biological cover and to help predict the likelihood of an autologous graft later in the course of treatment. Allograft usage for this indication has been most common in the management of deep electrical burns in the process of demarcation and escharotomy or fasciotomy sites although it can also be used to temporarily cover extensive open abdominal and soft tissue wounds. Adherence or vascularisation of the allograft is a reliable indication that the wound bed has sufficient blood supply to accept an autologous graft or flap.

2.1.5. Template for delayed application of keratinocytes

The clinical use of cultured epidermal autografts (CEA) in the care of burn patients was first described in 1981 (O'Connor *et al*, 1981). Since that time, there have been numerous reports supporting its use as a permanent skin replacement for patients with extensive full thickness burn injuries. This methodology has not been without problems, however, with many authors describing variable take rates and instability of the grafts. Cuono first advocated the use of allogeneic skin with CEA, allowing the allograft skin to vascularise before removing the antigenic epidermal layer by dermabrasion (Cuono *et al*, 1986). Hickerson reported his results on five burn patients demonstrating over 90% CEA take on the allogeneic dermis and supple, durable grafts up to four years post-operatively (Hickerson *et al*, 1994).

The past decade has also witnessed the development of an acellular dermal matrix (AlloDerm[R]) as a template for the simultaneous application of thin split thickness autografts (Livesey *et al*, 1995). The potential advantage of the dermal template is reasoned to be the use of a thinner autologous skin graft donor site with its resultant quicker healing time and reduced donor site scarring. A recently completed multicentre clinical trial demonstrated equivalence of this technique with a standard split thickness meshed autograft; however, autograft take rates were somewhat lower than that for controls and varied from centre to centre (Wainwright et al, 1996). In addition, the allogeneic dermal grafts measured only 36–116 cm^2 and were only evaluated up to 180 days post-grafting. AlloDerm^R has also been used as a template for CEA, however, there have only been anecdotal reports regarding the results of this potential application.

2.1.6. Micrografting techniques

Chinese surgeons have proposed the use of micrografts using both autologous and allogeneic skin (Zhang et al, 1988). This technique involves the mincing of autologous skin into pieces less than 1 mm in diameter. These micrografts are then used to seed the dermal surface of large sheets of allograft skin prior to transplantation onto the excised burn wound. As the autologous epidermal cells propagate on the wound surface, the allograft skin gradually separates in a manner similar to that observed with the overlay technique. This method, while resulting in an effective skin expansion ratio approaching 1:18, has been shown to be associated with severe wound contraction that is often worse than that noted with meshed skin grafts.

2.2. Potential disadvantages of allograft skin use

2.2.1. Infection

Allograft skin has been reported to cause bacterial infection (Monafo and Bradley, 1976), therefore, it is imperative that skin banks perform microbial cultures prior to release for transplantation (Table 4). Although White has suggested that cadaver allograft containing < 10^3 organisms/gram of tissue can be safely used for wound coverage (White et al, 1991), current American Association of Tissue Banks (AATB) Standards require that skin be discarded if pathogenic bacteria or fungi are present. This is particularly important given the immunocompromised status of the potential recipient and the likelihood of developing wound sepsis following such contamination.

Table 4. Disadvantages of human allograft skin use.

Potential infectious disease transmission
    Bacteria
    Viruses
        – HIV-1
        – CMV
Antigenicity
Rejection
Potential lack of availability

There have also been reports of viral disease transmission by skin allografts. In 1987, Clarke reported the transmission of HIV-1 to a burn patient from an HIV-positive donor (Clarke, 1987); results of donor testing were not known prior to skin use. To date, there have been no other reported cases of HIV or hepatitis transmission from skin allografts. Kealey has recently reported the transmission of cytomegalovirus (CMV) in cadaver skin allografts (Kealey *et al*, 1996). Because five of 22 CMV-negative patients (22.7%) seroconverted, the authors have recommended the use of CMV-negative allograft skin for seronegative burn patients. While there is good evidence to support the transmission of CMV by allograft in burn patients, there is little evidence that CMV seroconversion is clinically significant or affects outcome (Herndon and Rose, 1996). This is particularly important since approximately 60% of banked allograft skin is obtained from CMV-positive donors.

2.2.2. Rejection

While demonstrating many characteristics of an ideal wound covering, allograft skin contains Langerhans cells which express class II antigens on their surface. These cells reside in the epidermis of the skin and will ultimately result in an immunological rejection response. This typically results in an acute inflammatory reaction and may lead to the development of a deep wound infection. Vascularised allogeneic skin grafts typically remain intact on the wound of a burn patient for two to three weeks although there have been reports of allograft skin survival for up to 67 days due in part to the inherent immunosuppression of extensive burn injury (Ninnemann *et al*, 1978). Recent improvements in immunonutrition, critical care management, and a more aggressive surgical approach to definitive wound closure, however, have made the persistence of engraftment less predictable.

Efforts to prevent rejection have included methods that might reduce antigen expression by controlling Langerhans cell activity in the allograft skin. Treatment of the allografts with ultraviolet light irradiation and incubation of the skin in glucocorticoids has been reported to result in a modest prolongation of allograft survival compared to non-treated skin. However, these clinical trials were limited and the utility of this methodology has not been substantiated. In addition, investigators have studied the effects of pharmacological agents to induce immunosuppression in patients with major burn injuries (Burke *et al*, 1974). Initial clinical trials reported improved allograft and patient survival in children treated with azathioprine and antithymocyte globulin. This regimen was associated with azathioprine-induced neutropenia and patient outcome data has not been corroborated by others. More recently, the use of cyclosporin A has been demonstrated to prolong skin allograft survival in patients with extensive full thickness thermal injuries (Achauer *et al*, 1986; Sakabu *et al*, 1990). Allograft rejection is generally observed within a few days of discontinuing treatment; however, there have been instances where engraftment has persisted after the completion of therapy. Further studies of these and newer immune suppressive agents appear warranted.

2.3. The growth of skin banking

The widespread use of allograft skin in the management of patients with extensive burn, traumatic and soft tissue injuries has had a major impact on the number of skin banking facilities over the past two decades. Consequently, the majority of skin banks have been founded in close proximity to regional burn centres or within the burn centre hospitals themselves. Skin banks must therefore maintain a close working relationship with regional burn centres not only to meet the specific needs of the burn surgeon but also to help generate community support for skin donation through combined educational outreach programmes.

Between 1969 to 1988, there was a steady growth in the number of active skin banks in the United States, however this appears to have reached a plateau during the past ten years (Fig. 2). It is estimated that there are currently 44 operational skin banks in North America, however, data from these facilities indicates that there is insufficient allograft skin available to meet the estimated 32 000 ft^2 needed (DeClement and May, 1983) in burn and wound care centres. In fact,

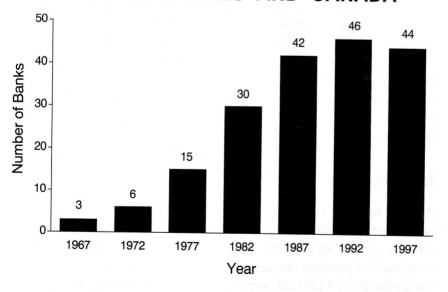

Fig. 2. Growth in the number of skin banks in the United States and Canada (from May (1990) and American Association of Tissue Banks).

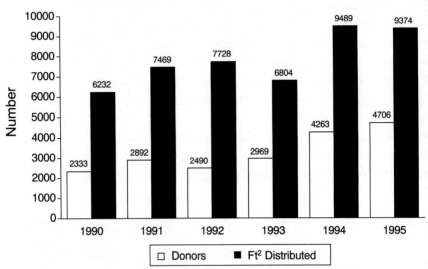

Fig. 3. Allograft skin donation and distribution from 1990–1995. (Source: American Association of Tissue Banks).

in 1995, only an estimated 9400 ft^2 was distributed (Fig. 3). Furthermore, because of the limited supply of allograft skin for transplantation, only skin that is not suitable for transplantation is available for scientific research.

2.4. Role of the american association of tissue banks

As skin banking facilities grew in number, it became apparent that policies and procedures required standardisation. This was quite difficult initially as there was insufficient data to develop a consensus regarding standards of practice. As early as 1976, the American Association of Tissue Banks (AATB) had begun to address this issue by the formation of the Skin Council. This provided a forum for the discussion of skin banking practices and was complimented by the activities of the

American Burn Association's Skin Banking Special Interest Group. The Standards and Procedures Committees were created in 1977 and produced the first "Guidelines" for tissue banking in 1979. The first *Standards for Tissue Banking* were published in 1984 and tissue-specific technical manuals (including skin) were developed in 1987. Since that time, the Standards have been modified and refined based upon consensus and, where available, supportive scientific research.

Shortly after the development and promulgation of its *Standards for Tissue Banking*, the AATB created an inspection and accreditation committee in 1982 and began conducting voluntary, peer-review inspections by 1986. To date, approximately 20 organisations involved in the banking of human skin have received accreditation, the majority of which are multi-tissue banking facilities.

2.5. Technical aspects of skin banking

2.5.1. Donor screening

It is vitally important that complete and accurate medical information about the potential donor be obtained to ensure the safety of the tissue for transplantation. The AATB and the US Food and Drug Administration (FDA) require a comprehensive medical and social history of the donor, a physical examination of the potential donor, and a panel of serologic screening tests for viral diseases (HIV-1/2, Hepatitis B and C, and HTLV-I). Recently, the AATB developed a "Donor Medical History and Behavioral Risk Assessment Questionnaire" with the cooperation and assistance of the FDA and other organ and tissue procurement organisations to help facilitate this process. It is also important that the time of death and body storage conditions be accurately documented as these have a significant bearing upon skin viability and microbial contamination. In addition, a thorough physical examination is necessary to determine the quality of the skin and the technical feasibility of skin retrieval by evaluating the donor's size, overall health status, and skin condition. Table 5 lists those conditions which are commonly associated with deferral of a potential skin donor.

Table 5. Disease states commonly associated with potential skin donor deferral.

Extensive dermatitis
Acute burn injuries
Cutaneous malignancy
Poor skin quality
Extensive tattoos
Collagen vascular disease
Toxic chemical exposure
Skin infections
Extensive skin lesions
Extensive skin or soft tissue trauma

2.5.2. Skin recovery

Once donor screening is complete and proper consents have been obtained, the recovery team must arrange the time and location for skin removal in an appropriate facility (i.e. hospital morgue or operating room, medical examiner's office, or the tissue bank). Skin retrieval should be performed expeditiously to minimise tissue deterioration and contamination. Current AATB Standards require that skin retrieval begin within 24 hours of death if the donor is refrigerated, within 12 hours of asystole or within 15 hours if refrigeration has not occurred.

In brief, the skin is removed under aseptic conditions. The areas from which the skin is taken are shaved of hair and cleansed with detergent solutions approved for use in operative procedures (i.e. povidone-iodine, chlorhexidine). This is usually followed by an iodophor prep and rinsing with 70% isopropanol. The retrieval technician puts on a cap and mask, performs a surgical scrub, and dons a sterile gown and gloves while the circulating technician prepares tissue and transport containers. The donor is then draped with sterile sheets and a blood sample is obtained by an intraventricular cardiac puncture. Following this, a thin layer of sterile mineral oil (or other sterile lubricant) is applied to the surfaces from which skin is to be removed. Split thickness skin grafts are then removed using an electric dermatome at a thickness of 0.012–0.018 inches. The width of the grafts generally range from 3–4 inches, but ideally should be determined by the preference of the transplanting surgeon. Skin retrieval sites are usually limited to the torso, hips, thighs, and upper calves. The amount of skin obtained per donor may vary depending on body habitus, skin defects or lesions, and body geometry. However, an average of 4–6 ft^2 per donor is not unusual. After tissue is obtained from the anterior surfaces, the donor is turned to the prone position, reprepped and draped prior to completing the retrieval process. The skin is then placed in tissue culture medium and maintained at 1–10°C during transport to the skin bank for processing.

2.5.3. Skin processing

2.5.3.1. Processing environment

Skin is processed under aseptic conditions. Current AATB Standards indicate the need for processing in a class 10 000 laminar flow environment, yet recent data from our skin bank suggests that this offers no benefit over processing in a class 100 000 clean room (Plessinger *et al*, 1997).

2.5.3.2. Microbiologic testing

After returning to the skin bank, the procurement team obtains microbiologic cultures for aerobic and anaerobic bacteria, yeast, and fungi. Samples are best obtained prior to exposure of the skin to antibiotics. It is generally recommended that a 1 cm^2 biopsy sample be taken for each 10% of the body surface area from which the skin has been removed (May and DeClement, 1981). Testing should be conducted in accordance with the National Committee on Clinical Laboratory Standards. Allograft skin should not be used for transplantation if it contains any of the following: (1) Coagulase-positive

Staphylococci, (2) Group A, beta-haemolytic *Streptococci,* (3) *Enterococci,* (4) gram-negative organisms, (5) *Clostridia sp.,* or (6) yeast or fungi. Contamination can be minimised by meticulous donor preparation and adherence to aseptic techniques. Incubation in antibiotics is somewhat controversial since many antibiotics are unable to effectively kill microorganisms at 4°C and there is the potential for exposing the recipient to resistant organisms. In addition, skin banking research has yet to determine which antibiotic combinations are effective against the commonly encountered organisms yet non-toxic to the cellular components of the skin.

2.5.3.3. Maintenance of viability

The maintenance of cell viability and structural integrity are keys to the engraftment and neovascularisation of allograft skin, yet there has been no quantification of the viability necessary for allograft "take". Post-mortem time lapse appears to have the single greatest effect on skin viability. May has demonstrated that the functional metabolic activity of the skin rapidly declines if the donor is not refrigerated within 18 hours of death (May and DeClement, 1981). The ideal nutrient tissue culture medium has not yet been identified. Eagle's MEM and RPMI-1640 continue to be generally accepted; however, Cuono has demonstrated the potential benefits of the University of Wisconsin's (UW) solution (Brown and Cuono, 1992). Lastly, it remains unclear which cryoprotectants offer the greatest preservation of cell viability and structural integrity. Glycerol (10–20%) and dimethylsulfoxide (10–15%) have been reported to maintain skin viability following incubation times ranging from 30 minutes to two hours, yet the optimal concentrations of these cryoprotectants have not been identified nor have these agents been compared for efficacy. Donor factors such as age and gender do not appear to influence skin viability.

Refrigeration

"Fresh" allograft skin is the preferred biological dressing for the temporary coverage of excised extensive full thickness burn wounds due to its more rapid adherence and vascularisation. The skin is stored at 4°C in tissue culture medium with or without antibiotics. Refrigeration slows the metabolic rate of the viable cells and the nutrient tissue culture medium supports cellular metabolic activity. The major shortcoming of this storage method is the limited time that viability can be maintained. May demonstrated that glucose metabolism declines at a rate of 10–15% each day during refrigerated storage (May and DeClement, 1982); therefore it has been common practice to cryopreserve skin within five to seven days of refrigeration. Recent studies (Robb *et al*, 1997; Rosenquist *et al*, 1988) suggest that skin viability can be maintained for up to two weeks at 4°C if the nutrient medium is changed every three to five days.

Cryopreservation

When skin is frozen for long-term storage, it is important that the methods utilised maintain cell viability and structural integrity. If the skin is not to be used "fresh," it should be cryopreserved within ten days of procurement. The skin is generally incubated in cryoprotectant solution for 30 minutes at 4°C. This is followed by slow cooling at a rate of approximately –1°C per minute. Although computer-assisted, control-rate freezing is thought to be optimal (Aggarwal *et al*, 1985), studies have demonstrated that cooling in a heat sink box at less than –2°C per minute is equally effective and does not compromise the metabolic activity of the skin (Cuono *et al*, 1988). The skin is frozen at –70 to –100°C prior to placement in either a mechanical freezer or liquid nitrogen. Although this methodology has been reported to result in 85% retention of viability (May and DeClement, 1981), there remains a need for research to determine the optimal technology for skin preservation.

2.5.4. Lyophilisation

Skin can also be lyophilised by freeze drying or incubation in glycerol. This process has been reported to decrease biological degradation and antigenicity. However, this also results in epidermal cell destruction and loss of barrier function. Moreover, lyophilised allograft skin has poor adherence to the excised wound bed, and is far less effective than "fresh" skin or cryopreserved skin in controlling microbial growth (Pruitt and Levine, 1984). Its clinical use has been further limited by its high cost of production compared to conventional allograft.

2.5.4.1. Skin storage

Refrigerated allograft skin should be stored in nutrient tissue culture medium at 4°C. The skin should be free-floating in an aseptic container with 300 ml of medium per square foot of skin. The medium should be changed twice weekly to maintain optimal viability (Robb *et al*, 1997). Skin that is to be frozen should be folded with fine mesh gauze or bridal veil covering the dermal surface prior to placement in a flat packet to ensure uniformity of the cooling process (May and DeClement, 1980). Skin stored in a mechanical freezer (−70 to −100°C) can be maintained for three to six months whereas storage in liquid nitrogen (−150 to −196°C) has been shown to maintain viability for up to ten years.

2.5.4.2. Transport

Refrigerated skin should be transported in tissue culture medium at wet ice temperatures (1–10°C) in an insulated container. Frozen allograft skin is transported on dry ice in an insulated container to prevent the skin temperature from rising to greater than −50°C. If the frozen skin is thawed at the tissue bank, it should be transported at wet ice temperatures.

2.5.4.3. Rewarming

Rewarming of frozen cryopreserved allograft skin must be performed in such a manner as to minimise cryodamage and preserve the structural integrity and viability of the skin. Early studies (Lehr *et al*, 1964) demonstrated that warming rates of 50–70°C/min resulted in 80–95%

graft survival. Subsequent research (May and DeClement, 1981) revealed that warming should be performed in less than two to four minutes at a temperature of 10–37°C (127–470°C/min). Rewarming in a microwave is not recommended due to uneven heating and excessive intracellular temperatures.

3. Skin Banking: Future

Skin banking must continue to evolve as engineered skin substitutes enter the clinical arena for the temporary and permanent coverage of partial and full thickness wounds. A number of skin substitutes have recently received FDA approval for use in the United States and have become part of the surgeon's armamentarium. Although they are generally more costly than allograft skin, such products possess a number of attributes including: (1) non-antigenicity, (2) ready availability, (3) sterility, and (4) the ability to provide a dermal equivalent as a template for the later application of thin (0.006 inch) split thickness autografts.

Allograft skin has the potential to play a major role in permanent skin reconstruction after extensive thermal injury; however this will require interactive research with the burn centres caring for these patients. In addition, skin banks must identify ways of increasing cadaveric skin donation, ensuring recipient safety from potential disease transmission, and reducing procurement and processing costs while optimising allograft viability. This will become increasingly difficult as it becomes necessary to perform additional and newer microbiological testing procedures. To accomplish these goals, it may become necessary for skin banking operations to become regionalised. Such an undertaking could enhance tissue supplies and availability and result in increased clinical use by surgeons.

3.1 Allograft-based skin products

There is tremendous potential for human allograft-based skin products to be developed in the upcoming years. However, it will become increasingly important for skin banks to perform basic science and clinical research (in conjunction with burn and wound healing centres) to demonstrate the clinical indications and efficacy of allograft skin products in various clinical applications. Technological advances may include modifications to reduce immunogenicity and/or the potential for disease transmission. Newer processing techniques could sterilise the skin without injuring the viable cellular elements or the structural integrity of the tissue. In addition, with continued research, de-epidermised allograft dermis could become (1) a source of growth factors and antimicrobial agents, (2) a permanent full thickness wound cover seeded with the patient's autologous keratinocytes and fibroblasts, and/or (3) a readily-available permanent wound cover preseeded with non-antigenic allogeneic keratinocytes, fibroblasts and melanocytes. Collaborative research efforts may be necessary to achieve these goals in a timely and cost-effective manner as skin banks find themselves competing with the bioengineering industry.

4. References

ACHAUER, B.M., HEWITT, C.W., BLACK, K.S., MARTINEZ, S.E., WAXMAN, K.S., OTT, R.A. and FURNAS, D.W. (1986). Long-term allograft survival after short-term cyclosporin treatment in a patient with massive burns, *Lancet* **1**, 14–15.

AGGARWAL, S.J., BAXTER, C.R. and DILLER, K.R. (1985). Cryopreservation of skin: An assessment of current clinical applicability, *J. Burn Care Rehabil.* **6**, 69–76.

ALEXANDER, J.W., MACMILLAN, B.G., LAW, E. and KITTUR, D.S. (1981). Treatment of severe burns with widely meshed skin autograft and meshed skin allograft overlay, *J. Trauma* **21**, 433–438.

BAXTER, H. and ENTIN, M.A. (1948). Experimental and clinical studies of reduced temperatures in injury an repair in man. III. Direct effect of cooling and freezing on various elements of the human skin, *Plast. Reconstr. Surg.* **3**, 303–334.

BETTMAN, A.G. (1938). Homogeneous Thiersch grafting as a life saving measure, *Am. J. Surg.* **39**, 156–162.

BILLINGHAM, R.E. and MEDAWAR, P.B. (1952). The freezing, drying, and storage of mammalian skin, *J. Exp. Bio.* **29**, 454–468.

BONDOC, C.C. and BURKE, J.F. (1971). Clinical experience with viable frozen human skin and a frozen skin bank, *Ann. Surg.* **174**, 371–382.

BROWN, J.B., FRYER, M.P., TANDALL, P. and LU, M. (1953). Post mortem homografts as 'biological dressings' for extensive burns and denuded areas, *Ann. Surg.* **138**, 618–623.

BROWN, W. and CUONO, C.B. (1992). Approaches to minimizing leakage of beneficial glycosaminoglycans in processing skin for cryopreservation. In: *Proc. Am. Burn Assoc.* **24**, 40.

BURKE, J.F., MAY, J.W., ALBRIGHT, N., QUINBY, W.C. and RUSSELL, P.S. (1974). Temporary skin transplantation and immunosuppression for extensive burns, *N. Engl. J. Med.* **290**, 269–271.

BURKE, J.F., QUINBY, W.C., BONDOC, C.C., COSIMI, A.B., RUSSELL, P.S. and SZYFELBEIN, S.K. (1975). Immunosuppression and temporary skin transplantation in the treatment of massive third degree burns, *Ann. Surg.* **182**, 183–197.

CLARKE, J.A. (1987). HIV transmission and skin grafts, *Lancet* **1**, 983.

COCHRANE, T. (1968). The low temperature storage of skin: A preliminary report, *Br. J. Plast. Surg.* **21**, 118–125.

CUONO, C., LANGDON, R. and McGUIRE, J. (1986). Use of cultured epidermal autografts and dermal allografts as skin replacement after burn injury, *Lancet* **1**, 1123–1124.

CUONO, C.B., LANGDON, R., BIRCHALL, N. and McGUIRE, J. (1988). Viability and functional performance of allograft skin preserved by slow, controlled, non-programmed freezing. In: *Proc. Am. Burn. Assoc.* **20**, 55.

DECLEMENT, F.A. and MAY, S.R. (1983). Procurement, cryopreservation and clinical application of skin. In: *The Preservation of Tissues and Solid Organs for Transplantation* Glassman, A. and Umlas, J., eds., American Association of Blood Banks, Arlington, VA, pp. 29–56.

EADE, G.G. (1958). The relationship between granulation tissue, bacteria, and skin grafts in burned patients, *Plast. Reconstr. Surg.* **22**, 42–55.

GIRDNER, J.H. (1881). Skin grafting with grafts taken from the dead subject, *Medical Record* **20**, 119–120.

HERNDON, D.N. and ROSE, J.K. (1996). Cadaver skin allograft and the transmission of human cytomegalovirus in burn patients: Benefits clearly outweigh risks, *J. Am. Coll. Surg.* **182**, 263–264.

HICKERSON, W.L., COMPTON, C., FLETCHALL, S. and SMITH, L.R. (1994). Cultured epidermal autografts and allodermis combination for permanent burn wound coverage, *Burns* **20**, S52–56.

JACKSON, D. (1954). A clinical study of the use of skin homografts for burns, *Br. J. Plast. Surg.* **7**, 26–43.

KEALEY, G.P., AGUIAR, J., LEWIS, R.W., ROSENQUIST, M.D., STRAUSS, R.G. and BALE, J.F. (1996). Cadaver skin allografts and transmission of human cytomegalovirus to burn patients, *J. Am. Coll. Surg.* **182**, 201–205.

LEHR, H.B., BERGGREN, R.B., LOTKE, P.A. and CORIELL, L.L. (1964). Permanent survival of preserved skin autografts, *Surgery* **56**, 742–746.

LIVESEY, S.A., HERNDON, D.N., HOLLYOAK, M.A., ATKINSON, Y.H. and NAG, A. (1995). Transplanted acellular allograft dermal matrix, *Transplantation* **60**, 1–9.

MATTHEWS, D.N. (1945). Storage of skin for autogenous grafts, *Lancet* **2**, 775–778.

MAY, S.R. (1990). The future of skin banking, *J. Burn Care Rehabil.* **11**, 484–486.

MAY, S.R. and DECLEMENT, F.A. (1980). Skin banking methodology: An evaluation of package format, cooling and warming rates, and storage efficiency, *Cryobiology* **17**, 34–45.

MAY, S.R. and DECLEMENT, F.A. (1981). Skin banking. Part II. Low contamination cadaveric allograft skin for temporary burn wound coverage, *J. Burn Care Rehabil.* **2**, 64–76.

MAY, S.R. and DECLEMENT, F.A. (1981). Skin banking. Part III. Cadaveric allograft skin viability, *J. Burn Care Rehabil.* **2**, 128–141.

MAY, S.R. and DECLEMENT, F.A. (1982). Development of a radiometric metabolic viability testing method for human and porcine skin, *Cryobiology* **19**, 362–371.

MONAFO, W.W., TANDON, S.N., BRADLEY, R.E. and CONDICT, C. (1976). Bacterial contamination of skin used as a biological dressing. A potential hazard, *JAMA* **235**, 1248–1249.

MORRIS, P.J., BONDOC, C. and BURKE, J.F. (1966). The use of frequently changed skin allografts to promote healing in the nonhealing infected ulcer, *Surgery* **60**, 13–19.

NINNEMANN, J.L., FISHER, J.C. and FRANK, H.A. (1978). Prolonged survival of human skin allografts following thermal injury, *Transplantation* **25**, 69–72.

O'CONNOR, N.E., MULLIKEN, J.B., BANKS-SCHLEGEL, S., KEHINDE, O. and GREENE, H. (1981). Grafting of burns with cultured epithelium prepared from autologous epidermal cells, *Lancet* **1**, 75–78.

O'DONAGHUE, M.N. and ZAREM, H.A. (1958). Stimulation of neovascularisation. Comparative efficacy of fresh and preserved skin grafts, *Plast. Reconstr. Surg.* **48**, 474–477.

PLESSINGER, R.T., ROBB, E.C. and KAGAN, R.J. (1997). Allograft Skin Cultures II: Should allograft skin be processed in a class 10,000 or better environment? In: *Proc. Am. Assoc. Tissue Banks* **21**, 62.

PRUITT, B.A., Jr. and LEVINE, N.S. (1984). Characteristics and uses of biologic dressings and skin substitutes, *Arch. Surg.* **119**, 312–322.

REVERDIN, J.L. (1871). Sur la greffe epidermique, *CR Acad. Sci. (Paris)* **73**, 1280.

REVERDIN, J.L. (1872). De la greffe epidermique, *Arch. Gen. Med. (Suppl.)* **19**, 276.

ROBB, E.C., BECHMANN, N., PLESSINGER, R.T., BOYCE, S.T. and KAGAN, R.J. (1997). A comparison of changed vs. unchanged media for viability testing of banked allograft skin. In: *Proc. Am. Assoc. Tissue Banks* **21**, 42.

ROSENQUIST, M.D., KEALEY, G.P., LEWIS, R.W. and CRAM, A.E. (1988). A comparison of storage viability of nonmeshed and meshed skin at 4°C, *J. Burn Care Rehabil.* **9**, 634–636.

SAKABU, S.A., HANSBROUGH, J.F., COOPER, M.L. and GREENLEAF, G. (1990). Cyclosporine A for prolonging allograft survival in patients with massive burns, *J. Burn Care Rehabil.* **11**, 410–418.

SHUCK, J.M., PRUITT, B.A., Jr., and MONCRIEF, J.A. (1969). Homograft skin for wound coverage. A study in versatility, *Arch. Surg.* **98**, 472–479.

TAYLOR, A.C. (1949). Survival of rat skin and changes in hair pigmentation following freezing, *J. Exp. Zoo.* **110**, 77–112.

THIERSCH, J.C. (1886). On skin grafting, *Verhandl 2nd Deutsch Ges Chir* **15**, 17–20.

WAINWRIGHT, D., MADDEN, M., LUTERMAN, A., HUNT, J., MONAFO, W., HEIMBACH, D., KAGAN, R., SITTIG, K., DIMICK, A. and HERNDON, D. (1996). Clinical evaluation of an acellular allograft dermal matrix in full-thickness burns, *J. Burn Care Rehabil.* **17**, 124–136.

WEBSTER, J.P. (1944). Refrigerated skin grafts, *Ann. Surg.* **120**, 431–439.

WENTSCHER, J. (1903). [A further contribution about the survivability of human epidermal cells], *Dtsch Z Chir* **70**, 21–44.

WHITE, M.J., WHALEN, J.D., GOULD, J.A., BROWN, G.L. and POLK, H.C., Jr. (1991). Procurement and transplantation of colonized cadaver skin, *Am. Surg.* **57**, 402–407.

WOODS, W.B. (1960). Phagocytosis with particular reference to encapsulated bacteria, *Bact. Rev.* **224**, 41.

ZAROFF, L.I., MILLS, W., Jr., DUCKETT, J.W., Jr., SWITZER, W.E. and MONCRIEF, J.A. (1966). Multiple uses of viable cutaneous homografts in the burned patient, *Surgery* **59**, 368–372.

ZHANG, M.L., CHANG, Z.D., WANG, C.Y. and FANG, C.H. (1988). Microskin grafting in the treatment of extensive burns: A preliminary report, *J. Trauma* **28**, 804–807.

7.2 BIOLOGICAL SKIN COVER: BANKING AND APPLICATION

P. MĚŘIČKA, L. KLEIN, H. STRAKOVÁ & D. ŠUBRTOVÁ

Tissue Bank, Department of Plastic Surgery
Department of Histology and Embryology
University Hospital and Medical Faculty
Charles University, Hradec Králové
Czech Republic

1. Introduction

Biological skin cover can be used as replacement of the skin in full thickness skin lesions or for stimulation of the wound healing in partial thickness skin lesions. The following types of covers are currently used: dermoepidermal autografts; dermoepidermal allografts; dermoepidermal xenografts; chorion-amnion; cultured epithelium; and composite grafts.

Permanent wound closure of full thickness skin lesions always requires either application of a skin autograft or application of cultured autologous keratinocytes. Skin allografts and xenografts as well as chorion-amnion can be used as biological dressings and changed at regular intervals until spontaneous epithelisation is completed in partial thickness burns or until autotransplantation is performed in full thickness burns (Winter, 1975). In these situations the grafts only adhere to the wound and the real take and/or vascularisation does not take place.

Skin allografts can also be used in temporary transplantation, i.e. the graft takes and temporary closure of the wound is achieved. The graft is surgically removed before spontaneous rejection and replaced by an autograft (Burke et al, 1974).

Cultured allogeneic keratinocyte sheets can be used to stimulate spontaneous epithelisation in burns, to cover donor sites and to treat chronic skin defects. The application of composite grafts increases the choice of the surgeon in the treatment of extensive full thickness burns.

2. Dermoepidermal Autografts

The early excision of a full thickness burn wound, followed by immediate autografting (Janzekovich, 1970), represents an ideal solution. Whereas the use of full thickness autografts is frequent in plastic surgery, the application of split skin autografts harvested by the Humby knife or dermatomes and meshed usually prevails in the treatment of burns (Fig. 3). The modern approaches to skin autografting are summarised in recent publications by Settle and Herndon (Settle, 1996; Herndon, 1996).

An alternative approach to the treatment of extensive burns by classic grafts is represented by autotransplantation of cultured epidermal keratinocytes (Rheinwald and Green, 1975; Green et al, 1979; O'Connor et al, 1981; Gallico et al, 1984; Matoušková et al, 1989; Königová et al, 1989). The epithelial sheets originating from secondary cultures are at the disposal of the surgeon within 21 days after the harvest of the skin sample. The culture techniques can accomplish expansion ratios which can exceed 1000-fold in three to four weeks. Thus the harvesting of a 4 cm × 4 cm section can result in 16000 cm^2 of cultured epithelium, which is sufficient to cover the entire body of a moderate-sized adult patient (Hansbrough, 1993).*

*Introduction of the method of culturing human epidermal keratinocytes in the Tissue Bank Hradec Králové was supported by the grant No. 1184-2, the research work on composite graft by the grant No. 3696-3, Internal Grant Agency of the Ministry of Health, establishing a bank of allogeneic keratinocytes by the grant "Keratinocyte", Ministry of Defence.

The interval between harvesting and application of keratinocytes can be shortened by the application of cells originating from primary cultures (Stark and Kaiser, 1994; Wood and Stoner, 1996).

In skin autotransplantation, the surgeon usually does not need the cooperation of a tissue bank. In the application of keratinocytes, it is sometimes necessary to preserve primary cultures for delayed preparation of keratinocyte sheets.

The disadvantages of using autologous keratinocyte sheets in full thickness burns are well described. These are the tendency to scarring due to the absence of the dermal layer and to the fragility of the epidermis, and blister formation as a consequence of a flat dermoepidermal junction and/or delayed formation of dermal papillae (Woodley *et al*, 1988; Compton *et al*, 1989). The take of cultured epithelial sheets in full thickness burns is sometimes problematic (Hansbrough 1993). We have observed incomplete take of keratinocytes in the case of toxic epidermal necrolysis in which full thickness skin loss developed (Klein *et al*, 1997). The take of keratinocytes is reported to be improved by using combination with allograft (Stark and Kaiser, 1994) or special artificial supporters, e.g. hyaluronic acid ester membranes (Andreassi *et al*, 1991, Donati *et al*, 1995).

3. Dermoepidermal Allografts

Hansbrough considers cadaveric skin allograft to be the present gold standard for excised burn wounds when sufficient autograft skin is not available or autografting is not clinically indicated (Hansbrough, 1993). Viable (fresh and/or hypothermically stored (4°C)) or cryopreserved skin as well as non-viable (deep frozen, freeze-dried and glycerolised) skin grafts are used. The advantages and disadvantages of viable and non-viable grafts have been intensively discussed. Viable grafts stimulate vascularisation, do not dissolve on the burn wound, and have a good ability in controlling infection of the burn wound. These cannot be sterilised, however. The risk of infection transmission can be lowered by proper screening and serological testing of the donor (Campagnari and O'Malley, 1994).

The immunogenicity of viable grafts is higher than that of non-viable grafts (Young and Wyatt, 1960; Hacket, 1975). For this reason, immunosuppresive drugs can be used to postpone the rejection phenomenon (Burke et al, 1974).

Non-viable grafts have a reduced ability to stimulate vascularisation, an increased tendency to dissolve on the burn wounds, and a reduced ability to control infection. These can be sterilised by pharmacopeial methods, and thus, the risk of infection transmission is minimised. The application of additional processing methods can reduce immunogenicity or modify degradability of the graft by cross-linking of collagen (Kearney, 1996).

The application of viable grafts is advisable if the real take of the graft is required, i.e. in temporary skin transplantation.

The cultured allogeneic epithelium is less antigenic than the classic dermoepidermal graft. It represents only a temporary cover (Phillips, 1991). It is a biologically active cover, releasing cytokines which can stimulate the healing process. For this reason it can be applied with success even in the treatment of chronic defects such as leg ulcers (Phillips et al, 1989). The application in partial thickness burns, donor sites or toxic epidermal necrolysis has also been described (Hansbrough, 1993). Neonatal foreskin is frequently used as a source for keratinocyte cultures (Phillips et al, 1989). In our practice the keratinocytes are cultured from skin removed either at surgical procedures or taken from cadavers (Straková et al, 1994; Měřička et al, in press).

4. Dermoepidermal Xenografts

Since the lack of allografts is a permanent problem in skin transplantation, the application of xenografts is frequently adopted. Pig skin is the most commonly used material (Moserová et al, 1974; Königová, 1990; Hansbrough, 1993). However, bovine, ovine, canine or even frog xenografts can also be used. Porcine xenografts are harvested from fresh porcine hides after shaving, washing, disinfection and removal using the Humby knife (Moserová et al, 1974; Moserová and Houšková, 1989) or a dermatome. The xenografts are especially suitable for covering extensive partial thickness burns and non-contaminated wounds. The grafts prevent evaporative fluid loss from the burn wound, dehydration and/or deepening of partial thickness burns, and/or assure favourable conditions for re-epithelisation.

In full thickness defects, the growth of granulations without overgrowth is stimulated. The disadvantage is a high demand of xenografts exceeding 1 m^2 per patient in severe burns (Měřička *et al*, 1989; Klein and Měřička, 1995).

From January 1986 to December 1995, a total of 95 m^2 of xenografts has been used by us in the treatment of 145 adult patients. The mechanisms of injury were as follows: direct flame: 79 cases, scalds caused by hot liquids: 44 cases, other mechanisms (electrical, chemical and contact burns): 22 cases. Partial thickness burns occurred in 96 patients. Correct and timely application of xenografts prevented further superficial damage due to wound surface dehydration. They promoted epithelisation at the wound edges, but simultaneously suppressed overgrowth of granulations in the centre. In full thickness burns (49 patients) necrectomy and wound preparation for autografting were carried out. Xenografts were changed every three to four days, usually two to four times to prevent infection of the wound or the real take and vascularisation of the graft. These frequent dressing changes facilitated debridement of the wound and prepared it for a successful permanent closure with autografts.

Case history: A 49-year old man sustained extensive burn injury while extinguishing a housefire. He had full thickness burns on the dorsal side of the trunk, buttocks and lower extremities covering 27% of the total body surface area (TBSA) (Fig. 1). Previously, he had been suffering from ischaemic cardiac disease including a heart attack. After necrectomy the wound was covered with xenografts (Fig. 2). For the definitive cover, autotransplantation was performed when the necrectomised wound bed was prepared to take in the autoskin graft (Fig. 3). All grafts took within seven days (Fig. 4) and the patient was discharged from the burn unit for home convalescence after another ten days.

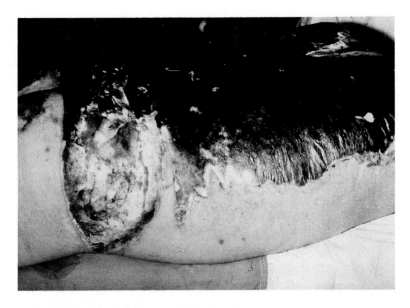

Fig. 1. Status of the patient at the admission to the burn unit.

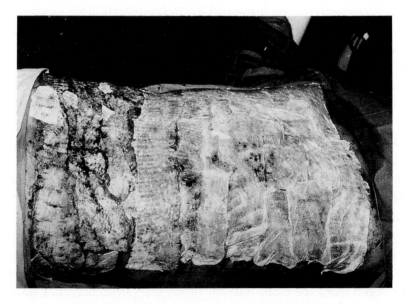

Fig. 2. Necrectomised area covered with xenografts.

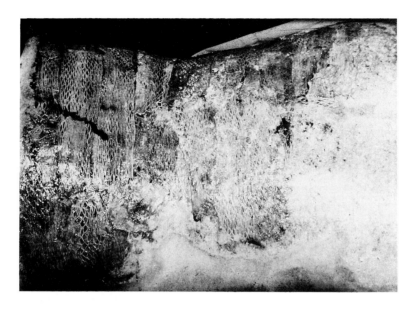

Fig. 3. Meshed autografts on the wound surface.

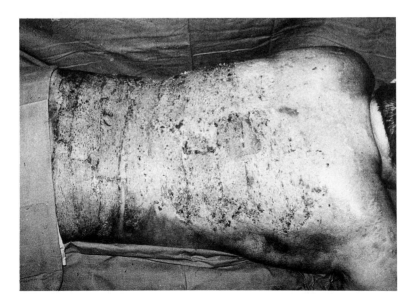

Fig. 4. Healed area seven days after autografting.

5. Skin Banking Technologies

A review of early skin banking technologies was published by Perry more than 30 years ago (Perry, 1966). The problem was later reviewed by Baxter (Baxter *et al*, 1985), and recently by Kearney (Kearney, 1996) and McCauley (McCauley, 1996). The modern technology of preservation of viable skin allografts was elaborated by May and DeClement (May and DeClement, 1980, 1981).

The classic method of moist chamber preservation or preservation in tissue culture media leads to continuous decrease in viability (May and DeClement, 1981). Moreover, the bacterial growth may be significant in longer storage (Klen and Heger, 1969). For this reason the shelf-life of skin preserved at 4°C is limited. Storage for seven to eight days is recommended by Kearney (Kearney, 1996). The problem of bacterial growth is excluded in deep freezing or cryopreservation of skin. The cryopreservation methods use either: (1) controlled rate freezing in programmable freezers usually followed by storage in a liquid nitrogen container, or (2) uncontrolled freezing by placing the skin samples covered by an insulation layer to the constant temperature achieved using a mechanical freezer (May and DeClement, 1980), or cooling in liquid nitrogen vapour (Praus *et al*, 1980). Glycerol or dimethylsulphoxide in concentrations of 10–15% are used as cryo-protectants. The freezing rate should not exceed −5 K/min (May and DeClement, 1980; Campagnari and O'Malley, 1994). The thin sample format (achieved by wrapping skin into disposable plastic bags) can assure rapid thawing by immersion of the bag with the graft into warm water (37°C). The methods assure the post-thaw viability of the skin as high as 85% of initial values. Controlled-rate freezing at the rate −1 K/min until −15°C, −5 K/min until −60°C, plunging into liquid nitrogen was used by us for skin allografts wrapped in laminated foil bags, and uncontrolled freezing for preservation of xenografts stored in Petri dishes at −70°C (Měřička *et al*, 1987). Now we use wrapping of grafts in double disposable plastic bags, a cooling rate of −1 K/min and storage at −80°C

Human keratinocytes can be cryopreserved in suspension in ampoules or as whole sheets. Our freezing protocol for primary cultures is as follows: The trypsinised primary cultures are mixed with the cryoprotective mixture consisting of foetal calf serum with 10% of sterile and endotoxine-tested dimethylsulphoxide to achieve the cell density 2–4×10^6 /ml. The suspension is filled to 1.8 ml cryotubes and frozen at the rate of -1 K/min until $-40°$C, -5 K/min until $-80°$C and -10 K/min until $-150°$C. Only a one-day delay was observed in the growth of secondary cultures originating from the thawed cells in comparison with unfrozen controls (Straková *et al*, 1994). The methodology of cryopreservation of whole keratinocyte sheets is based on similar principles as cryopreservation of conventional dermoepidermal grafts and has been described, for example by Kostadinow (Kostadinow *et al*, 1991). The preservation methods which do not maintain the viability of the skin are as follows: deep freezing ($-50°$C and below), freeze drying and dehydration in concentrated glycerol.

Deep freezing and freeze drying followed by radiation sterilisation are commonly used in preparing porcine xenografts. The same methods also can be applied in allograft preservation (Klen and Skalská, 1978; Měřička *et al*, 1986).

Glycerolisation of the skin has become very popular in western Europe due to the activity of the Euroskin Bank in Bewerwijk, the Netherlands. The grafts are stored in 85% glycerol at 4°C. The storage life of the product is two years (Kreis *et al*, 1989). After rehydration in isotonic saline, the product is ready for surgical use. van Baare *et al* (1994) described the following advantages of the glycerolised skin: technically simple procedure, low cost storage, unchanged "take" of the skin (if compared to fresh or deep frozen skin) and decreased antigenicity (Kreis *et al*, 1990; van Baare *et al*, 1994). The antibacterial (Basile, 1982) and virucidal effects of concentrated glycerol are also described (van Baare *et al*, 1994).

The long shelf-life of cryopreserved, deep frozen, freeze-dried or glycerolised skin makes it possible to establish the stock of grafts available at extraordinary situations (Měřička *et al*, 1989, 1995; Tosinska-Okroj *et al*, 1994–1995).

6. Composite Grafts

Composite grafts represent combinations of autologous cultured epithelium with allogeneic dermis, xenogeneic dermis or artificial dermal substitutes. The classic method of application of the composite graft was elaborated by Cuono et al (Cuono et al, 1986, 1987). The excised burn wound is covered by the classic allograft which is surgically removed before spontaneous rejection and replaced by autologous keratinocyte sheets.

Later, in vitro investigations proved the importance of seeding the reticular dermis with fibroblasts and/or maintaining the basement membrane zone of the papilllary dermis for good attachment of keratinocytes (Woodley et al, 1988; Krejci et al, 1991). Using the methods described by Krejci and Cuono, it is possible to prepare dermal grafts in which collagen and elastic fibres and some components of the dermal-epidermal junction are preserved [Figs. 5(a)–(c)].

The possibility of combining cultured keratinocytes with bioartificial dermal matrix seeded by cultured fibroblasts has also been investigated (Hansbrough 1993).

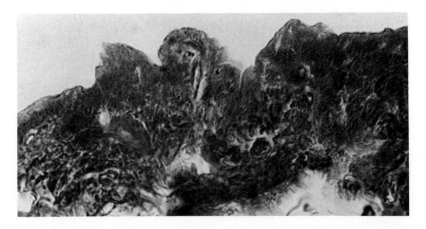

Fig. 5(a). Acellular de-epidermised frozen dermis prepared as a substrate for cultured keratinocytes. Paraffin-embedded section. Collagen fibres demonstrated with Masson's trichrome stain (× 490).

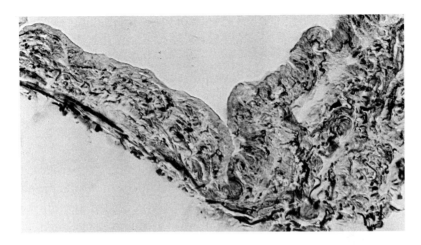

Fig. 5(b). Elastic fibres in the same dermis. Parafin embedded section, resorcin/fuchsin (× 320).

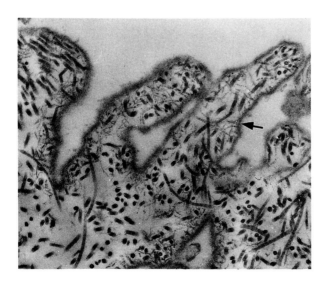

Fig. 5(c) Transmission electron micrograph of de-epidermised frozen dermis revealing the preserved complex of lamina densa and poorly distinguishable anchoring fibrils on the dermal papillary surface (arrow), approx. (× 21 000).

The composite of autologous keratinocytes and porcine xenografts, used upside-down, was applied with success in the Prague Burns Centre (Czech Republic). In this case, the xenograft serves as the protection of the keratinocyte layer and the graft is easier to handle than the keratinocyte sheet alone (Matoušková et al, 1993).

7. Conclusions

1. Current banking technologies make it possible to provide biologically an active and safe skin allografts and xenografts prepared according to nationally or internationally accepted standards.
2. The skin banks contribute substantially to the improvement of the quality of burn care.
3. The problem of a permanent wound closure in case of the lack of donor sites in extensive burns is still unsolved.
4. Combining autologous cultured cells with allogeneic dermal components or dermal substitutes seems to provide the adequate solution.

8. References

ANDREASSI, L., CASINI, I., TRABUCCHI, E., DIAMANTINI, S., RASTELLI, A., DONATI, L., TENCHINI. M.I. and MALCOVATI, M. (1991). Human keratinocyte culture on membranes composed of benzyl ester of hyaluronic acid, Wounds 3, 116–126.

BASILE, A.R.D. (1982). A comparative study of glycerinized and lyophilized porcine skin in dressings for third degree burns, Plastic Reconstr. Surg. 69, 969–974.

BAXTER, C., AGGARWAL, S. and DILLER, K.R. (1985). Cryopreservation of skin. A review, Transplant. Procs. XVII, Suppl., pp 112–120.

BRYCHTA, P., SUCHÁNEK, J., ŘÍHOVÁ, H., ADLER, J. and KOMÁRKOVÁ J. (1995). Cultured epidermal allografts for the treatment of deep dermal burns, Acta Chir. Plast. 37, 20–24.

BURKE, J.P., MAY, J.W., Jr., ALBRIGHT, N., QUINBY, W.C. and RUSSELL, P.S.(1974). Temporary skin transplantation and immunosuppression for extensive burns, *N. Engl. J. Med.* **31**, 269–271.

CAMPAGNARI, D. and O'MALLEY, J.P.O., eds. (1994). Standards of the American Red Cross Tissue Services, 6th edition, Washington, DC.

COMPTON, C.C., GILL, J.M., BRADFORD, D.A., REGAUER, S., GALLICO, G.G. and O'CONNOR, N.E. (1989). Skin regenerated from cultured epithelial autografts on full-thickness burn wounds from 6 days to 5 years after grafting. A light, electron microscopic and immunohistochemical study, *Lab. Invest.* **60**, 600–612.

CUONO, C.B., LANGDON, R. and McGUIRE, J. (1986). Use of cultured epidermal autografts and dermal allografts as skin replacement after burn injury, *Lancet* **1**, 1123–1124.

CUONO, C.B., LANGDON, R., BIRCHALL, N., BARTTLBORT, S. and McGUIRE, J. (1987). Composite autologous, allogeneic skin replacement: Development and clinical application, *Plast. Reconstr. Surg.* **80**, 626–635.

DONATI, L. (1985). Development and clinical application of keratinocytes cultured on hyaluronic ester membrane in burned patients. In: *The Management of Burns and Fire Disasters: Perspectives 2000.* M. Maselis and Gunn, S.W.A. eds., Kluwer Academic Publishers, Dordrecht, Boston, London, pp 357–361.

GALLICO, G.G., O'CONNOR, N.E., COMPTON, C.C., KEHINDE, O. and GREEN, H. (1984). Permanent coverage of large burn wounds with autologous cultured human epithelium, *N. Eng. J. Med.* **311**(7), pp 448–451.

GREEN, H., KEHINDE, O. and THOMAS, J. (1979). Growth of cultured epidermal cells into multiple epithelia suitable for grafting. In: *Proc. Nat. Acad. Sci. USA* **76**, pp 5665–5668.

HACKET, M.E.J. (1975). Preparation, storage and use of homograft, *Br. J. Hosp. Med.* **13**, 272–284.

HANSBROUGH, J.F. (1993). *Wound coverage with Biological Dressings and Cultured Skin Substitutes.* R.G. Landes Company, Austin, Second Printing, 152 p.

HERNDON, D.N., ed. (1996). *Total Burn Care.* W.B. Saunders Co. Ltd., London, Philadelphia, Toronto, Sydney, Tokyo.

JANZEKOVIC, Z. (1970). A new concept in the early excision and immediate grafting of burns, *J. Trauma* **10**, 1103–1108.

KEARNEY, J. (1996). Banking of skin grafts and biological dressings, In: *Principles and Practice of Burns Management.* J.A.D. Settle, ed., Churchill Livingstone, New York, Edinburgh, London, Madrid, Melbourne, San Francisco, Tokyo, pp 329–351.

KLEIN, L., MĚŘIČKA, P., STRAKOVÁ, H., JEBAVÝ, L., NOŽIČKOVÁ, M., BLÁHA, M., TALÁBOVÁ, Z. and HOŠEK, F. (1997). Biological skin covers in treatment of two cases of the Lyell's syndrome, *Ann. Transplant.* **2**, 45–48

KLEIN, L. and MĚŘIČKA, P. (1995). Clinical experience with skin xenografts in burned patients. In: *Management of Burns and Fire Disasters: Perspectives 2000.* M. Masellis and Gunn, S.W.A., eds., Kluwer Academic Publishers, Dordrecht, Boston, London, pp 343–345.

KLEN, R. and HEGER, J. (1969). A contribution to the degradation of skin and cornea preserved hemibioticaly in the temperature near 0°C, *Acta Chir. Plast.* **11**, 47–55.

KLEN, R. and SKALSKÁ, H. (1976). A comparison of dermoepidermal and chorioamniotic grafts in the treatment of burns, *Acta Chir. Plast.* **18**, 225–232.

KÖNIGOVÁ, R., KAPOUNKOVÁ, Z., VOGTOVÁ, D., VESELÝ, P. and MATOUŠKOVÁ, E. (1989). First experiences with clinical application of cultured auto-epithelium grafts, *Acta Chir. Plast.* **31**, 193–200.

KÖNIGOVÁ, R. (1990). The extensive burns trauma. (in Czech) Avicenum Prague.

KOSTADINOW, A., MÜHLBAUER, W., HARTINGER, A. and von DONNERSMARCK, G.G.H. (1991). Skin banking: A simple method for cryopreservation of split-thickness skin and cultured human epidermal keratinocytes, *Ann. Plast. Surg.* **26**, 89–97.

KREIS, R.W., VLOEMANS, A.F.P.M., HOEKSTRA, M.J., MACKIE, D.P. and HERMANS, R.P. (1989). The use of non-viable glycerol-preserved cadaver skin combined with widely expanded autografts in the treatment of extensive third-degree burns, *J. Trauma* **29**, 51–54.

KREJCI, N.C., CUONO, Ch.B., LANGDON, R.C. and McGUIRE, J. (1991). *In vitro* reconstitution of skin: Fibroblasts facilitate keratinocyte growth and differentiation on acellular reticular dermis, *J. Invest. Dermatol.* **97**, 843–848.

MATOUŠKOVÁ, E., VESELÝ, P. and KÖNIGOVÁ, R. (1989). Modified method of *in vitro* cultivation of human keratinocytes suitable for grafting, *Folia Biol. (Prague)* **35**, 267–271.

MATOUŠKOVÁ, E., NEMCŎVÁ, D., VOGTOVÁ, D. and KÖNIGOVÁ, R. (1993). Healing effect of recombined human-pig skin on dermal defects. In: *Burn Symposium on Occasion of the 40th Anniversary of the Prague Burns Centre (with international participation)*, Abstracts, Prague, Czech Republic, 29 September–1st October, pp 22.

MAY, S.R. and DECLEMENT, F.A. (1980). Skin banking methodology: An evaluation of package format, cooling and warming rates and storage efficiency, *Cryobiology* **17**, 33–45.

MAY, S.R. and DECLEMENT, F.A. (1981). Skin banking. Part I. Procurement of transplantable cadaveric allograft skin for burn wound coverage, *J. Burn. Care Rehab.* **2**, 7–23.

MAY, S. R. and DECLEMENT, F.A. (1981). Skin banking. Part II. Low contamination of dermal allograft for temporary burn wound coverage, *J. Burn Care Rehab.* **2**, 64–76.

MAY, S. R. and DECLEMENT, F.A. (1981). Skin banking. Part III. Cadaveric allograft skin viability, *J. Burn Care Rehab.* **2**, 128–141.

McCAULEY, R.L. (1996). The skin bank. In: *Total Burn Care.* W.B. Saunders Co. Ltd., London, Philadelphia, Toronto, Sydney, Tokyo, pp 159–163.

MĚŘIČKA, P., LEVÍNSKÁ, M., KEREKEŠ, Z., POZLEROVÁ, E., DVOŘÁČEK, I., VÁVRA, L., STRAKOVÁ, H. and HUŠEK, Z. (1986). Unsere Erfahrungen mit der Anwendung von abiotisch konservierten dermoepidermalen und Chorion-Amnion Transplantaten bei Heilung von Verbrennungen, *Probl. Hematol. Transf. Transplant.* **13**, 361–369.

MĚŘIČKA, P., HUŠEK, Z., STRAKOVÁ, H., VÁVRA, L., VINŠ, M., SCHUSTER, P. and DUDEK, A. (1987). Cryopreservation of dermoepidermal grafts for treatment of burns. In: *Proceedings of the 27th International Congress of Refrigeration*, Vienna, Austria, 24–29 August, 1987. International Institute of Refrigeration, Paris, 1987, pp 1–8.

MĚŘIČKA, P., KLEIN, L., PREIS, J., STRAKOVÁ, H., HUŠEK, Z., POZLEROVÁ, E., MORÁVKOVÁ, V., ŠTĚPÁNOVÁ, V. and ACHOVÁ, P. (1989). Problems encountered in banking biological coverings for treatment of burns. In: *Progress in Burn Injury Treatment, Proceedings of the 3rd Congress of European Burns Association*, Prague, October 4–7, 1989. W. Boeckx and J. Moserová, eds., Acco Leuven/Amersfoort, pp 85–87.

MĚŘIČKA, P., KLEIN, L., PREIS, J. and ETTLEROVÁ, E. (1995). The role of the tissue bank in disaster planning. In: *The Management of Burns and Fire Disasters: Perspectives 2000*. M. Masellis and Gunn, S.W.A., eds., Kluwer Academic Publishers, Dordrecht, Boston, London, pp 73–83.

MĚŘIČKA, P., STRAKOVÁ, H., KLEIN, L. and ŠUBRTOVÁ, D. (in press). Practical aspects of establishing an allogeneic keratinocyte bank. Roczniki Oparzen, *Ann. Burns*.

MOSEROVÁ, J., PÁVKOVÁ, L., PELLAR, F. and VRABEC, R. (1974). Bacteriological control of dermoepidermal grafts from porcine hides, *Rozhl. Chir.* **53**, 631–634 (In Czech).

MOSEROVÁ, J. and HOUŠKOVÁ, E. (1989). The healing and treatment of skin defects. Karger, Basel, Munchen, Paris, London, New York, New Delhi, Singapore,Tokyo, Sydney 163 pp.

PERRY, V.P. (1966). A review of skin preservation, *Cryobiology*, 192–230.

PHILLIPS, T.J. (1991). Cultured epidermal allografts. A temporary or permanent solution, *Transplantation* **51**, 937–941.

PHILLIPS, T.J., KEHINDE, O., GREEN, H. and GILCHREST, B. (1989). Treatment of skin ulcers with cultured epidermal allografts, *J. Am. Acad. Dermatol.* **21**, 191–199.

PRAUS, R., BÖHM, F., DVOŘÁK, R. *et al* (1980). Skin Cryopreservation I: Incorporation of radioactive sulphate as a criterion of pigskin graft viability after freezing to −196°C in the presence of cryoprotectants, *Cryobiology* **17**, 130–134.

RHEINWALD, J.G. and GREEN, H. (1975). Serial cultivation of strains of human epidermal keratinocytes. The formation of keratinizing colonies from single cells, *Cell* **6**, 331–343.

RHEINWALD, J.G. and GREEN, H. (1977). Epidermal growth factor and multiplication of cultured human epidermal keratinocytes, *Nature* **265**, 421–424.

SETTLE, J.A.D., ed. (1996). *Principles and Practice of Burns Management.* Churchill Livingstone, New York, Edinburg, London, Madrid, Melbourne, San Francisco, Tokyo, 496 pp.

STARK, G.B. and KAISER, H.W. (1994). Cologne Burn Centre experience with glycerol preserved allogeneic skin. Part II: Combination with autologous cultured keratinocytes, *Burns* **20**, 34–38.

STRAKOVÁ, H., MĚŘIČKA, P., ČERVINKA, M., KEREKEŠ, Z. and ŠUBRTOVÁ, D. (1995). Cultivation of epithelial sheets from cryopreserved keratinocyte primocultures, *J. Exp. Clin. Cancer Res.* **Suppl. 14**, 99–101.

ŠUBRTOVÁ, D., MOKRÝ, J., MĚŘIČKA, P. and STRAKOVÁ, H. (1995). Light and electron microscopy of cultured keratinocyte sheets designed to be used for burn treatment, *Surg. Radiol. Anat.* **17**, pp 230.

TOSINSKA-OKROJ, H., GROBELNY, I., RENKIELSKA, A., MIRON-KLEIN, E., HONORY, M., JANKAU, J. and MURASZKO-KUZMA, M. (1994–1995) Analysis of procedures, trauma severity and methods of treatment in the mass burn in the entertainment of the Gdansk Shipyard. Roczniki Oparzen — *Ann. Burns* **5–6**, 103–110 (In Polish).

van BAARE, J., BUITENWERF, J., HOECKSTRA, M.J. and duPONT, J.S. (1994). Virucidal effect of glycerol as used in donor skin preservation, *Burns* **20**, 77–80.

WINTER, C.D. (1975). Temporary skin cover. In: *Basic Problems in Burns.* R. Vrabec, Z. Koníěková, J. Moserová, eds., Springer Verlag, Berlin Heidelberg, New York, Avicenum, Czechoslovak Medical Press, Prague, pp. 19–24.

WOOD, F.M. and STONER, M. (1996). Implication of basement membrane development on the underlying scar in partial thickness burn injury, *Burns* **22**, 459–462.

WOODLEY, D.T., PETERSON, M.D., HERZOG, S.R., STRICKLIN, G.P., BURGESON, R.E., BRIGGAMAN. R.A., CRONCE, D.J. and O'KEEFE, E.J. (1988). Burn wounds resurfaced by cultured epidermal autografts show abnormal reconstitution of anchoring fibrils, *JAMA* **259**, 2566–2571.

YOUNG, J.M. and WYATT, G.W. (1960). Stored skin homografts in extensively burned patients, *Arch. Surg.* **80**, 208–213.

7.3 EVALUATION OF COLLAGEN MEMBRANES AS BIOLOGICAL DRESSINGS

J. GRZYBOWSKI

Department of Microbiology
Military Institute of Hygiene and Epidemiology
Kozielska 4, 01-163 Warsaw, Poland

J. SIKORSKI & J. KURMANOW

Division of Trauma and Burn, Second Department of Surgery
University Hospital No 1
Karol Marcinkowski University of Medical Sciences
Ul. Długa 1/2, 61-848 Poznań, Poland

1. Introduction

Bovine collagen membranes have been successfully used as a biological dressing in many cases (Yang, 1960). This follows from a growing use of biomaterial in clinical practice.

The bovine collagen membranes which we have been using are manufactured in Poland by COLLDRES Ltd., Warsaw, together with Ravimed Ltd. from Lajsk near Legionów. They are prepared from bovine collagen fibres which are cross-linked in the final stage of production. They are thin (0.02–0.03 mm) sheets cut into pieces of 100 mm × 150 mm, packed within a laminated paper and sterilised by radiation. The product is rigid, but after immersion in normal saline for a short duration of time — about 0.5 min — it becomes soft and easy to shape on the wounded surface. It has satisfactory adhesive properties and good elasticity. It also has sufficient transparency which allows wound control without dress changing (Grzybowski and Sakiel, 1995).

We have used collagen membranes as dressings for covering partial-thickness burn wounds (2a° and 2b°), for care of donor sites after split thickness skin excision, for grafting, and finally for the care of places after dermabrasion.

2. Patients and Methods

Between 1994–1996, three trials were conducted at three different Burn Centres in Poland: (a) Burn Unit, Siemianowice, where we evaluated the usefulness of collagen membranes as dressings for covering partial thickness burns (2a° and 2b°); (b) The Clinic of Plastic Surgery, Polanica Zdrój, where collagen membranes were used as dressings for healing the donor sites after harvesting split thickness skin grafts; and (c) the Burn Unit at Pozna ½, where clinical trials were conducted on 35 donor places after harvesting split thickness skin grafts and on ten surfaces after dermabrasion.

While using collagen membranes for covering partial thickness burns we monitored the rate of wound healing, possible infection, pain, and transparency. Our results were compared to that of a group of patients treated with porcine skin covering 2a° and 2b° burn wounds, and with traditional dressings composed of gauze saturated with paraffin when covering donor places after harvesting split thickness skin grafts and for surfaces after dermabrasion.

3. Results

At the Burn Unit at Siemianowice, the application of perforated collagen membranes as dressings for covering partial thickness burn wounds (2a° and 2b°) gave similar therapeutic results to those of biological dressings prepared from perforated xenogenic porcine skin.

The results showed that when treating 2a° and 2b° burns without signs of infection, collagen membranes are good biological dressings (Tables 1 and 2). They adhere to the wound and, therefore, no additional fixation is necessary, and since they are transparent wound inspection is easy. The overlying bandage does not stick to the collagen membranes, which makes dressing changes easy. The healing time of collagen membranes and porcine skin was proximately the same. The advantage of biological dressings is the possibility of permanent wound cover, except in the few cases where bacterial infection (mostly G-negative) occurred under the membrane. In such cases either collagen membranes or porcine skin were digested by bacterial protease and before then could be easily removed. Superficial necrotic tissues were excised and dressing (collagen membranes or porcine skin) was applied again on the wound up to epithelisation.

Table 1. 2a° burns.

Dressing	Number of Patients	Time of Healing (Days)	Infection	Pain	Transparency
CM PERFORATED	10	9 ± 3.5	0	–	+
PARAFFIN DRESSING	7	10 ± 3.2	2		±

Table 2. 2b° burns.

Dressing	Number of Patients	Time of Healing (Days)	Infection	Pain	Transparency
CM PERFORATED	10	29 ± 6.1	3	–	+
PARAFFIN DRESSING	10	30 ± 5.4	6	±	–

Collagen membranes also induce pain relief.

As is well known, the basic management of deep burns is the early removal of dead tissues (necrectomy) and rapid covering of the wound using the patient's own skin graft. After the graft procedure, the burn patient suffers an additional wound. In a severely burned patient there is need for several split thickness skin grafts to be harvested from the same donor area, so the donor site must be protected from infection and receive the best conditions for fast healing. For this, a tight dressing of paraffin gauze with addition of antibiotics is widely used. The inconvenience of this dressing is that it soaks up blood from the donor site and often becomes infected. Therefore, we have searched for a better product which would protect donor sites, and we believe that we have found this in collagen membranes.

Recently, a clinical trial utilising collagen membranes "COLLDRES" was conducted at the Division of Trauma, Burn Unit, Clinical Hospital, University of Medical Sciences in Pozna½. The collagen membranes were used on 35 donor sites after harvesting a split thickness skin graft which measured between 100–600 cm^2, and on ten surfaces after dermabrasion of post-burn scars which measured between 100–200 cm^2. Traditional dressings and collagen membranes were given to the same patients on different sites to compare the results. We monitored (1) time of healing, (2) haemostatic properties, (3) contamination, (4) patients' feelings, and (5) time of possible graft reharvesting. We also evaluated the results of using collagen membranes and paraffin dressings (Tables 3 and 4).

The healing time using the collagen membranes was established at 9–10 days for donor sites where split thickness skin grafts were harvested and at 7–10 days for sites after dermabrasion (Photograph 1).

The traditional dressings in 70% of the cases achieved healing donor sites after 10–15 days and in 30% of the cases, the healing time was even longer (more than 15 days). Thus, using collagen membranes as a biological dressing resulted in the acceleration of the healing time.

Collagen membranes were applied on 20 surfaces after the haemostase was carried out using warm normal saline (Photograph 2),

Table 3. 35 donor sites.

Dressing	Number of Patients	Time of Healing (Days)	Infection	Pain	Transparency	Reharvesting Time (Days)
CM	10	9–10	1	–	+	10–11
PERFORATED PARAFFIN DRESSING	7	10–15	4	+	–	13–15

Table 4. 10 sites after dermabrasion.

Dressing	Number of Patients	Time of Healing (Days)	Infection	Pain	Transparency	Haemostatic Properties
CM	10	7–10	1	–	+	GOOD
PERFORATED PARAFFIN DRESSING	10	for 7 patients, 10–15 for 3 patients, > 15	4	+	–	BAD

and on 15 surfaces without any haemostatic action, directly on to point bleeding surfaces (Photograph 3). Covering the bleeding surfaces with collagen membranes after harvesting split thickness skin grafts confirmed the good haemostatic properties of this dressing (Antiszko and Braczko, 1995; Browder and Litwin, 1986). A small amount of fluid accumulation with blister formation does not interfere with healing.

The collagen membranes also induced pain relief when compared with traditional dressings. On 35 donor sites covered by collagen membranes, only in one case did we observed infection (Trafny and Grzybowski, 1996), whereas when using paraffin dressing, four cases of infection were observed. When an infection occurred the collagen membranes were digested by bacterial protease and the wound was covered by a dressing containing Betadine.

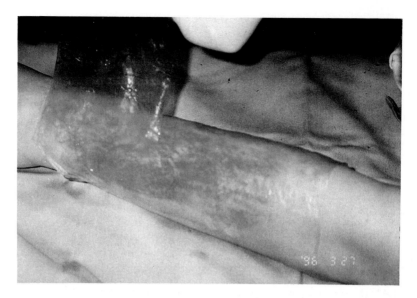

Photograph 1. The collagen membranes used to cover the places after dermabrasion.

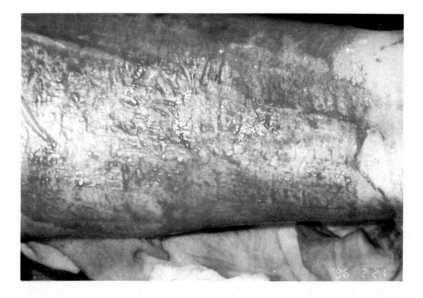

Photograph 2. The collagen membranes used to cover the sites after harvesting the split thickness skin graft with haemostatic action.

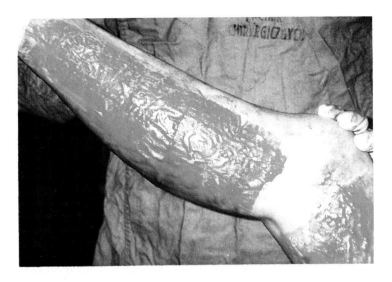

Photograph 3. The collagen membranes used to cover the sites after harvesting the split thickness skin graft without haemostatic action.

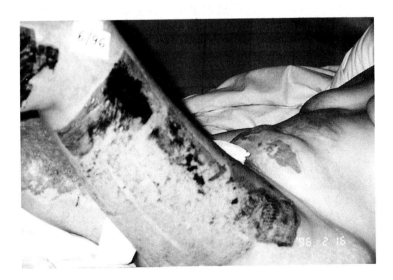

Photograph 4. Ten days after harvesting the split thickness skin graft, the wound is completely healed.

It was necessary to reharvest the skin for split thickness skin grafts in eight cases. At the time of second harvesting of the skin grafts, healing was estimated at between 10–11 days for collagen membranes and 13–15 days for the gauze paraffin dressings. After the scale-off of collagen membranes, or after their removal using the normal saline rinses, we received a very smooth surface of healed skin (Photograph 4).

4. Conclusions

- Collagen membranes are good biological dressings for covering clean partial thickness burn wounds, donor sites after harvesting split thickness skin grafts, and sites after dermabrasion.
- The use of collagen membranes resulted in the acceleration of wound healing compared to the application of traditional dressings composed of gauze saturated with paraffin.
- The use of this dressing does not require haemostasis.
- Collagen membranes induce pain relief.
- Collagen membranes are sufficiently transparent for observation of the wounds. Infection can be recognised as a result of loss of transparency.
- Collagen membranes are always sterile, and easy to use and store.
- They are a good barrier against infection.
- They protect the wound against drying up.
- They have satisfactory adhesive properties and, therefore, no additional fixation is necessary.

5. References

ANTISZKO, M., BRACZKO, M., GRZYBOWSKI, J. and JETHON, J. (1995). The comparative investigation of haemostatic properties of xenogenic collagenic biomaterials, *Polim. Med.* **3–4**, 37–45.

BROWDER, I. and LITWIN, M. (1986). Use of absorbable collagen for hemostatis in general surgical patients, *Am. J. Surg.* **52**, 492.

GRZYBOWSKI, J. and SAKIEL, S. (1995). Clinical application of new bovine collagen membranes as a partial-thickness burn wound dressing, *Polim. Med.* **3–4**, 19–24.

TRAFNY, E.A., GRZYBOWSKI, J., OLSZOWSKA-GOLEC, M., ANTOS, M. and STRUŻYNA, J. (1996). Antipseudomonal activity of collagen sponge with liposomal polymyxin B, *Pharmacol. Res.* **33**, 19.

YANG, J.Y. (1990). Clinical application of collagen sheet, YCWM, as a burn wound dressing, *Burns* **16**, 457–463.

7.4 EXPERIENCE IN THE USE OF FOETAL MEMBRANES FOR THE TREATMENT OF BURNS AND OTHER SKIN DEFECTS

J. KOLLER & E. PANÁKOVÁ

Center for Burns and Reconstructive Surgery
Central Tissue Bank
Ruzinov General Hospital
Bratislava, Slovakia

1. Introduction

Human foetal membranes (HFMs), from an anatomical point of view, represent two loosely connected membranes: the amnion and the chorion. The processing of human foetal membranes for use as biological skin substitutes or dressings was first practiced more than 80 years ago by Davis (1910) and Sabella (1913).

In clinical practice, HFMs are used mainly as biological dressings. In addition to their barrier properties and good adherence to wound surfaces due to the fibrin-elastin bond mechanism, HFMs contain a range of biologically active substances such as angiogenetic factors, allantoin, immunoglobulins, lysozyme, progesterone, etc. (Burgos, 1983; Faulk, 1980). The role of HFMs in scarless foetal wound healing is not yet fully understood (Longaker and Adzick, 1991).

The method of HFM harvesting, processing and storage in the Bratislava Central Tissue Bank was introduced in 1990 (Panáková *et al*, 1991) and a review of the subject has been given (Panáková and Koller, 1997).

2. Materials and Methods

HFMs are collected after obtaining informed consent from healthy mothers (exclusion criteria are identical for the tissue donation exclusion criteria of the European Association of Tissue Banks) during cesarean sections under aseptic conditions. The samples of cord blood are collected for serological testing (HBsAg, HIV-1/-2, syphilis), and the grafts are transported in cold sterile saline solution to the Tissue Bank for further processing.

The processing of HFMs in the tissue bank is performed under aseptic conditions in laminar air flow boxes. The processing itself starts with thorough cleaning of the grafts from blood remnants by rinsing them several times in saline solution. This is followed by incubation in antibiotic solutions twice during 20 minutes. After this incubation, the grafts are again rinsed in saline, and then one of the following three preservation methods is chosen:

(a) short-term storage by refrigeration
(b) long-term storage by freezing to −85°C
(c) long-term storage by glycerolisation.

The details of preservation methods have been described previously (Panáková and Koller, 1997). The majority of HFMs were preserved by deep freezing (Table 1). HFMs were used in 45 patients as temporary biological skin substitutes by four clinical departments of the Ruzinov General Hospital: the Department of Burns, the Department of Dermatology, the Department of Plastic Surgery, and the Department of General Surgery.

3. Results

The clinical indication for the use of foetal membranes were as follows:

Table 1. Indications for application of human foetal membranes.

Indication	Number of Patients
Skin defects of various origin not suitable for immediate skin autografting	25
Skin defects after superficial dermabrasion of scars	8
Crural ulcers in preparation for skin grafting	12
Total number of patients	**45**

- skin defects of various origin not suitable for immediate skin autografting (25 patients)
- skin defects after superficial dermabrasion of scars (8 cases)
- crural ulcers in preparation for skin grafting (12 cases)

The grafts were applied to the defects with slight overlapping of the defects' margins. After applications, the grafts were covered with tulle gras and compressive dressing to achieve good adherence to the wound surface. Dressing changes were performed every other day by changing only the outer layers of the dressing and leaving the tulle gras undisturbed.

In heavily discharging wounds, such as crural ulcers, or chronic skin defects, it was necessary to cope first with massive microbial colonisation of the wounds. This was performed by intensive local care with frequent dressing changes, hydrotherapy, and the use of topical anti-microbial agents. Even after this preparation, the grafts were often digested after several days by bacterial enzymes and virtually "disappeared" from the wound surface. In these cases, they were replaced several times by new membranes until the expected effects were achieved. Repeated application of HFMs to chronic atrophic, non-healing wounds resulted in gradual improvement of the character of the wounds: better vascularisation, enhancement of formation of granulations, and finally, enhancement of epithelisation in smaller wounds, and enabling or improving the graft take in larger defects treated by skin grafting. HFMs were also used as a kind of "test" graft before planned autografting.

In clean wounds, such as after dermabrasion, the grafts were left in place until the raw areas were covered by new epithelium. This usually took place in an average of five to seven days; the grafts were found to be dry, forming a type of crust which was then gradually peeled off leaving a well-healed wound surface.

In all applications, no adverse effects were observed. The results of applications were less satisfactory in wounds where the primary cause was insufficient blood supply due to atherosclerosis or diabetic angiopathy.

4. Discussion

HFMs were reported to be used in many different clinical circumstances, such as the treatment of superficial burns (Douglas, 1952; Pigeon, 1960; Bose, 1979; Quinby *et al*, 1982; Goebel and Schubert, 1990), coverage of split thickness skin graft donor sites (Colocho *et al*, 1974; Unger and Roberts, 1976), and the treatment of chronic granulating wounds (Dlabalová *et al*, 1972; Trelford *et al*, 1976; Bennett *et al*, 1980; Salisbury *et al*, 1980; Ward *et al*, 1989). Except for the treatment of fresh burns and donor sites, our indications were very similar. The advantages of HFMs compared to other biological skin substitutes are availability, simple harvesting and processing, low antigenicity, and relatively low costs.

The beneficial effects observed after the application of HFMs were prevention of desiccation of the wounds, cleaning of wounds by repeated graft changes, enhancement of the growth of new granulation tissue, improvement of the vascularity of the wounds, enhancement of epithelisation from the wound margins, and preparation of the wounds for better "take" of autografts. In painful wounds the pain disappeared very soon after the application of the graft, and the comfort of the patient was much improved. In covering the post-dermabrasion defects, the post-operative pain was almost completely absent during the entire healing time, and the need for several painful post-operative dressing changes was eliminated.

5. Summary

In conclusion, HFMs proved to be very beneficial in treating both clean and problem wounds due to their availability, low antigenicity, low cost, and potential for enhancing the wound healing process, including diminution of pain, prevention of wound desiccation, and shortening of the healing time.

6. References

BENNETT, J.P., MATTHEWS, R. and FAULK, W.P. (1980). Treatment of chronic ulceration of the legs with human amnion, *Lancet* **1**, 1153.

BOSE, B. (1979). Burn wound dressing with human amniotic membrane, *Ann. Roy. Coll. Surg. Engl.* **61**, 444–447.

BURGOS, H. (1983). Angiogenetic and growth factors in human amnio-chorion and placenta, *Euro. J. Clin. Invest.* **13**, 289–296.

COLOCHO, G., GRAHAM, W.P., GREENE, A.E., *et al* (1974). Human amniotic membrane as a physiologic wound dressing, *Arch. Surg.* **109**, 370–373.

DAVIS, J.S. (1910). Skin transplantation with a review of 550 cases at the Johns Hopkins Hospital, *JHH Report* **15**, 307.

DLABALOVÁ, H., KLEN, R. and JANDOVÁ, E. (1972). Treatment of leg ulcers with chorion grafts (In Czech), *Ès. Dermatol.* **47**(1), 42.

DOUGLAS, B. (1952). Homografts of fetal membranes as a covering for large wounds especially those from burns, *J. Tennessee Med. Assoc.* **45**, 230.

FAULK, W.P., STEVENS, P.J., BURGOS, H., *et al* (1980). Human amnion as an adjunct in wound healing, *Lancet* **1**, 1156–1158.

GOEBEL, P. and SCHUBERT, W. (1990). Personal experiences with covering burns in children with amnion, *Brit. Orthop. Traumatol.* **37**, 495–498.

LONGAKER, M.T. and ADZICK, N.S. (1991). The biology of fetal wound healing: A review, *Plast. Reconstr. Surg.* **87**, 788–798.

PANÁKOVÁ, E. and KOLLER, J. (1997). Utilisation of foetal membranes in the treatment of burns and other skin defects. In: *Advances in Tissue Banking, Vol. I*, G.O. Phillips, R. von Versen, D.M. Strong and A. Nather, eds., World Scientific, Singapore, pp. 165–181.

PANÁKOVÁ, E., KOLLER, J. and BURSOVÁ, M. (1991). Experience with the retrieval, processing, storage and distribution of biological temporary skin substitutes in the Tissue Bank of the Burn Department in Bratislava, *1st Conference on Tissue Banking and Clinical Application*, Oct. 24–26, 1991, Berlin.

PIGEON, J. (1960). Treatment of second degree burns with amniotic membranes, *Can. Med. Assoc. J.* **83**, 844.

QUINBY, W.C., HOOVER, H.C., SCHEFFLAN, M., *et al* (1982). Clinical trials of amniotic membranes in burn wound care, *Plast. Reconstr. Surg.* **70**, 711–716.

SABELLA, N. (1913). Use of fetal membranes in skin grafting, *Med. Rec. N. Y.* **83**, 478.

SALISBURY, T.E., CAINES, R. and McCARTHY, R. (1980). Comparison of the bacterial clearing effects of different biologic dressings on granulating wounds following thermal injury, *Plast. Rec. Surg.* **66**, 596.

TRELFORD, J.D., HANSON, F.W. and ANDERSON, D.G. (1976). Wound healing and the amniotic membrane, *J. Med. Clin. Exp. Theoret.* **6**, 383–386.

UNGER, M.G. and ROBERTS, M. (1976). Lyophilised amniotic membranes on graft donor sites, *Brit. J. Plast. Surg.* **29**, 99–101.

WARD, D.J., BENNETT, J.P, BURGOS, H. and FABRE, J. (1989). The healing of chronic venous ulcers with prepared human amnion, *Brit. J. Plast. Surg.* **42**, 463–467.

7.5 ACELLULAR HUMAN DERMIS FOR *IN VITRO* AND *IN VIVO* SKIN GRAFTING

H.O. RENNEKAMPFF, N. PALLUA & A. BERGER

The Department of Plastic,
Hand and Reconstructive Surgery
Medical School Hannover
Hannover, Germany

V. KIESSIG & J.F. HANSBROUGH

The Department of Surgery
University of California
San Diego Medical Center
San Diego, California

1. Introduction

Timely and permanent wound closure in patients with extensive burns may improve patient survival (Wolfe *et al*, 1983). Although meshed split thickness skin autografts can provide wound closure, in extensive burns autologous skin for grafting is limited. An approach to accelerate the availability of graftable tissue is the expansion of autologous epidermis by culturing human keratinocytes in the laboratory (Rheinwald and Green, 1977; O'Conner *et al*, 1981).

In an effort to improve the quality of healed skin, dermal replacements can be utilised beneath cultured epithelial grafts. This approach is in line with various reports addressing the importance of dermal structure for adherence, survival and maturation of keratinocytes (Briggaman and Wheeler, 1968; Donjacour and Cunha, 1991; Leary et al, 1991; Meredith et al, 1993; Gailit and Clark, 1994; Gil et al, 1994).

In an attempt to meet the demand for a durable dermal substrate which can be used for allogeneic grafting, an acellular dermal matrix has been produced from fresh human cadaver skin utilising a carefully controlled process (Livesey et al, 1995). This process involves the removal of immunogenic cells from isolated dermis without altering the extracellular matrix structure or the basement membrane complex. The processing avoids extended fluid incubation which reduces the original glycosaminoglycan content of the dermis.

2. Materials And Methods

2.1. Cell culture

Human keratinocytes (HK) were isolated from cadaveric donor skin obtained from the University of California San Diego Regional Tissue Bank. After reduction of the epidermis into single cells, HK were resuspended and expanded in culture using Keratinocyte-SFM medium (Gibco BRL Life Technologies, Grand Island, NY).

2.2. AlloDerm® Dermal matrix

AlloDerm® dermal matrix (commercially available from LifeCell Corp., The Woodlands, TX) is produced from fresh human cadaver skin obtained in accordance with the guidelines of the American Association of Tissue Banks. The epidermis is removed and then decellularised via incubation in 0.5% sodium dodecyl sulfate. The resultant acellular dermal grafts are then freeze dried. The rapid processing procedure (< 72 hours to the time of freezing) is designed to minimise the loss of important biochemical components of the dermis, including glycosaminoglycans.

2.3. Keratinocyte/AlloDerm® dermal matrix *in vitro* coculture

After trypsinisation, cultured keratinocytes were seeded (5×10^4) on rehydrated AlloDerm® and incubated at 37°C, 5% CO_2 for two to 15 days.

2.4. Preparation of polyurethane-HK grafts

Human keratinocytes were seeded at a density of 5×10^4 cells/cm² onto a synthetic hydrophilic dressing, Hydroderm® (Wilshire Medical Inc., Dallas, TX), as previously described (Rennekampff *et al*, 1996).

Seeded keratinocytes were fed every two days with Keratinocyte-SFM medium. After two to three days when the cells had just become confluent, forming a single layer of keratinocytes, the membrane was transplanted.

2.5. Athymic mouse grafting model

Animal experiments were performed with the approval of the University of California, San Diego Animal Research Committee, and in accordance with guidelines prepared by the Committee on Care and Use of Laboratory Animals of the Institute of Laboratory Animal Resources, National Research Council. Full thickness skin defects (2 cm × 2 cm) were created on athymic mice (CD1-nu/nu) to a depth sparing the panniculus carnosis.

One group of animals ($n = 11$) received Hydroderm® (2 cm × 2 cm) seeded with human keratinocytes (Hydroderm-HK). In a second group ($n = 9$), a 2 cm × 2 cm piece of AlloDerm® dermal matrix was sutured into the defect with the basement membrane side facing up. The dermal matrix graft was immediately covered with a section of Hydroderm-HK, inverted onto the processed dermal matrix to achieve cell contact with the exposed basement membrane of the AlloDerm® dermal matrix.

At 21 days post-grafting the wound areas were excised through the dorsal muscle bed for histological and ultrastructural evaluation. Wound surface area measurements were obtained by tracing the perimeter of the wound with a planimetre (Planix 7, Tamaya Inc., Japan). The wound size was measured immediately post-operatively and on day 21. The data for wound contraction were expressed as the mean percentage of the original wound size.

2.6. Histological analysis of tissues

For light microscopy, tissue samples were stained with haematoxylineosin.

Immunohistochemical identification of human involucrin in healed wounds on athymic mice followed instructions as described in the Histostain-SP Kit (Zymed Laboratories Inc., San Francisco, CA). Human involucrin was detected with a primary antibody (rabbit anti-human involucrin; Biomedical Technologies Inc., Stoughton, MA).

Additional specimens were incubated with the human collagen type IV primary antibody (rabbit anti-human collagen IV; Chemicon, Temecula, CA), human laminin primary antibody (rabbit anti-human laminin-1; Chemicon) or rat laminin-5 primary antibody (a gift from V. Quaranta, The Scripps Research Institute, LaJolla, CA), which cross-reacted with human laminin-5.

2.7. Electron microscopic analysis

Specimens were processed as previously described (Livesey et al, 1995).

3. Results

3.1. Histology of AlloDerm matrix prior to grafting

AlloDerm dermal matrix retains the normal architecture of human dermis and sparse anchoring fibrils can be visualised by electron microscopy (not shown). Immunohistochemical studies exhibited retention of human collagen types IV, laminin-1 and laminin-5 at the epidermal side.

3.2. AlloDerm/HK composite *in vitro* graft

As shown in Fig. 1, keratinocytes formed a multi-layered epithelium on the dermal matrix.

3.3. Gross appearance of grafted wounds

Keratinocyte-seeded Hydroderm was adherent to the wound bed after post-operative day 2. Re-epithelialisation preceded spontaneous separation of Hydroderm from the healing epithelium. Wounds were re-epithelialised in all groups after 21 days and a silvery pink appearance of the wound surface was observed (Fig. 2).

3.4. Wound contraction

Statistical analysis of the planimetric data showed significantly lesser wound contraction ($p = 0.016$) in the group of animals which received the processed acellular dermis placed beneath cultured human keratinocytes (23% ± 5.5%) as compared to controls without AlloDerm matrix (48% ± 6.8%).

3.5. Histological examination of healed wounds

Examination of biopsies from animals receiving Hydroderm seeded with human keratinocytes (Hydroderm-HK) overlaid onto the dermal matrix revealed a differentiated layer of human epidermal cells attached to the repopulated dermal matrix. At day 21 a well vascularised dermis was observed with a moderate number of stellate-shaped fibroblasts. The repopulated dermal matrix was less cellular than the wound bed of animals which did not receive a dermal replacement.

Immunohistochemical analysis with the anti-human involucrin antibody revealed persistence of human keratinocytes on the murine

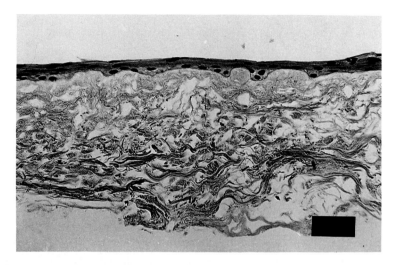

Fig. 1. *In vitro* reconstitution of a composite graft prior to lifting at the air-liquid interface. Multilayer of keratinocytes resting on AlloDerm matrix ten days after seeding. (Original magnification × 100, Bar = 100 mm)

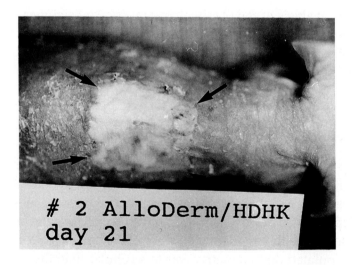

2 AlloDerm/HDHK
day 21

Fig. 2. *In vivo* application of AlloDerm matrix. Twenty-one days after application of Hydroderm-HK overlaid on the processed dermal graft on excised wound a silvery epidermis is visible (arrows). Only a small amount of contraction was noticeable.

wounds at 21 days post-grafting. Animals which received Hydroderm-HK without the dermal matrix showed positive "take" of human keratinocytes in 63.6% of the animals compared to 100% for the dermal matrix grafts in combination with Hydroderm-HK ($p < 0.05$).

3.6. Ultrastructural findings

Basal layer keratinocytes exhibited hemidesmosome formation with a mature basement membrane. Anchoring fibrils were also observed spanning the basement membrane complex. In contrast, ultrastructural analysis of biopsies from animals receiving only Hydroderm-HK revealed a thin, less mature basement membrane complex.

4. Discussion

Timely wound closure in extensive burns has been shown to reduce patient morbidity (Wolfe *et al*, 1983). Wound coverage can be achieved by the meshing and expansion of harvested autograft skin, or by cultured epithelium. However, time requirements for culturing and technical obstacles impart significant limitations on this grafting procedure (Poumay *et al*, 1991).

We have developed a new technique for the delivery of a single layer of cultured human keratinocytes which may permit earlier delivery of autologous cultured keratinocytes and which may eliminate some of the technical problems associated with the use of cultured epithelial sheets (Rennekampff *et al*, 1995). This technique was used to apply a single layer of cultured human keratinocytes to full thickness wounds.

However, absence of dermis is a serious deficiency when attempting to achieve clinically successful replacement of human skin. Delayed attachment to the wound bed, variable graft take, breakdown of the grafted epithelium and significant wound contracture have been reported in clinical applications of cultured epithelial sheet grafts (Kumagai *et al*, 1988; DeLuca *et al*, 1989; Rue III *et al*, 1993).

Here, we demonstrated that a single layer of keratinocytes delivered in combination with an acellular dermal matrix can achieve a reconstituted skin in an athymic mouse model. Indeed, we showed a reduced wound contraction after the application of a dermal replacement. In a pilot study a similar take of autologous keratinocytes was seen in severely injured patients.

The importance of the basement membrane has previously been demonstrated (Briggaman and Wheeler, 1968; Donjacour and Cunha, 1991; Eady *et al*, 1994; Gailit and Clark, 1994). Laminin-5, a major component of the basement membrane, was shown to be critically involved in keratinocyte adherence to the basement membrane and cell signalling (Gil *et al*, 1994; Rousselle and Aumailley, 1994). Rete ridge formation at the dermal-epidermal junction provides increased surface area for attachment of the epidermis to the dermis and increases resistance to shear forces. Therefore, this unique acellular dermal matrix with preserved basement membrane architecture and biomolecules such as laminin-5 and collagen IV should promote keratinocyte engraftment and persistence of newly-formed epithelium.

Keratinocytes seeded and cultured on Hydroderm express integrin subunits $\alpha 3$ and $\alpha 6$ similar to keratinocytes cultured in flasks (Hertle *et al*, 1991). The integrin $\alpha 3$ preferentially binds to laminin-5, while the integrin subunit $\alpha 6$ recognizes laminin-1 and laminin-5 (Rouselle and Aumailley, 1994), all of which are found in the basement membrane complex of the skin and AlloDerm matrix. The keratinocytes adhere most efficiently on laminin-5 (Hormia *et al*, 1995) and the integrin $\alpha 3$ is involved in this early adhesion process. This may explain the superior adherence and engraftment of cultured keratinocytes to the preserved basement membrane complex of the acellular dermal matrix *in vitro* and *in vivo*.

Hemidesmosome formation was common in keratinocytes resting on AlloDerm at three weeks post-grafting. In contrast, keratinocytes transplanted without the dermal replacement exhibited a very flat dermal-epidermal junction with an immature basement membrane. Consistent with these findings, it has been reported that basement membrane complex formation in the absence of a dermal component may take several months (Woodley *et al*, 1988). The number of fibroblasts observed in the dermal matrix at three weeks post-grafting was much less than that seen in granulation tissue. It is tempting to speculate that the observed small number of fibroblasts and a normal matrix environment may have contributed to the reduced contraction observed in wounds grafted with the dermal matrix.

The development and use of an effective dermal replacement appears necessary in order to achieve functional skin replacements. A variety of reports emphasise the roles which extracellular matrices play in tissue engineering (Bell, 1995; Donjacour and Cunha, 1991). While the importance of growth factors and the epithelium is well recognised in skin regeneration, extracellular matrix may need more clinical attention.

5. Acknowledgement

H.O. Rennekampff was supported by a grant from "Deutsche Forschungsgemeinschaft", and partial funding was received from LifeCell Corporation.

6. References

BELL, E. (1995). Deterministic models for tissue engineering, *Cellular Engineering* **1**, 28–34.

BRIGGAMAN, R.A. and WHEELER, C.E. (1968). Epidermal-dermal interactions in adult human skin: Role of dermis in epidermal maintenance, *J. Invest. Dermatol.* **51**, 454–465.

DELUCA, M., ALBANESE, E., BONDANAZA, S., MEGNA, M., UGOZZOLI, L., MOLINA, F., CANCEDDA, R., SANTI, P.L., BORMIOLI, M., STELLA, M. and MAGLIACANI, G. (1989). Multicentre experience in the treatment of burns with autologous and allogenic cultured epithelium, fresh or preserved in a frozen state, *Burns* **15**, 303–309.

DONJACOUR, A.A. and CUNHA, G.R. (1991). Stromal regulation of epithelial function, *Cancer Treat. Res.* **53**, 335–364.

EADY, R.A.J, McGRATH, J.A. and McMILLAN, J.R. (1994). Ultra-structural clues to genetic disorders of skin: The dermalepidermal junction, *J. Invest. Dermatol.* **103**, 13S–18S.

GAILIT, J. and CLARK, R.A.F. (1994). Wound repair in the context of extracellular matrix, *Curr. Opinion. Cell Biol.* **6**, 717–725.

GIL, S.G., BROWN, T.A., RYAN, M.C. and CARTER, W.G. (1994). Junctional epidermolysis bullosis: Defects in expression of epiligrin/nicein/kalinin and integrin β4 that inhibit hemidesmosome formation, *J. Invest. Dermatol.* **103**, 31S–38S.

HERTLE, M.D., ADAMS, J.C. and WATT, F.M. (1991). Integrin expression during epidermal development *in vivo* and *in vitro*, *Development* **112**, 193–206.

HORMIA, M., FALK-MARZILLIER, J., PLOPPER, G., JONES, J.C.R. and QUARANTA V. (1995). Rapid spreading and mature hemidesmosome formation in HaCat keratinocytes induced by incubation with soluble laminin-5, *J. Invest. Dermatol.* **105**, 557–561.

LEARY, T., JONES, P.L., APPLEBY, I., BLIGHT, A., PARKINSON, K. and STANLEY, M. (1991). Epidermal keratinocyte self-renewal is dependent upon dermal integrity, *J. Invest. Dermatol.* **99**, 422–430.

LIVESEY, S.A., HERNDON, D.N., HOLLYOAK, M.A., ATKINSON, Y.H. and NAG, A. (1995). Transplanted acellular allograft dermal matrix, *Transplantation* **60**, 1–9.

MEREDITH, J.E., FAZELI, B. and SCHWARTZ, M.A. (1993). The extracellular matrix as a cellular survival factor, *Mol. Bio. Cell* **4**, 953–961.

O'CONNOR, N.E., MULLIKEN, J.B., BANKS-SCHLEGEL, S., KEHINDE, O. and GREEN, H (1981). Grafting of burns with cultured epithelium prepared from autologous epidermal cells, *Lancet* **1**, 75–78.

POUMAY, Y., BOUCHER, F., DEGEN, A. and LELOUP, R. (1991). Inhibition of basal cell proliferation during storage of detached cultured epidermal keratinocyte sheets, *Acta Dermatol-Venerol* (*Stockh.*) **71**, 195–198.

RENNEKAMFF, H.O., HANSBROUGH, J.F., KIESSIG, V., ABIEZZI, S. and WOODS, V. JR (1996). Wound closure with human keratinocytes cultured on a polyurethane dressing overlaid on a cultured dermal replacement, *Surgery* **120**, 16–22.

RHEINWALD, J.G. and GREEN, H. (1977). Epidermal growth factor and the multiplication of cultured human epidermal keratinocytes, *Nature* **265**, 421–424.

ROUSSELLE, P. and AUMAILLEY, M. (1994). Kalinin is more efficient than laminin in promoting adhesion of primary keratinocytes and some other epithelial cells and has a different requirement for integrin receptors, *J. Cell Bio.* **125**, 205–214.

RUE, L.W. III, CIOFFI, W.G., McMANUS, W.F. and PRUITT, B.A. JR (1993). Wound closure and outcome in extensively burned patients treated with cultured autologous keratinocytes, *J. Trauma* **34**, 662–667.

WOLFE, R.A., ROI, L.D., FLORA, J.D., FELLER, I. and CORNELL, R.G. (1983). Mortality differences and speed of wound closure among specialised burn care facilities, *J. Am. Med. Assoc.* **250**, 763–766.

WOODLEY, D.T., PETERSON, H.D., HERZOG, S.R., STRICKLIN, G.P., BURGESON, R.E., BRIGGAMAN, R.A., CRONCE, D.J. and O'KEEFE, E.J. (1988). Burn wounds resurfaced by cultured epidermal autografts show abnormal reconstitution of anchoring fibrils, *J. Am. Med. Assoc.* **259**, 2566–2571.

WOOD, R.A., KEIL, K.H., PALME, H.L., FREDRIKSSON, K.V.(1970),
S.O. (1968) Modelling differences in the physical of various chemical
among chondrites meteorites. Meteoritic. J. Am. Meteorit Soc. 236-
38-386.

WOODWORTH, J.B., RAY, K.H., HERSCHEL, S.K., STRAUSS, S.L.,
BURKHART, H.M., BRODZAMAN, R.A., GRENCH, H.D., and
DREISTI, F.V. (1968) High volume resistance of colloidal
electronic assembly. Same structural test reactions as suggestions.
Juma. J. Am. Acad. Assoc. 284. pp. 4472.